T0250164

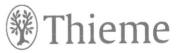

The Jefferson Manual for Neurocritical Care

Jack I. Jallo, MD, PhD
Professor and Vice-Chair for Academic Services;
Director
Division of Neurotrauma and Critical Care
Department of Neurological Surgery
Sidney Kimmel Medical College
Thomas Jefferson University
Philadelphia, Pennsylvania, USA

Jacqueline S. Urtecho, MD
Assistant Professor of Neurology and Neurological Surgery
Department of Neurological Surgery
Division of Neurotrauma and Critical Care
Sidney Kimmel Medical College
Thomas Jefferson University
Philadelphia, Pennsylvania, USA

78 illustrations

Thieme
New York • Stuttgart • Delhi • Rio de Janeiro

Library of Congress Cataloging-in-Publication Data is available from the publisher.

Important note: Medicine is an ever-changing science undergoing continual development. Research and clinical experience are continually expanding our knowledge, in particular our knowledge of proper treatment and drug therapy. Insofar as this book mentions any dosage or application, readers may rest assured that the authors, editors, and publishers have made every effort to ensure that such references are in accordance with **the state of knowledge at the time of production of the book.**

Nevertheless, this does not involve, imply, or express any guarantee or responsibility on the part of the publishers in respect to any dosage instructions and forms of applications stated in the book. **Every user is requested to examine carefully** the manufacturers' leaflets accompanying each drug and to check, if necessary in consultation with a physician or specialist, whether the dosage schedules mentioned therein or the contraindications stated by the manufacturers differ from the statements made in the present book. Such examination is particularly important with drugs that are either rarely used or have been newly released on the market. Every dosage schedule or every form of application used is entirely at the user's own risk and responsibility. The authors and publishers request every user to report to the publishers any discrepancies or inaccuracies noticed. If errors in this work are found after publication, errata will be posted at www.thieme.com on the product description page.

Some of the product names, patents, and registered designs referred to in this book are in fact registered trademarks or proprietary names even though specific reference to this fact is not always made in the text. Therefore, the appearance of a name without designation as proprietary is not to be construed as a representation by the publisher that it is in the public domain.

Thieme Medical Publishers, Inc.
333 Seventh Avenue, 18th Floor
New York, NY 10001, USA
www.thieme.com
+1 800 782 3488, customerservice@thieme.com

Cover design: Thieme Publishing Group
Typesetting by Ditech, India

Printed in USA by King Printing Company, Inc.   5 4 3 2

ISBN 978-1-62623-494-9
Also available as e-book:
eISBN 978-1-62623-495-6

FSC
www.fsc.org
100%
Paper from well-managed forests
FSC® C103101

Contents

Preface xv

Contributors xvi

1.   Encephalopathy and Delirium 1
        Catriona M. Harrop

1.1   **Encephalopathy** 1

1.1.1 Definition 1
1.1.2 Causes of Encephalopathy 1
1.1.3 Diagnosis of Encephalopathy 1
1.1.4 Treatment of Encephalopathy 3
1.1.5 Relationship to Delirium 3

1.2   **Delirium** 3

1.2.1 Definition 3
1.2.2 Duration of Symptoms 4
1.2.3 Level of Activity 4
1.2.4 Risk Factors for Delirium 5
1.2.5 Clinical Assessment 5

1.3   **Treatment** 8

1.3.1 Medications for Agitation 8
1.3.2 Pharmacologic Management of Hyperactive Delirium and Agitation 8
1.3.3 Nonpharmacologic Treatments for Delirium 8

2.   Cerebrovascular Emergency: Acute Stroke Diagnosis and
        Management 11
        Maria Carissa C. Pineda, Sridhara S. Yaddanapudi, and Norman Ajiboye

2.1   **Epidemiology** 11

2.2   **Etiology** 11

2.2.1 Nonmodifiable Risk Factors 11
2.2.2 Modifiable Risk Factors 11
2.2.3 Stroke Subtypes 12

2.3   **Common Clinical Presentations** 12

2.4   **Differential Diagnosis for Acute Ischemic Stroke** 12

2.5   **Acute Stroke Diagnosis, Treatment, and Management** 13

2.5.1   Stroke Activation.. 13

2.6   **Criteria for Endovascular Therapy** 18

2.6.1   Neurocritical Care Management of Ischemic Stroke 23

2.7   **Stroke Workup and Management** 26

2.7.1   Post Stroke Complication 28

3.   **Cerebrovascular Emergency: Spontaneous Intracerebral Hemorrhage (ICH)** 33

Syed Omar Shah

3.1   **Epidemiology** 33

3.2   **Etiologies/Differential Diagnosis** 33

3.3   **Common Clinical Presentations** 34

3.4   **Neuroimaging** 35

3.5   **Treatment**.. 35

3.5.1   Aggressive Reduction in SBP to Goal of 140 37
3.5.2   Seizures 37
3.5.3   Intracranial Pressure 37
3.5.4   Medical Issues 37
3.5.5   Coagulopathies 38
3.5.6   Surgical Options 38
3.5.7   Craniotomy... 38
3.5.8   Craniectomy.. 38
3.5.9   Minimally Invasive Surgical Evacuation 40

3.6   **Prognosis** 40

4.   **Cerebrovascular Emergencies: Aneurysmal Subarachnoid Hemorrhage (SAH)** 45

Norman Ajiboye, Yu Kan Au, and Syed Omar Shah

4.1   **Epidemiology** 45

4.2   **Risk Factors** 45

4.3   **Diagnosis** 45

4.4   **Grading System** 46

4.4.1   Hunt and Hess Grade.. 46

4.4.2	World Federation of Neurological Surgeons Grade	47
4.4.3	Modified Fischer Scores	47
4.5	**Management of Subarachnoid Hemorrhage**	47
4.5.1	Early Phase	48
4.5.2	Late Phase	51
4.6	**Vasospasm, Delayed Neurologic Deterioration (DND), and Delayed Cerebral Ischemia (DCI)**	53
4.6.1	Detection and Management of Vasospasm and DCI	54
4.7	**Hyponatremia and Endocrine Dysfunction**	56
4.7.1	Hyponatremia	56
4.7.2	Endocrine Dysfunction	56
5.	**Transfusion Medicine and Anticoagulation**	58
	Bhuvanesh Govind and Matthew Vibbert	
5.1	**Introduction**	58
5.2	**Anemia in the ICU**	58
5.3	**Red Cell Transfusion**	59
5.3.1	Leukocyte Reduction Indications	59
5.3.2	Washed RBC	59
5.3.3	Irradiation	59
5.3.4	Complications of Red Blood Cell Transfusion	59
5.3.5	Benefits to Transfusion	60
5.4	**Hemoglobin "Triggers"**	60
5.5	**Thrombocytopenia**	61
5.6	**Prophylaxis Thresholds**	62
5.6.1	Treatment of Bleeding	62
5.7	**Antiplatelet Reversal in Intracranial Hemorrhage**	62
5.8	**Coagulation Cascade and Anticoagulants**	64
5.9	**Anticoagulants**	64
5.9.1	Warfarin	64
5.10	**Oral Factor Xa Inhibitors**	66
5.10.1	Apixaban, Rivaroxaban, Edoxaban	66
5.11	**Thrombin Inhibitors**	67

5.11.1	Oral	67
5.11.2	Intravenous	69
5.12	**The Heparins**	70
5.12.1	Unfractionated Heparin	70
5.12.2	Low-Molecular-Weight Heparin (LMWH)	70
5.12.3	Fondaparinux	71
5.13	**Deep Vein Thrombosis (DVT) Prophylaxis**	72
6.	**Cerebral Edema and Elevated Intracranial Pressure**	75
	Anna Karpenko and Michelle Ghobrial	
6.1	**The Basics**	75
6.1.1	Monro-Kellie Doctrine	75
6.1.2	ICP and Cerebral Perfusion Pressure (CPP)	75
6.1.3	Intracranial Compliance	76
6.1.4	ICP Waveforms and Herniation Syndromes	76
6.2	**Cerebral Edema**	81
6.3	**Stepwise Approach to the Management of Elevated ICP**	82
6.4	**Management of Increased Intracranial Pressure**	84
6.4.1	Tier 1	84
6.4.2	Tier 2	84
6.4.3	Tier 3	86
7.	**Fevers and Infections in the Neuro-ICU**	91
	Deena M. Athas, Amna Sheikh, and Jacqueline S. Urtecho	
7.1	**Brain**	91
7.1.1	Meningitis	91
7.1.2	Acute Bacterial Meningitis	92
7.1.3	Aseptic Meningitis	96
7.1.4	Viral Meningitis	96
7.1.5	Fungal Meningitis	97
7.1.6	Ventriculitis	97
7.1.7	HIV-Related Infections	99
7.1.8	Empyema	103
7.2	**Spine**	104
7.2.1	Epidural Abscess	104
7.2.2	Osteomyelitis	106
7.3	**Central Fever**	108

8. Treatment of Status Epilepticus in Adults........................... 111
    James Park, Alan Wang, Andres Fernandez, and Sara Hefton

8.1 **Overview and Definitions** 111

8.2 **Convulsive Status Epilepticus Management** 112

8.3 **Nonconvulsive Status Epilepticus (NCSE)**................................ 115

8.4 **Refractory Status Epilepticus (RSE)**...................................... 116

8.5 **Super Refractory Status Epilepticus (SRSE)**............................. 116

9. Trauma... 119
    Ravichandra Madineni and Christian Hoelscher

9.1 **Acute Spinal Cord Injury** 119

9.1.1 Introduction 119
9.1.2 Medical Treatment of Acute SCI 119
9.1.3 Surgical Management of Acute SCI... 121

9.2 **Traumatic Brain Injury** 122

9.2.1 Introduction 122
9.2.2 Management of Elevated ICP... 125
9.2.3 Other Post-TBI Considerations 126

9.3 **Paroxysmal Sympathetic Hyperactivity (PSH)**............................ 127

10. Neuromuscular and Other Neurologic Emergencies 132
     Danielle Wilhour and Alison L. Walsh

10.1 **Guillain-Barré Syndrome (GBS)/Acute Inflammatory Demyelinating
       Polyradiculoneuropathy (AIDP)**... 132

10.1.1 Definition 132
10.1.2 Epidemiology... 132
10.1.3 Differential Diagnosis.. 133
10.1.4 Common Clinical Presentation 133
10.1.5 Diagnosis.. 133
10.1.6 GBS Variants... 133
10.1.7 Ancillary Testing 134
10.1.8 Complications of GBS... 134
10.1.9 Management 135
10.1.10 Prognosis.. 135

10.2 **Myasthenia Gravis** 136

10.2.1 Definition 136

Contents

10.2.2   Epidemiology..   136

10.2.3   Differential Diagnosis...   136

10.2.4   Clinical Presentation of Generalized Myasthenia Gravis   136

10.2.5   Diagnosis..   137

10.2.6   Management of Myasthenic Crisis..   137

10.2.7   Prognosis..   138

10.3   Botulism   139

10.3.1   Definition   139

10.3.2   Epidemiology...   139

10.3.3   Pathophysiology   139

10.3.4   Differential Diagnosis...   139

10.3.5   Clinical Presentation   139

10.3.6   Diagnosis..   140

10.3.7   Management   140

10.3.8   Prognosis..   140

10.4   Organophosphate Toxicity..   141

10.4.1   Definition   141

10.4.2   Epidemiology...   141

10.4.3   Pathophysiology   141

10.4.4   Differential Diagnosis...   141

10.4.5   Clinical Presentation   141

10.4.6   Diagnosis..   141

10.4.7   Management   142

10.4.8   Prognosis..   142

10.5   Neuroleptic Malignant Syndrome (NMS) and Serotonin Syndrome (SS)   142

10.5.1   Definition   142

10.5.2   Epidemiology...   143

10.5.3   Pathogenesis...   143

10.5.4   Differential Diagnosis...   143

10.5.5   Clinical Presentation   143

10.5.6   Diagnosis..   143

10.5.7   Management   144

10.5.8   Complications   145

10.5.9   Prognosis..   146

11.   Brain Tumor Postoperative Management...   149

Richard F. Schmidt, Nikolaos Mouchtouris, Muaz Qayyum, James J. Evans, and Christopher Farrell

11.1   Introduction   149

11.1.1   Clinical Presentation   150

11.1.2   Tumor Classification...   151

11.2 Postoperative Care and Complications 152

11.2.1 Airway Management 152
11.2.2 Blood Pressure Control and Postoperative Hemorrhage 156
11.2.3 Seizure Prophylaxis 156
11.2.4 Venous Thromboembolism Prophylaxis...................................... 157
11.2.5 Antibiotic Prophylaxis and Postoperative Infection 158
11.2.6 Cerebral Edema 159
11.2.7 CSF Leak... 160

11.3 Specific Concerns for Sellar and Parasellar Tumors 162

11.3.1 Hormonal Dysregulation 162
11.3.2 Pituitary Apoplexy 164

11.4 Conclusion 165

12. Brain Death in Adults 169
Rodney D. Bell, Norman Ajiboye, and Yu Kan Au

12.1 Definition of Brain Death 169

12.2 Clinical Evaluation 169

12.2.1 Establishing the Proximate Cause of Coma 170
12.2.2 Clinical Examination to Establish Irreversibility 170

12.3 Ancillary Tests 171

12.4 Legal 171

12.5 Management of the Brain-Dead Patient for Organ Donation 172

13. Sodium Dysregulation 178
M. Kamran Athar and Christian Bacheler

13.1 Terminology 178

13.2 Hyponatremia Classification 178

13.2.1 Causes of Hyponatremia... 179
13.2.2 Symptomatic Hyponatremia 179

13.3 SIADH versus CSW 181

13.3.1 Syndrome of Inappropriate Antidiuretic Hormone Secretion (SIADH) 181
13.3.2 Cerebral Salt Wasting (CSW) 181
13.3.3 SIADH and CSW Diagnosis 182

13.4 Diagnostic Approach to Hyponatremia 183

13.4.1 Hyponatremia Treatment: General Principles 184

13.4.2 Acute Symptomatic Moderate to Severe Hyponatremia 184
13.4.3 Acute Asymptomatic Moderate Hyponatremia 185
13.4.4 Severe Chronic Mild-Moderate Hyponatremia................................ 185
13.4.5 SIADH Treatment 186
13.4.6 CSW Treatment 186
13.4.7 Treatment of Hyponatremia in Patients with Subarachnoid Hemorrhage 186
13.4.8 Treatment of Hyponatremia in Patients with Heart Failure 187

13.5   Hypernatremia... 187

13.5.1 Central (Neurogenic) Diabetes Insipidus 187
13.5.2 Nephrogenic Diabetes Insipidus 189

13.6   Diagnostic Approach to Hypernatremia................................ 189

13.6.1 Treatment 190
13.6.2 Central DI Treatment 192
13.6.3 Nephrogenic DI Treatment.. 192

14.   Nutrition.. 194
         Stephanie Dobak and Jacqueline S. Urtecho

14.1   Glucose Utilization.. 194

14.2   Nutrition in Critical Care.. 194

14.3   Nutrition Status... 196

14.3.1 Malnutrition 196
14.3.2 Refeeding Syndrome 198
14.3.3 Nutrition-Related Laboratory Tests 198

14.4   Nutrition Assessment.. 198

14.4.1 Calorie Needs... 198
14.4.2 Protein Needs... 199
14.4.3 Nutrition Support 200
14.4.4 Enteral Nutrition.. 200

14.5   Specific EN Considerations 204

14.5.1 Parenteral Nutrition... 204

14.6   Therapy-Specific Considerations.. 204

14.7   Conclusion 208

15.   Sedation 210
         Akta Patel and Michelle Ghobrial

15.1   Introduction 210

15.2	**Indications for Sedation**	210
15.3	**Complications of Sedation**	211
15.4	**Assessment of Sedation**	211
15.5	**Choice of Sedative**	212
15.5.1	Propofol (Diprivan)	216
15.5.2	Midazolam (Versed)	217
15.5.3	Dexmedetomidine (Precedex)	218
15.5.4	Fentanyl (Sublimaze)	219
15.5.5	Ketamine (Ketalar)	220

16.	**Pain Management in the Neuro-Intensive Care Unit (ICU)**	222
	Amy Shah, David A. Wyler, and Andrew Ng	
16.1	**Introduction**	222
16.2	**Modern Strategy of Pain Management in ICU Liberation**	223
16.3	**Challenges of Pain Management in Neuro-ICU**	224
16.4	**Individualizing Therapy in NICU**	224
16.4.1	Pharmacologic Interventions of Pain	224
16.4.2	Nonpharmacologic Approach	233
16.5	**Neuro-specific Diseases at Risk for Pain**	233
16.5.1	Pain with SAH	233
16.5.2	Spondylosis and Disk Herniation	233
16.5.3	Spasticity	234
16.6	**Ongoing Continuous Pain Monitoring in NICU**	234
16.6.1	Pain Scales	234

17.	**Advanced Hemodynamic and Neurological Monitoring in the Neuro-ICU**	238
	David F. Slottje and John W. Liang	
17.1	**Hemodynamic Monitoring**	238
17.1.1	Invasive Monitoring: Pulmonary Thermodilution	240
17.1.2	Less Invasive: Transpulmonary Thermodilution	241
17.1.3	Minimally Invasive Monitoring: Pulse Contour Analysis	245
17.1.4	Noninvasive Hemodynamic Monitoring	247
17.2	**Neurological Monitoring**	249
17.2.1	Noninvasive Monitors	249

17.2.2   Invasive Monitors: Cerebral Oximetry 254
17.2.3   Cerebral Blood Flow Monitors... 260
17.2.4   Intracranial Pressure Monitoring 261

18.   Neuroimaging 266
         Michael J. Lang

18.1   Introduction 266

18.2   Types of Imaging.. 266

18.2.1   Brain Imaging.. 266
18.2.2   Spine Imaging 266

18.3   Advantages and Limitations 267

18.3.1   Brain Imaging.. 267
18.3.2   Spine Imaging 279
18.3.3   Systemic... 281

19.   Ventilation Strategies in Neuro-ICU 285
         Amandeep S. Dolla and M. Kamran Athar

19.1   Introduction 285

19.2   Respiratory Failure.. 285

19.2.1   Noninvasive Oxygenation and Ventilation................................. 285
19.2.2   Invasive Mechanical Ventilation.. 289
19.2.3   Basic Principles of Mechanical Ventilation 291
19.2.4   Modes of Ventilation 292
19.2.5   Initial Ventilator Settings 294
19.2.6   For Pressure Ventilation 295
19.2.7   Common Ventilator Problems... 295
19.2.8   Weaning from Ventilator 295
19.2.9   WHEANS NOT Mnemonic... 295
19.2.10 Extubation Procedure 297

         Index 299

Preface

Everything we do, every thought we've ever had, is produced by the brain. But exactly how it operates remains one of the biggest unsolved mysteries, and it seems the more we probe its secrets, the more surprises we find.

Neil deGrasse Tyson

This book was developed out of a desire to share our knowledge and experience in neurocritical care from Thomas Jefferson University Hospitals. The brain continues to be a "black box" for many practitioners and the need for expertise is greater than ever in this evolving field. As a large quaternary hospital with 40 dedicated neurocritical care beds and 8 board-certified neurointensivists, we have extensive experience with both common and rare neurological and neurosurgical diseases (ischemic stroke, intracerebral hemorrhage, subarachnoid hemorrhage, acute spinal cord injury, traumatic brain injury, encephalitis/meningitis, myasthenia gravis, Guillain-Barré syndrome). Using current guidelines and Thomas Jefferson University protocols, we map out a process for the diagnosis and treatment of the more common diseases managed in the neuro-ICU. We chose a format that would be user-friendly so that any practitioner could use at the bedside. As we continue to discover more of the brain's secrets and advance the field of neurocritical care, we will continue to update this handbook.

We would like to acknowledge and thank all the contributors to this book. Without their dedication and hard work, this book wouldn't have been possible.

Jack I. Jallo, MD, PhD
Jacqueline S. Urtecho, MD

Contributors

Norman Ajiboye, MD
Assistant Professor of Neuroendovascular
  Surgery
Department of Surgery
Texas Chrisitan University
University of North Texas School of Medicine
Dallas-Fort Worth, Texas USA;
Co-Medical Director
Neuroendovascular Surgery Fellowship,
Texas Stroke Institute
Dallas, Texas, USA

M. Kamran Athar, MD
Assistant Professor of Medicine and
  Neurological Surgery
Department of Neurological Surgery
Division of Neuro-Trauma and Critical Care
Sidney Kimmel Medical College
Thomas Jefferson University
Philadelphia, Pennsylvania, USA

Deena M. Athas, MD
Infectious Disease Specialist
Gundersen Health System
La Crosse, Wisconsin, USA

Yu Kan Au, MD
Assistant Professor of Neurology
University of Connecticut
Hartford, Connecticut, USA

Christian Bacheler, MD
Neurohospitalist, Vascular Neurologist
Memorial Healthcare System
Hollywood, Florida, USA

Rodney D. Bell, MD
Professor of Neurology
Lynne and Harold Honickman
Vice Chairman (Hospital Affairs)
Department of Neurology
Sidney Kimmel Medical College
Thomas Jefferson University
Philadelphia, Pennsylvania, USA

Stephanie Dobak, MS, RD, LDN, CNSC
Clinical Dietitian III
Jefferson Weinberg ALS Center
Philadelphia, Pennsylvania, USA

Amandeep S. Dolla, MBBS, MD
Clinical Assistant Professor
Department of Neurology/Division of
  Neurocritical Care
Sidney Kimmel Medical College
Thomas Jefferson University
Philadelphia, Pennsylvania, USA

James J. Evans, MD
Professor of Neurological Surgery and
  Otolaryngology
Department of Neurological Surgery
Sidney Kimmel Medical College
Thomas Jefferson University
Philadelphia, Pennsylvania, USA

Christopher Farrell, MD
Assistant Professor
Department of Neurological Surgery
Sidney Kimmel Medical College
Thomas Jefferson University
Philadelphia, Pennsylvania, USA

Andres Fernandez, MD, MSEd
Assistant Professor
Department of Neurology
Sidney Kimmel Medical College
Thomas Jefferson University
Philadelphia, Pennsylvania, USA

Michelle Ghobrial, MD
Neurointensivist
Novant Health
Winston Salem, North Carolina, USA

Bhuvanesh Govind, MD
Staff Neurointensivist
Medical City Plano
Plano, Texas, USA

Catriona M. Harrop, MD, SFHM, FACP
Associate Chief Medical Officer, South
   Philadelphia
Medical Co-Director for Pre Admission
   Testing
Associate Professor of Clinical Medicine
Sidney Kimmel Medical College
Thomas Jefferson University
Philadelphia, Pennsylvania, USA

Sara Hefton, MD
Assistant Professor of Neurology and
   Neurological Surgery
Department of Neurological Surgery
Division of Neurotrauma and Critical Care
Sidney Kimmel Medical College
Thomas Jefferson University
Philadelphia, Pennsylvania, USA

Christian Hoelscher, MD
Clinical Assistant Professor of Neurosurgery
Sidney Kimmel Medical College
Thomas Jefferson University
Philadelphia, Pennsylvania, USA

Anna Karpenko, MD
Assistant Professor
Department of Neurology
Dartmouth Hitchcock Medical Center
Lebanon, New Hampshire, USA

Michael J. Lang, MD
Assistant Professor
Department of Neurosurgery
University of Pittsburgh Medical Center
Pittsburgh, Pennsylvania, USA

John W. Liang, MD
Director
Neurosciences ICU
Mount Sinai West;
Assistant Professor
Departments of Neurosurgery & Neurology
Mount Sinai Health System
New York, New York, USA

Ravichandra Madineni, MD
Neurosurgeon
Main Line Health Jefferson Neurosurgery
Bryn Mawr Hospital
Bryn Mawr, Pennsylvania, USA

Nikolaos Mouchtouris, MD
Resident Physician in Neurological Surgery
Sidney Kimmel Medical College
Thomas Jefferson University
Philadelphia, Pennsylvania, USA

Andrew Ng, MD
Assistant Professor of Anesthesiology and
   Physical Medicine and Rehabilitation
Program Director Pain Medicine Fellowship
Department of Anesthesiology, Jefferson Pain
   Center
Thomas Jefferson University
Philadelphia, Pennsylvania, USA

James Park, DO
Epileptologist
Pickup Family Neuroscience Institute
Hoag Hospital
Newport Beach/Irvine, California, USA

Akta Patel, PharmD, BCPS
Advanced Practice Pharmacist, Critical Care
Department of Pharmacy
Thomas Jefferson University
Philadelphia, Pennsylvania, USA

Maria Carissa C. Pineda, MD
Associate Professor
Department of Neurosciences
University of the Philippines
Manila, Philippines

Muaz Qayyum, MBBS
Research Fellow
Department of Neurological Surgery
Sidney Kimmel Medical College
Thomas Jefferson University
Philadelphia, Pennsylvania, USA

Richard F. Schmidt, MD
Clinical Assistant Professor
Department of Neurological Surgery
Sidney Kimmel Medical College
Thomas Jefferson University
Philadelphia, Pennsylvania, USA

Amy Shah, MD
Physician Neurosurgical Anesthesiologist
Valley Anesthesiology Consultants
Envision Physician Services
Phoenix, Arizona, USA

Syed Omar Shah, MD, MBA
Assistant Professor of Neurology and
    Neurological Surgery
Associate Fellowship Director,
    Neurocritical Care
Department of Neurological Surgery
Sidney Kimmel Medical College
Thomas Jefferson University
Philadelphia, Pennsylvania, USA

Amna Sheikh, MBBS, MD
Intensivist
Department of Critical Care
Winchester Medical Center
Winchester, Virgina, USA

David F. Slottje, MD
Neurosurgeon
Sentara Martha Jefferson Neurosciences
Charlottesville, Virginia, USA

Jacqueline S. Urtecho, MD
Assistant Professor of Neurology and
    Neurological Surgery
Department of Neurological Surgery
Division of Neurotrauma and Critical Care
Sidney Kimmel Medical College
Thomas Jefferson University
Philadelphia, Pennsylvania, USA

Matthew Vibbert, MD
Assistant Professor
Neurology and Neurological Surgery;
Director, Neurocritical Care
Sidney Kimmel Medical College
Thomas Jefferson University
Philadelphia, Pennsylvania, USA

Alison L. Walsh, MD
Assistant Professor
Morsani College of Medicine
University of South Florida
Tampa, Florida, USA;
Division of Neurology
Lehigh Valley Health Network
Allentown, Pennsylvania, USA

Alan Wang, MD
Clinical Assistant Professor of Neurology
Department of Neurology
University of Arizona College of Medicine –
    Phoenix
Phoenix, Arizona, USA

Danielle Wilhour, MD
Assistant Professor
Department of Neurology
University of Colorado
Aurora, Colorado, USA

David A. Wyler, MD
Assistant Professor
Anesthesiology and Neurological Surgery
Director of Anesthesiology Neurocritical Care
Assistant Program Director
Anesthesiology Residency Program
Sidney Kimmel Medical College
Thomas Jefferson University
Philadelphia, Pennsylvania, USA

Sridhara S. Yaddanapudi, MBBS, MD
Neurohospitalist
ChristianaCare Medical Center
Newark, Delaware, USA

1 Encephalopathy and Delirium

Catriona M. Harrop

Abstract

Encephalopathy is characterized by the National Institute of Neurological Disorders and Stroke as "any diffuse disease of the brain that alters brain function or structure,"[1] and can be classified as acute or chronic. The definition, diagnosis, and treatment of encephalopathy is reviewed here, along with one of its most common symptoms, delirium.

Keywords: encephalopathy, delirium, confusion, agitation, arousability, Ramsay score, Riker score

1.1 Encephalopathy

1.1.1 Definition

The National Institute of Neurological Disorders and Stroke (NINDS) defines encephalopathy as "a term for any diffuse disease of the brain that alters brain function or structure"[1] with the hallmark of encephalopathy being an altered mental state. Encephalopathy can be categorized by chronicity[2]:

- Acute
  - Toxic: due to medications, illicit substances, or toxins
  - Metabolic: due to a metabolic disturbance
  - Toxic-metabolic: due to a combination of both
- Chronic: characterized by a slowly progressive alteration in mental status resulting from permanent structural changes within the brain[2]

1.1.2 Causes of Encephalopathy[3]

See ▶ Table 1.1.

1.1.3 Diagnosis of Encephalopathy

Diagnosis is guided by the history and physical examination of the patient. It is considered on a case-by-case basis.

- Laboratory testing
  - Serum electrolytes
  - Renal function
  - Glucose

- ○ Calcium
- ○ Complete blood count
- ○ Urinalysis
- ○ Hepatic function
- ○ Thyroid function
- ○ Drug levels (if applicable), i.e., phenytoin
- ○ Drugs of abuse screen
- ○ Vitamin levels—B-12, folate
- ○ Arterial blood gas
- Imaging
  - ○ Computed tomography (CT) of brain
  - ○ Magnetic resonance imaging (MRI) of brain

Table 1.1 Common causes of encephalopathy

Drugs and toxins	Idiopathic
	Withdrawal states
	Medication side effects
	Poisons
Infections	Sepsis
	Systemic infections
	Fever
Metabolic derangements	Electrolytes
	Endocrine disturbance
	Hypercarbia
	Hyperglycemia and hypoglycemia
	Hyperosmolar and hypo-osmolar states
	Hypoxemia
	Inborn errors of metabolism
	Nutritional
Brain disorders	CNS infection
	Seizures
	Head injury
	Hypertensive encephalopathy
	Psychiatric disorders
Systemic organ failure	Cardiac failure
	Hematologic
	Hepatic encephalopathy
	Pulmonary disease
	Renal failure

Abbreviation: CNS, central nervous system.

- Evaluation for infections
  - Lumbar puncture
  - Blood cultures
- Seizure evaluation
  - Electroencephalography (EEG)

1.1.4 Treatment of Encephalopathy

- Acute encephalopathy
  - Based on treatment of the underlying pathophysiology, i.e., treatment of sepsis and hypothyroidism with the potential for reversal of encephalopathy.
- Chronic encephalopathy
  - Often not amenable to treatment as the inciting insult has caused permanent brain changes, i.e., anoxic encephalopathy.

1.1.5 Relationship to Delirium

Delirium can be characterized as the symptom of the underlying abnormal brain function, i.e., encephalopathy.[2]

1.2 Delirium

Delirium is a common disorder in hospitalized patients that has significant societal and economic impact.[4] In-hospital mortality rates reportedly associated with delirium range from 22 to 33%.[5,6] Currently patients aged 65 years and older account for more than 48% of hospital care; therefore, the impact of delirium on hospitalized patients will continue to grow as our population ages.[4]

1.2.1 Definition

The Diagnostic and Statistical Manual of Mental Disorders (DSM) 5 defines delirium under Neurocognitive Disorders[7] which encompasses "the group of disorders in which the primary clinical deficit is in cognitive function, and that are acquired rather than developmental." The diagnostic criteria are as follows:

- A disturbance in attention (i.e., reduced ability to direct, focus, sustain, and shift attention) and awareness (reduced orientation to the environment).
- The disturbance develops over a short period of time (usually from hours to a few days), represents a change from baseline attention and awareness, and tends to fluctuate in severity during the course of a day.
- An additional disturbance in cognition (e.g., memory deficit, disorientation, language, visuospatial ability, or perception).

- The disturbances are not explained by another pre-existing, established, or evolving neurocognitive disorder and do not occur in the context of a severely reduced level of arousal, such as coma.
- There is evidence from the history, physical examination, or laboratory findings that the disturbance is a direct physiologic consequence of another medical condition, substance intoxication or withdrawal (i.e., due to a drug of abuse or a medication), or exposure to a toxin, or is due to multiple etiologies.

As outlined in the DSM 5, Delirium can be further subdivided into:
- Substance intoxication
- Substance withdrawal
- Medication induced
- Another medical condition
- Multiple etiologies

1.2.2 Duration of Symptoms

- **Acute:** Lasting for a few hours or days
- **Persistent:** Lasting for weeks or months

1.2.3 Level of Activity (▶ Table 1.2)

- **Hyperactive:** The individual has a hyperactive level of psychomotor activity that may be accompanied by mood lability, agitation, and/or refusal to cooperate with medical care.
- **Hypoactive:** The individual has a hypoactive level of psychomotor activity that may be accompanied by sluggishness and lethargy that approaches stupor.
- **Mixed level of activity:** The individual has a normal level of psychomotor activity even though attention and awareness are disturbed. Also includes individuals whose activity level rapidly fluctuates.

Table 1.2 Types of delirium

	Description	RASS score	Prevalence[8]
Hyperactive	Agitation and restlessness	1 + to 4 +	Rare (1.6%)
Hypoactive	Decreased responsiveness, withdrawal, apathy	0 to 3	Common in ICU (43.5%)

Abbreviations: ICU, intensive care unit; RASS, Richmond Agitation Sedation Scale.

Table 1.3 Risk factors for delirium

Predisposing factors[10]	Precipitating factors[11]	Targeted interventions[12]
• Cognitive impairment • Severe underlying illness • Advanced age • Functional impairment • Chronic renal insufficiency • Dehydration • Malnutrition • Depression • Substance abuse • Vision or hearing impairment	• Use of physical restraints • Malnutrition • More than three medications • Use of bladder catheter • Psychoactive medication use • Any iatrogenic event • Immobilization • Dehydration	• Noise reduction • Reality orientation program • Early mobilization • Minimize medications • Provision of visual and hearing aids • Volume repletion and proper nutrition • Optimize nonpharmacologic protocols

A description of a patient in terms of the DSM 5 criteria could look like "acute, hypoactive delirium due to sepsis."

1.2.4 Risk Factors for Delirium

Delirium involves a multifactorial etiology ranging from patient vulnerability to delirium at the time of admission and the occurrence of noxious insults during hospitalization.[9] See ▶ Table 1.3.

1.2.5 Clinical Assessment

Assessment begins in the intensive care unit (ICU) setting for the level of arousability, ranging from sedation to agitation, prior to assessing level of consciousness and subsequent delirium.[13]

Arousability Assessment Tools

- **Richmond Agitation Sedation Scale (RASS):** See ▶ Table 1.4. A 10-point scale ranging from +4 to −5, created to assess sedation and agitation in the adult patient admitted to the ICU. An RASS score of 0 denotes a calm and alert patient. Positive RASS scores indicate positive or aggressive symptoms. Negative RASS scores differentiate between response to verbal commands (−1 to −3) and physical stimulus (−4 to −5).[3]
- **Ramsay score:** See ▶ Table 1.5. It defines the conscious state from a level 1: the patient is anxious, agitated, or restless, through to the continuously sedated level 6: the patient is completely unresponsive.[14]
- **Riker Sedation Agitation Scale (SAS):** See ▶ Table 1.6. It was developed in 1999 with the goal of clearly defining and providing more inclusive levels of sedation and agitation than the Ramsay score.[15]

Table 1.4 Richmond Agitation Sedation Scale

Richmond Agitation Sedation Scale	Description
+ 4 Combative	Overtly combative, violent, danger to staff
+ 3 Very agitated	Pulls or removes tubes or catheters; aggressive
+ 3 Agitated	Frequent nonpurposeful movement, fights ventilator
+ 1 Restless	Anxious, but movements not aggressive or vigorous
0 Alert and calm	
−1 Drowsy	Not fully alert, but has sustained awakening (eye opening/eye contact) to voice (> 10 s)
−2 Light sedation	Briefly awakens with eye contact to voice (< 10 s)
−3 Moderate sedation	Movement or eye opening to voice (but no eye contact)
−4 Deep sedation	No response to voice, but movement or eye opening to physical stimulation
−5 Unable to rouse	No response to voice or physical stimulus

Table 1.5 Ramsay Sedation Scale

Ramsay Sedation Scale	Description
1	Anxious, agitated, restless
2	Cooperative, oriented, tranquil
3	Responsive to commands only
4	Brisk response to light glabellar tap or loud auditory stimulus
5	Sluggish response to light glabellar tap or loud auditory stimulus
6	No response to light glabellar tap or loud auditory stimulus

Delirium Assessment

Confusion Assessment Method for the ICU (CAM-ICU): See ► Fig. 1.1. Four features assess fluctuation in mental status, inattention, disorganized thinking, and altered level of consciousness.[16]

Table 1.6 Riker Sedation Scale

Riker Sedation Agitation Scale	Description
7 Dangerous agitation	Pulling at ET tube, trying to remove catheters, climbing over bedrail, striking at staff, thrashing side to side
6 Very agitated	Requiring restraint and frequent verbal reminding of limits, biting ET tube
5 Agitated	Anxious or physically agitated, calms to verbal instruction
4 Calm and cooperative	Calm, easily arousable, follows commands
3 Sedated	Difficult to arouse but awakens to verbal stimuli or gentle shaking, follows simple commands but drifts off again
2 Very sedated	Arouses to physical stimuli but does not communicate or follow commands, may move spontaneously
1 Unarousable	Minimal to no response to noxious stimuli, does not communicate or follow commands

Abbreviation: ET, endotracheal.

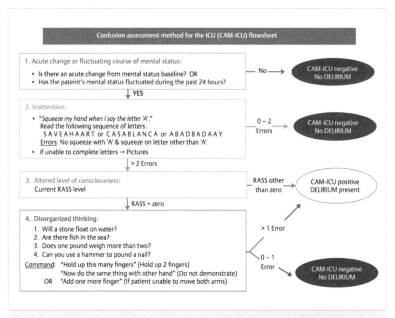

Fig. 1.1 Confusion assessment method for the intensive care unit (CAM-ICU) flowsheet. Copyright © 2002, E. Wesley Ely, MD, MPH and Vanderbilt University, all rights reserved.

Table 1.7 Medications used to treat agitation

Agent	Mechanism	Advantage	Adverse effects
Midazolam	Increases GABA activity	Rapid onset of action with high metabolic clearance	Respiratory depression, hypotension
Lorazepam	Increases GABA activity	Intermediate onset of action with mid-range metabolic clearance	Respiratory depression, hypotension; propylene glycol-related acidosis, nephrotoxicity
Diazepam	Increases GABA activity	Rapid onset of action with long half-life (10–20 hours)	Respiratory depression, hypotension, phlebitis
Propofol	Increases GABA activity	Rapid onset of action with high metabolic clearance	Pain on injection, hypotension, respiratory depression, hypertriglyceridemia, pancreatitis, allergic reactions, propofol infusion syndrome
Dexmedetomidine	Alpha 2 adrenergic receptor agonist	Provides sedation without respiratory depression risk	Bradycardia, hypotension; hypertension with loading dose; loss of airway reflexes

Abbreviation: GABA, gamma aminobutyric acid.

1.3 Treatment

1.3.1 Medications for Agitation[3]

See ▶ Table 1.7.

1.3.2 Pharmacologic Management of Hyperactive Delirium and Agitation

See ▶ Table 1.8

1.3.3 Nonpharmacologic Treatments for Delirium[21]

- Frequent reorientation with signs, clocks, and calendars
- Address dehydration and constipation
- Assess for hypoxia and optimize oxygen saturation
- Assess for underlying infection
- Avoid unnecessary catherization
- Early mobilization

- Address pain
- Review medications
- Nutrition assessment
- Address reversible sensory impairment with glasses and hearing aids
- Promote good sleep hygiene

Table 1.8 Medications used to treat delirium

	Mechanism	Advantage	Adverse effects
Typical antipsychotics Haloperidol Chlorpromazine Thioridazine	Postsynaptic blockade of dopamine D2 receptors with varying effect on neuronal 5-HT2a, alpha-1, histaminic, and muscarinic receptors[17]	Fewer anticholinergic effects, few active metabolites, minimally sedating, amelioration of hallucinations, delusion, and unstructured thought patterns[18]	Significant risk of extrapyramidal side effects and tardive dyskinesia; cognitive numbness and dysphoria, extrapyramidal side effects, neuroleptic malignant syndrome, dystonic reactions, ventricular arrhythmias, torsades de pointe, cardiac arrest, QT prolongation[17]
Atypical antipsychotics Olanzapine Risperidone Quetiapine Ziprasidone	Postsynaptic blockade of D2 receptors with varying effect on neuronal 5-HT2a, alpha-1, histaminic, and muscarinic receptors; *serotonin 5-HT2 receptor binding exceeds its loose affinity for dopamine D2*	Generally they have lower risk of extrapyramidal side effects and tardive dyskinesia compared with first-generation antipsychotics[19]	Weight gain and related metabolic effects, hypotension, sedation, anticholinergic symptoms, hyperprolactinemia, extrapyramidal symptoms (EPS), cardiac effects, cardiomyopathies, cataracts, and sexual dysfunction; *anticholinergic effects most prominent with olanzapine, quetiapine, and clozapine*
Benzodiazepines Midazolam Lorazepam Diazepam	Bind to specific receptors in the gamma aminobutyric acid (GABA) receptor complex, which enhances the binding of this	Anxiolysis is achieved at low doses; rapid effect; duration varies and can be given via continuous infusion for stability	Sedation, respiratory and cardiovascular depression; *paradoxical reaction characterized by agitation, restlessness, and hostility*[20]

References

[1] Encephalopathy Information Page | National Institute of Neurological Disorders and Stroke. https://www.ninds.nih.gov/Disorders/All-Disorders/Encephalopathy-Infomation-Page. Published 2018. Accessed

[2] Pinson, R. Encephalopathy: Clinicians often struggle with the distinction between delirium and encephalopathy. Coding Corner, 2015. https://acphospitalist.org/archives/2015/01/coding.htm

[3] Barr J, Fraser GL, Puntillo K, et al. American College of Critical Care Medicine. Clinical practice guidelines for the management of pain, agitation, and delirium in adult patients in the intensive care unit. Crit Care Med. 2013; 41(1):263–306

[4] Leslie DL, Marcantonio ER, Zhang Y, Leo-Summers L, Inouye SK. One-year health care costs associated with delirium in the elderly population. Arch Intern Med. 2008; 168(1):27–32

[5] Pandharipande P, Jackson J, Ely EW. Delirium: acute cognitive dysfunction in the critically ill. Curr Opin Crit Care. 2005; 11(4):360–368

[6] Inouye SK, Schlesinger MJ, Lydon TJ. Delirium: a symptom of how hospital care is failing older persons and a window to improve quality of hospital care. Am J Med. 1999; 106(5):565–573

[7] Diagnostic and Statistical Manual of Mental Disorders, Fifth Edition. https://dsm.psychiatryonline.org/doi/book/10.1176/appi.books.9780890425596

[8] Peterson JF, Pun BT, Dittus RS, et al. Delirium and its motoric subtypes: a study of 614 critically ill patients. J Am Geriatr Soc. 2006; 54(3):479–484

[9] Inouye SK. Prevention of delirium in hospitalized older patients: risk factors and targeted intervention strategies. Ann Med. 2000; 32(4):257–263

[10] Dubois MJ, Bergeron N, Dumont M, Dial S, Skrobik Y. Delirium in an intensive care unit: a study of risk factors. Intensive Care Med. 2001; 27(8):1297–1304

[11] Girard TD, Pandharipande PP, Ely EW. Delirium in the intensive care unit. Crit Care. 2008; 12 Suppl 3:S3

[12] Elie M, Cole MG, Primeau FJ, Bellavance F. Delirium risk factors in elderly hospitalized patients. J Gen Intern Med. 1998; 13(3):204–212

[13] Khan BA, Guzman O, Campbell NL, et al. Comparison and agreement between the Richmond agitation-sedation scale and the Riker sedation-agitation scale in evaluating patients' eligibility for delirium assessment in the ICU. Chest. 2012; 142(1):48–54

[14] Ramsay MA, Savege TM, Simpson BR, Goodwin R. Controlled sedation with alphaxalone-alphadolone. BMJ. 1974; 2(5920):656–659

[15] Jacobi J, Fraser GL, Coursin DB, et al. Task Force of the American College of Critical Care Medicine (ACCM), of the Society of Critical Care Medicine (SCCM), American Society of Health-System Pharmacists (ASHP), American College of Chest Physicians. Clinical practice guidelines for the sustained use of sedatives and analgesics in the critically ill adult. Crit Care Med. 2002; 30(1):119–141

[16] Inouye SK, van Dyck CH, Alessi CA, Balkin S, Siegal AP, Horwitz RI. Clarifying confusion: the confusion assessment method. A new method for detection of delirium. Ann Intern Med. 1990; 113 (12):941–948

[17] Skrobik YK, Bergeron N, Dumont M, Gottfried SB. Olanzapine vs haloperidol: treating delirium in a critical care setting. Intensive Care Med. 2004; 30(3):444–449

[18] Kalisvaart KJ, de Jonghe JF, Bogaards MJ, et al. Haloperidol prophylaxis for elderly hip-surgery patients at risk for delirium: a randomized placebo-controlled study. J Am Geriatr Soc. 2005; 53 (10):1658–1666

[19] Schwartz TL, Masand PS. The role of atypical antipsychotics in the treatment of delirium. Psychosomatics. 2002; 43(3):171–174

[20] Pandharipande P, Shintani A, Peterson J, et al. Lorazepam is an independent risk factor for transitioning to delirium in intensive care unit patients. Anesthesiology. 2006; 104(1):21–26

[21] O'Mahony R, Murthy L, Akunne A, Young J, Guideline Development Group. Synopsis of the National Institute for Health and Clinical Excellence guideline for prevention of delirium. Ann Intern Med. 2011; 154(11):746–751

2 Cerebrovascular Emergency: Acute Stroke Diagnosis and Management

Maria Carissa C. Pineda, Sridhara S. Yaddanapudi, and Norman Ajiboye

Abstract

Stroke is one of the leading causes of disability in the USA. Timely acute interventions in the form of tPA and endovascular therapy have changed the landscape of acute stroke care. Having an organized and efficient system of care is extremely important for delivering acute stroke care. This chapter details the components of acute stroke care from the emergency room to the neurocritical care unit. The chapter covers pre- and post-tPA and endovascular care as well as post stroke complication management in the neurocritical care unit.

Keywords: acute stroke, tPA, endovascular therapy, neurocritical care

2.1 Epidemiology

- Stroke is the fifth leading cause of death in North America
- It is the leading cause of disability
- 795,000 people/year have a stroke in North America

2.2 Etiology

2.2.1 Nonmodifiable Risk Factors

- Age
- Sex
- Race
- Family history

2.2.2 Modifiable Risk Factors

- Hypertension
- Diabetes mellitus
- Hyperlipidemia
- Smoking
- Excessive alcohol use
- Obstructive sleep apnea

2.2.3 Stroke Subtypes

According to TOAST[9] classification there are five subtypes of ischemic stroke:
1. Large artery atherosclerosis
2. Cardioembolism
3. Small vessel occlusion (lacunar stroke)
4. Stroke of other determined etiology
   - Mechanical valves
   - Atrial fibrillation/flutter
   - Left atrial (LA) appendage thrombus
   - Left ventricular (LV) thrombus
   - Recent myocardial infarction (MI)
   - Dilated cardiomyopathy
   - Endocarditis/infection
   - Patent foramen ovale
   - Atrial septal aneurysm
   - Congestive heart failure
   - Vasculopathies
   - Hypercoagulable state
5. Stroke of undetermined etiology/cryptogenic

2.3 Common Clinical Presentations

Presentation depends on the vascular territory. See ▶ Table 2.1.

F.A.S.T. is the acronym most associated with recognition of early stroke signs:
F = Facial weakness
A = Arm weakness
S = Speech difficulty
T = Time to call 9–1-1

Once in the emergency department a more thorough examination using the National Institutes of Health Stroke Scale (NIHSS) is completed (▶ Table 2.2).

2.4 Differential Diagnosis for Acute Ischemic Stroke

- Intracerebral hemorrhage (ICH)
- Subarachnoid hemorrhage (SAH)
- Migraine with aura (most auras DO NOT last beyond 60 minutes nor present with loss of function)
- Transient global amnesia
- Postictal Todd's palsy (history of epilepsy or prior Todd's palsy, short duration with improvement)
- Hypoglycemia (rapid improvement with glucose correction)[2]

Table 2.1 Common clinical presentation by vascular territory

Vascular territory	Symptoms
Middle cerebral artery	Contralateral facial droop, weakness and sensory loss (arm > leg), aphasia, neglect, contralateral homonymous hemianopia, ipsilateral gaze deviation
Anterior cerebral artery	Contralateral hemiplegia (leg >> face and arm), abulia, rigidity, gait apraxia, urinary incontinence
Posterior cerebral artery	Contralateral homonymous hemianopia, alexia, contralateral sensory loss, cortical blindness, visual hallucinations, optic ataxia, gaze apraxia
Subcortical	Contralateral hemiplegia or hemisensory loss (usually face = arm = leg), no cortical features (aphasia, neglect), thalamic strokes may have aphasia, delirium, other cortical features
Basilar artery	Cranial nerve palsy, crossed sensory deficits, dizziness, diplopia, dysarthria, dysphagia, vertigo, nausea/vomiting, hiccups, contralateral weakness, ataxia, nystagmus, coma

2.5 Acute Stroke Diagnosis, Treatment, and Management[4]

2.5.1 Stroke Activation (▶ Fig. 2.1)

- **ABC**: airway, breathing, circulation
  - O_2 saturation > 94% (supplemental oxygen is not recommended if the patient is not hypoxic)
  - Finger-stick glucose should be > 50
- Intravenous (IV) access
- **History:** Past medical, surgical, and medication (ask about antiplatelet and anticoagulant agents)
- Check electrocardiogram (ECG)—rule out acute ST-elevation myocardial infarction (STEMI)
- **Send STAT labs:** Coagulation panel and platelet
- Perform focal stroke examination using NIHSS (▶ Table 2.2 *shows the pictures and sentences used for questions 9 and 10 on the scale.*)

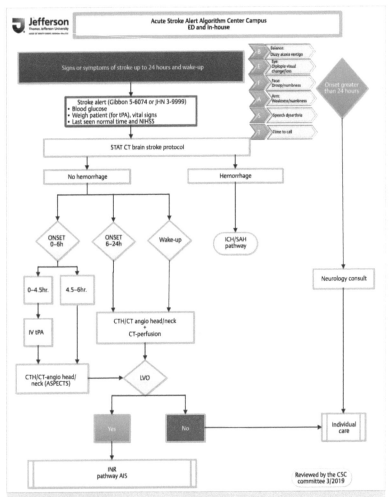

Fig. 2.1 Thomas Jefferson University acute stroke algorithm for in-house and emergency room activation.

Table 2.2 **(a)** NIH stroke scale. **(b)** Supplement to questions 9 and 10 on the National Institutes of Health Stroke Scale (NIHSS) used to determine deficits in language and speech. **(1–3)** Assessment of aphasia: **(1)** describing the picture, **(2)** reading the short sentences, and **(3)** naming the objects listed. **(4)** Words repeated by the patient to assess dysarthria. (Reproduced with permission from National Institute of Neurological Disorders and Stroke (NINDS).)

NIH stroke scale		
Category	**Description**	**Score**
1a. Level of consciousness (LOC)	0 = Alert 1 = Drowsy 2 = Stuporous 3 = Coma	
1b. LOC questions	0 = Answers both correctly 1 = Answers one correctly 2 = Answers neither correctly	
2. Best gaze	0 = Normal 1 = Partial gaze palsy 2 = Forced deviation	
3. Visual	0 = No visual loss 1 = Partial hemianopia 2 = Complete hemianopia 3 = Bilateral hemianopia	
4. Facial palsy	0 = No facial palsy 1 = Minor facial palsy 2 = Partial facial palsy 3 = Complete facial palsy	
5a. Motor left arm	0 = No drift 1 = Drift 2 = Can't resist gravity 3 = No effort against gravity 4 = No movement UN = Amputation/Joint fusion	
5b. Motor right arm	0 = No drift 1 = Drift 2 = Can't resist gravity 3 = No effort against gravity 4 = No movement UN = Amputation/Joint fusion	

(*Continued*)

Table 2.2 (*Continued*) **(a)** NIH stroke scale. **(b)** Supplement to questions 9 and 10 on the National Institutes of Health Stroke Scale (NIHSS) used to determine deficits in language and speech. **(1–3)** Assessment of aphasia: **(1)** describing the picture, **(2)** reading the short sentences, and **(3)** naming the objects listed. **(4)** Words repeated by the patient to assess dysarthria. (Reproduced with permission from National Institute of Neurological Disorders and Stroke (NINDS).)

Category	Description	Score
6a. Motor left leg	0 = No drift 1 = Drift 2 = Can't resist gravity 3 = No effort against gravity 4 = No movement UN = Amputation/Joint fusion	
6b. Motor right leg	0 = No drift 1 = Drift 2 = Can't resist gravity 3 = No effort against gravity 4 = No movement UN = Amputation/Joint fusion	
7. Limb ataxia	0 = Absent 1 = Present in one limb 2 = Present in two limbs	
8. Sensory	0 = Normal 1 = Partial loss 2 = Severe loss	
9. Best language[a]	0 = No aphasia 1 = Mild to moderate aphasia 2 = Severe aphasia 3 = Mute	
10. Dysarthria[b]	0 = Normal articulation 1 = Mild to moderate dysarthria 2 = Near to unintelligible 3 = Intubated or other barrier	
11. Extinction and inattention	0 = No neglect 1 = Partial neglect 3 = Complete neglect	
	Total	

(*Continued*)

Table 2.2 (*Continued*) (a) NIH stroke scale. (b) Supplement to questions 9 and 10 on the National Institutes of Health Stroke Scale (NIHSS) used to determine deficits in language and speech. (1–3) Assessment of aphasia: (1) describing the picture, (2) reading the short sentences, and (3) naming the objects listed. (4) Words repeated by the patient to assess dysarthria. (Reproduced with permission from National Institute of Neurological Disorders and Stroke (NINDS).)

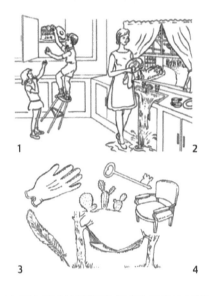

You know how.

Down to earth.

I got home from work.

Near the table in the dining room.

They heard him speak on the radio last night.

Mama
Tip–top
Fifty–fifty
Thanks
Huckleberry
Baseball player

See ▶ Table 2.2(a) ᵃAsk patient to name items, describe the picture, read a sentence, intubated patients should write response if able.
ᵇEvaluate speech clarity by asking patient to repeat the listed words
Abbreviations: LOC, level of consciousness; NIHSS, National Institute of Health Stroke Scale.

- Check STAT computed tomography (CT) of head (▶ Fig. 2.2)
  - Rule out hemorrhage
  - Rule out large completed ischemic stroke
  - Identify acute middle cerebral artery (MCA) or basilar occlusion
- Assess eligibility for *IV tPA* (▶ Table 2.3 and ▶ Fig. 2.3)
  - If eligible, dosing for tPA is 0.9 mg/kg with a maximum dose of 90 mg.
  - A bolus of 10% is given over the first minute followed by the remaining dose over 1 hour.
  - If a patient is ineligible for tPA then administer 325 mg aspirin orally or 300 mg aspirin rectally (provided no hemorrhage on CT of head).

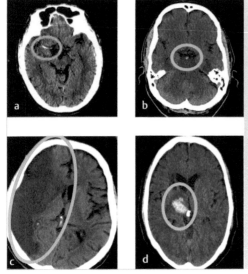

Fig. 2.2 (a, b) Examples of a dense occlusion of an artery due to acute thrombus: **(a)** Dense occluded right middle cerebral artery (MCA). **(b)** Dense occluded basilar artery. **(c, d)** Examples of computed tomography (CT)scan finding that would exclude a patient from receiving intravenous (IV) tPA. **(c)** A completed right middle cerebral artery (MCA) stroke. **(d)** A right thalamic hemorrhage.

- Blood pressure goals (▶ Fig. 2.4):
    - Blood pressure must be controlled prior to administering IV tPA to minimize the bleeding risk. Goal is < 185/110.
    - With tPA administration, maintain a blood pressure (BP) goal of < 180/105.
    - If tPA is NOT given then the BP goal should be < 220/110 during the first 24 hours.
    - Avoid agents like hydralazine, nitroprusside, and nitroglycerin due to their vasodilatory effect.
- ▶ Fig. 2.1 outlines the pathway for further imaging in patients with suspected large vessel occlusion or dense vessel on plain CT head. CT angiogram (CTA) of head and neck to identify artery occlusion and CT perfusion to evaluate size of core infarct and penumbra (▶ Fig. 2.5).

2.6 Criteria for Endovascular Therapy

Early studies published in 2013 (IMS-III, SYNTHESIS, and MR RESCUE) failed to show benefit of endovascular treatment of acute ischemic stroke.[6,7,8]

Between 2015–2018, multiple studies have shown the benefit of endovascular treatment with or without tPA.[1,10,11,12] Based on the findings of these studies, the American Heart Association/American Stroke Association published new guidelines in 2018 supporting endovascular treatment with stent retriever provided the following criteria are met:[4]

Table 2.3 Eligibility criteria, warnings, and contraindications to intravenous tPA (Alteplase)

Eligibility criteria within the 3 hours window	
	Recommended for both severe stroke and for mild but disabling strokes
	Age ≥ 18 years; equally recommended for ages < 80 and > 80 years under 3 hours of onset
Warnings for IV tPA within the 3 hours window	
	Clinical syndrome not consistent with ischemic stroke
	Recent history of intracranial hemorrhage
Contraindications for IV tPA within the 3 hours window	
	Active intracranial hemorrhage (i.e., subdural hematoma, epidural hematoma, subarachnoid hemorrhage, or spontaneous intracerebral hemorrhage)
	Active internal bleeding
	Clinical presentation suggesting cerebral aneurysm rupture and/or subarachnoid hemorrhage
	Delay in patient arrival, unknown time of onset and/or "wake up" stroke
	Current severe uncontrolled hypertension (SBP > 185 mm Hg or DBP > 110 mm Hg) despite aggressive treatment
	Presence of intracranial conditions that may increase the risk of bleeding (neoplasm either primary or metastatic; cerebral arteriovenous malformation, etc.)
	Ischemic stroke in the setting of infective endocarditis
	Recent intracranial or intraspinal surgery within prior 3 months (lumbar puncture within 7 days does **NOT** apply)
	Recent severe head trauma or history of post-traumatic stroke within 3 months
	History of structural gastrointestinal malignancy or recent gastrointestinal hemorrhage within 3 weeks
	Known or suspected aortic dissection

(*Continued*)

Table 2.3 (*Continued*) Eligibility criteria, warnings, and contraindications to intravenous tPA (Alteplase)

	Bleeding diathesis/coagulopathy or thrombocytopenia including but not limited to: • Known INR > 1.7 and/or elevated PT > 15 seconds • Known administration of therapeutic doses of heparin or low-molecular-weight heparin within 24 hours of presentation or elevated aPTT > 40 seconds • Known platelet count < 100,000/mm³ • Known use of direct thrombin inhibitors or factor Xa inhibitors (BOACs) within 48 hours of stroke symptoms assuming normal renal function
Eligibility criteria for the 3 to 4.5 hours window	
	Age < 80 years
	NO history of both stroke and diabetes mellitus
	NIHSS < 25
	Not on oral anticoagulant agents
	No evidence of ischemia of > 1/3 of the MCA territory
Additional **warnings** within the 3 to 4.5 hours window[a]	
	Age > 80 years
	History of prior stroke and diabetes mellitus
	NIHSS > 25
Additional **contraindications** within the 3 to 4.5 hours window	
	Current use of oral anticoagulant and/or INR > 1.7
	Patients with imaging evidence of ischemic injury involving more than one-third of the MCA territory

[a]Deemed Class IIb (possible benefit > risk) so it may be considered.

Adapted from the AHA/ASA 2018 Guideline for the Early Management of Acute Ischemic Stroke[3]
Abbreviations: aPTT, activated partial thromboplastin time; DBP, diastolic blood pressure; INR, international normalized ratio; MCA, middle cerebral artery; NIHSS; PT, prothrombin time; SBP, systolic blood pressure.

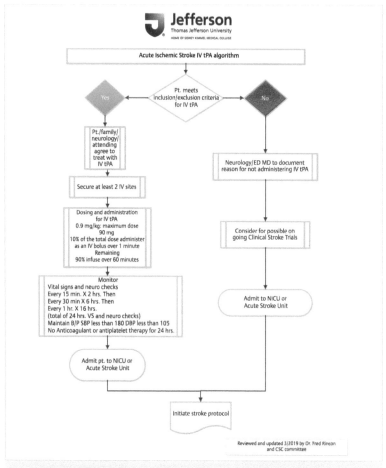

Fig. 2.3 Thomas Jefferson University algorithm for Ischemic Stroke and Assessment for intravenous tPA (Alteplase).

- Age ≥ 18 years
- Pre-stroke modified Rankin score (mRS) is 0–1
- Causative occlusion is in the internal carotid or proximal middle cerebral vessel (M1). CT angiogram (CTA) or magnetic resonance angiogram (MRA) should be completed to look for large vessel occlusion in the internal carotid artery ot proximal middle cerebral artery (M1)
- NIHSS ≥ 6

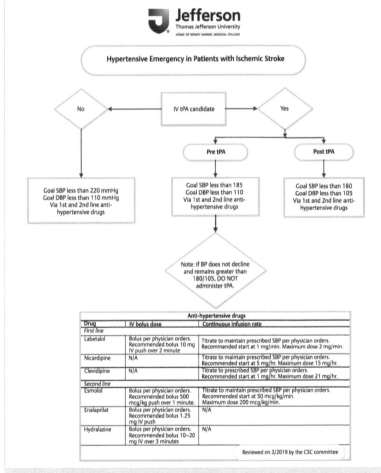

Fig. 2.4 Thomas Jefferson University algorithm for the management of hypertensive emergency in patients with acute ischemic stroke.

- Alberta Stroke Program Early CT Score (ASPECTS) ≥ 6
- Endovascular treatment should be initiated with 6 hours of symptom onset

Furthermore, the most recent guidelines recommend mechanical thrombectomy for select patients whose last known well time was within 16 to 24 hours, who have signs of anterior circulation large vessel occlusion, and who meet the eligibility criteria defined in the clinical trials of DAWN[11] and DEFUSE 3.[12]

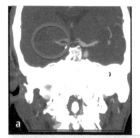 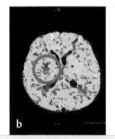 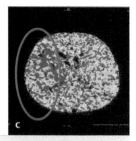

Fig. 2.5 Advanced imaging obtained for patients suspected of large vessel occlusions. **(a)** Computed tomography (CT) angiogram demonstrating occlusion of the right middle cerebral artery with a "cutoff" of contrast. **(b, c)** Represent CT perfusion images. **(b)** Cerebral blood flow showing decreased flow within the right basal ganglia. **(c)** Mean transit time (MTT) demonstrating prolonged perfusion time. MTT helps to distinguish tissue "at risk" (penumbra) from ischemic nonviable tissue.

2.6.1 Neurocritical Care Management of Ischemic Stroke

After administration of the appropriate acute stroke therapy, there are important medical management issues that need to be addressed. Studies have shown that acute care in a stroke unit or a neurocritical care unit has shown better outcomes especially with the utilization of stroke protocols.

- Post tPA complications
- Post tPA management
- Post thrombectomy management
- Stroke workup and risk factor management
- Post stroke complications
- Surgical management of stroke

Post-tPA Complication

- Bleeding
  - ○ 6.4% risk of symptomatic bleed from IV tPA
  - ○ Patients acutely develop worsening neurologic examination (increase of NIHSS by 4 or more points), headache, nausea/vomiting, or acute hypertension
  - ○ Management of post tPA bleeding
    - – Stop IV tPA infusion
    - – Reduce blood pressure to < 140/90
    - – Send stat complete blood count (CBC), coagulation panel, fibrinogen, and type and screen
    - – Check STAT CT head

- If bleeding is present on the CTH (CT head) transfuse
  - ► Cryoprecipitate 10 units over 10 to 30 minutes if fibrinogen < 200 give
  - ► Tranexamic acid (TXA) 1 gm IV over 10 minutes or
  - ► E-aminocaproic acid (EACA) 5 gm over 1 hour followed by 1 gm IV until bleeding controlled.
- Follow serial fibrinogen levels goal > 200
- STAT neurosurgical consultation
- Angioedema
  - Although relatively rare, angioedema and anaphylaxis have occurred post-tPA administration. Angioedema has been estimated to occur in approximately 5% of patients (those taking ACE inhibitors are at increased risk). If needed treat with:
    - IV diphenhydramine or
    - IV methylprednisolone or
    - IV ranitidine
    - Epinephrine can be used for severe anaphylaxis

Post tPA Management

- BP goal 140–180/105. Avoiding extremes in either direction, blood pressure which can cause bleeding or increased ischemia.
- No antiplatelet, anticoagulant, or chemoprophylaxis for deep vein thrombosis (DVT) prophylaxis for 24 hours.
- Repeat CT or magnetic resonance imaging (MRI) of brain 24 hours post TPA administration to look for hemorrhagic transformation[13] or large territory stroke that would delay initiating antiplatelet or anticoagulation therapy (► Table 2.4).

Table 2.4 Subtypes of hemorrhagic transformation of ischemic stroke

Radiographic classification of hemorrhage transformation of ischemic stroke	
Hemorrhagic classification	Radiographic appearance
Hemorrhagic infarct type 1 (HI1)	Petechial hemorrhage at the margins
Hemorrhagic infarct type 2 (HI2)	Petechial hemorrhages throughout the infarct without mass effect
Parenchymal hematoma type 1 (PH1)	Hemorrhage of ≤ 30% of the stroke volume with mild mass effect due to the hematoma
Parenchymal hematoma type 2 (PH2)	Hemorrhage of > 30% of stroke volume with substantial mass effect due to the hematoma

Adapted from Demaerschalk BM, Kleindorfer DO, Adeoye OM, et al.[5]

Post Thrombectomy Care (▶ Fig. 2.6)

- Femoral artery site: Monitor for hematoma formation and loss of distal pulses.
  - Check distal pulses every 15 minutes for the first hour, every 30 minutes for next 4 hours then hourly for 24 hours.
  - If there is loss of pulses, notify endovascular team and consider vascular surgery for possible thrombectomy.

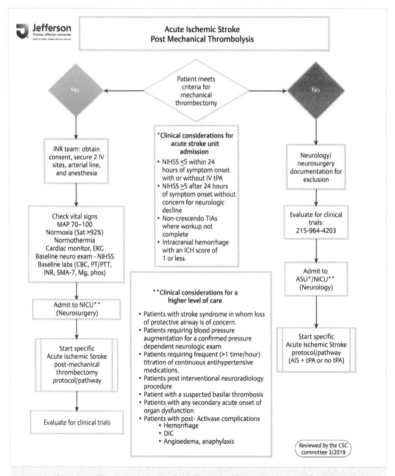

Fig. 2.6 Thomas Jefferson University algorithm for the management of post-thrombectomy patients.

- o If there is groin hematoma, check CT of abdomen/pelvis to rule out retro-peritoneal hemorrhage.
- Radial artery site: Monitor radial artery band.
  - o Continue full inflation for 1 hour post procedure.
  - o Slowly deflate radial band by 5 cc every 10 minutes after the first hour.
- Blood pressure:
  - o Successful thrombectomy with TICI (Thrombolysis in cerebral infraction) ≥ 2b[10]
    - – Keep systolic blood pressure (SBP) within 140–160 mm Hg or mean arterial pressure (MAP) 70–90 mm Hg
  - o Unsuccessful thombectomy with TICI ≤ 2a[11]
    - – Blood pressure goal should be in accordance with the acute ischemic stroke guidelines
      - ► < 220/110 if IV tPA is not given
      - ► < 180/105 if IV tPA is given

2.7 Stroke Workup and Management

Stroke workup may include any of the following based on specific risk factor management:

- MRI of head/MR angiography (MRA) of head and neck (if no CTA was performed)
- Transthoracic echocardiogram with bubble study
- Transesophageal echocardiogram in certain patient populations
- MR venogram if venous stroke is suspected
- Lower extremity Dopplers
- Carotid ultrasound for patients who cannot get CTA or MRA
- Bedside dysphagia screen followed by formal swallow evaluation if bedside screening fails.
  - o Consider placing nasogastric tube for enteral access if unable to obtain formal swallow evaluation in a timely manner
  - o Percutaneous gastrostomy tube may be indicated during the hospitalization but would allow time for improvement of swallowing function before preceding
- Anemia
  - o Avoid unnecessary transfusion
  - o Transfuse for hemoglobin of ≤ 7 mg/100 mL[3] unless there are significant cardiac risk factors in which case consider goal of Hgb > 8 mg/dL
- BP management
  - o During the first 24 hours blood pressure is managed to preserve the stroke penumbra.

- Once the workup is completed and the etiology identified, it is reasonable to slowly lower the blood pressure (to normotension) over days to weeks to allow for collateral vessel formation.
- For patients with poor collateral vessels and/or with significant intracranial stenosis, the examination may worsen with normalization of blood pressure. When that occurs induced hypertension may be needed to allow for cerebral perfusion.
- When induced hypertension is implemented the goal is to increase the SBP by 25% and follow the examination. If there is no improvement in the examination within 1 to 2 hours the blood pressure can return to baseline and obtain a repeat CTH to evaluate for stroke progression.
- If the examination improves with induced hypertension then continue the methods used to maintain the new blood pressure for 3 to 5 days and then slowly lower while monitoring for worsening symptoms.
- BP should be individualized by patient noting pertinent comorbidities.
- There are occasions when BP must be augmented after the first 24 hours in order to maintain cerebral perfusion. Induced hypertension can be used with a goal of increasing the SBP by 25% and following the examination. If there is improvement in the exam then maintain that new goal. If there is no improvement then the patient can revert to baseline.
- Lipids
  - All acute stroke patients should be started on a high intensity statin
    - Atorvastatin 40 mg or Rosuvastatin 20 mg
    - Long-term goal for low-density lipoprotein (LDL) is < 100 and < 70 in high-risk atherosclerotic cardiovascular disease (ASCVD) patients. If LDL is controlled on admission it is reasonable to continue the outpatient dose.
- Antiplatelet or anticoagulation
  - Medication choice should be based on the patient's prior medication history and stroke etiology (embolic vs. thrombotic). Aspirin or Plavix or Aggrenox.
- **Anticoagulation:** There is no consensus on timing. It depends on:
  - Size of stroke
    - 24 to 48 hours for lacunar stroke with minimal deficit
    - 3 to 7 days for moderate size strokes without hemorrhage
    - 14 to 21 days for large stroke
  - Hemorrhagic conversion of current stroke
    - 3 to 5 days for petechial hemorrhage
    - 5 to 7 days for moderate bleed
    - ≥ 14 days for significant blood within the stroke bed
  - Risk of further stroke with atrial fibrillation
  - Risk of bleeding with anticoagulation
  - Heparin infusion is usually started prior to oral agents as it can be tightly controlled and reversed

- **Newer oral anticoagulants** (**NOAC**): Rivaroxaban, apixaban, Pradaxa, and edoxaban are only approved for nonvalvular atrial fibrillation and DVT/PE
  - Lovenox is preferred over warfarin in strokes in cancer patients and in pregnant women
- DVT prophylaxis
  - All patients must be screened appropriately for chemoprophylaxis
  - Intermittent pneumatic compression devices to all patients
  - Without tPA or with unsuccessful thrombectomy, chemoprophylaxis can be started on admission
  - With tPA or successful thrombectomy, chemoprophylaxis is held for 24 hours until significant hemorrhage is ruled out on repeat imaging
- Glucose control
  - Maintain serum glucose of 140 to 180 mg/dL[3]
  - Dextrose containing fluids should be avoided
  - Insulin infusion may be needed if serial Accu-Cheks have glucose > 250 mg/dL

2.7.1 Post Stroke Complication

- Cerebral edema
  - There is little evidence showing that prophylactic treatment of cerebral edema improves outcomes
  - Cerebral edema generally peaks 3 to 5 days post stroke
  - Malignant edema[14] refers to edema that causes brain compression or midline shift with change in examination
  - Malignant edema is the leading cause of early death post stroke[14]
  - Risk factors for developing malignant edema include[14]:
    - Younger age
    - Higher NIHSS at admission
    - Large hypodensity > 50% on initial CT of head
  - Cerebellar strokes pose a particularly high risk with swelling compressing the fourth ventricle causing obstructive hydrocephalus. These patients need to be followed closely by neurosurgery for possible suboccipital craniectomy.
- Management of malignant edema
  - Intubation for anyone with decreased level of consciousness (Glasgow coma score [GCS] ≤ 8) or with significant bulbar weakness
  - Head of bed is tilted by 30 degrees
  - Hyperosmolar therapy[15] avoid prophylactic use
    - Hypertonic saline (HTS) for cerebral edema
      - ►Need central venous access
      - ►HTS 3% used to maintain Na^+ goal of 145 to 155 mEq/L

- ► Bolus with 250 cc of 3% or followed by infusion starting rate of 30 mL/hour
- ► Follow serum Na^+ every 6 hours. If not at goal, rebolus and increase infusion rate
- ► Avoid other isotonic fluids
- ► If there are clinical signs of herniation, 30 mL of 23.4% can be given in slow IVP (if given too fast, will cause profound bradycardia and hypotension)
- ► Note: HTS is a volume expander and can exacerbate heart failure
  - – Mannitol
    - ► Dosing of 0.25 to 1 gm/kg every 4 to 6 hours as needed
    - ► Hold for SOsm of > 320 mOsm or Osm Gap > 10
    - ► Follow Chem 7, SOsm and/or osmolar gap every 6 hours
      - - Calculated osmolality = 2(Na) + glucose/18 + BUN (blood urea nitrogen)/2.8
      - - Increased gap may be caused by alcohol, lorazepam, diazepam, midazolam, phentobarbital, or phenobarbital (propylene glycol carrier)
    - ► Can cause hypotension and hypovolemia, replace volume with isotonic fluids (0.9NSS or Plasmalyte™)
- • Fever
  - ○ Common after large strokes and impacts mortality and outcome
  - ○ Infectious cause of fever should be ruled out
  - ○ Goal should be to maintain normothermia of 37 °C
  - ○ Aggressive fever management is indicated for temperatures > 38 °C
    - – Standing acetaminophen
      - ► Dosing: 650 mg po every 4 to 6 hours, 975 mg po every 6 hours or 1 gm IV every 6 hours
    - – Surface cooling
      - ► Arctic Sun® or BrainCool® allow for therapeutic temperature management
    - – Intravascular cooling
      - ► Thermogard XP® offers a variety of catheters for upper body and lower body which can be very effective at maintaining normothermia
    - – With any surface or intravascular cooling device, protocols to counteract shivering must be maintained.
- • Seizures
  - ○ Prophylactic treatment is not indicated
  - ○ Incidence of seizure is most often related to hemorrhagic transformation with an incidence of 4 to 8%
  - ○ Start antiseizure medication with clinical or electrographic seizure
- • Cardiac events
  - ○ Poststroke patients with and without coronary artery disease are at risk for adverse cardiac events: Acute MI, acute heart failure, arrhythmias
  - ○ All stroke patients should have troponins sent along with admission ECG

- ○ Common ECG changes seen in acute stroke include[16]
  - – T wave abnormalities
  - – Prolonged QTc
  - – U waves
  - – ST depression or change
- ○ Arrhythmias[17]
  - – Atrial fibrillation
  - – Sinus tachycardia
  - – Premature ventricular contractions
  - – Mobitz Type II AV Block
- ○ Elevated troponin
  - – Marker of ischemic heart disease
  - – Poor prognostic indicator[18]
  - – Associated with possible embolic source of stroke[19]
- ○ Management
  - – Following serial troponins
  - – Early cardiology consultation to discuss long-term management of risk factors
  - – Medications like beta-blockers or calcium channel blockers are usually restarted slowly to allow for permissive hypertension post stroke. If needed due to malignant arrhythmia or concern for STEMI they can be started within the first 24 hours paying special attention to blood pressure.
  - – Anticoagulation should be avoided in the acute stage (see above)
- • Surgical management of stroke
  - ○ Decompressive hemicraniectomy[20,21]
    - – Life-saving procedure but patients are left with significant disability (hemiplegia, need assistance with all activities of daily living [ADLs])
    - – Patients who benefit the most:
      - ► < 60 years
      - ► > 50% stroke volume
      - ► NIHSS > 16
      - ► Surgery < 48 hours from symptom onset
    - – No benefit if surgery performed > 48 hours from symptom onset
    - – Does not improve outcome for patients > 60 years
    - – No difference in outcome between dominant and nondominant hemisphere craniectomy
  - ○ Suboccipital craniectomy
    - – Surgical decompression should be addressed prior to signs of clinical deterioration:
      - ► Headache, nausea, vomiting, lethargy

- ► Nonreactive pupil (fixed and dilated)
- ► New cranial nerve palsy
  - External ventricular drainage (EVD) can be considered along with craniectomy and cerebellectomy
  - STAT head CT findings of:
    - ► Effacement of the fourth ventricle
    - ► Obstructive hydrocephalus
    - ► Brainstem compression
- ○ Carotid endarterectomy[22]
  - Symptomatic stenosis > 70%
  - Revascularization should be delayed by more than 48 hours post stroke
  - Delaying surgery to post stroke days 8 to 14 decreases odds of postoperative stroke and death

References

[1] Mozaffarian D, Benjamin EJ, Go AS, et al. American Heart Association Statistics Committee and Stroke Statistics Subcommittee. Heart disease and stroke statistics—2015 update: a report from the American Heart Association. Circulation. 2015; 131(4):e29–e322

[2] Fernandes PM, Whiteley WN, Hart SR, Al-Shahi Salman R. Strokes: mimics and chameleons. Pract Neurol. 2013; 13(1):21–28

[3] Powers WJ, Rabinstein AA, Ackerson T, et al. American Heart Association Stroke Council. 2018 Guidelines for the early management of patients with acute ischemic stroke. A guideline for healthcare professionals from the American Heart Association/American Stroke Association. Stroke. 2018; 49:e46–e99

[4] Powers WJ, Derdeyn CP, Biller J, et al. et al. 2015 American Heart Association/American Stroke Association focused update of the 2013 guidelines for the early management of patients with acute ischemic stroke regarding endovascular treatment. A guideline for healthcare professionals from the American Heart Association/American Stroke Association. Stroke. 2015; 46:3020–3035

[5] Demaerschalk BM, Kleindorfer DO, Adeoye OM, et al. American Heart Association Stroke Council and Council on Epidemiology and Prevention. Scientific rationale for the inclusion and exclusion criteria for intravenous alteplase in acute ischemic stroke: a statement for healthcare professionals from the American Heart Association/American Stroke Association. Stroke. 2016; 47(2):581–641

[6] Broderick JP, Palesch YY, Demchuk AM, et al. Interventional Management of Stroke (IMS) III Investigators. Endovascular therapy after intravenous tPA versus tPA alone for stroke. N Engl J Med. 2013; 368(10):893–903

[7] Ciccone A, Valvassori L, Nichelatti M, et al. SYNTHESIS Expansion Investigators. Endovascular treatment for acute ischemic stroke. N Engl J Med. 2013; 368(10):904–913

[8] Kidwell CS, Jahan R, Gornbein J, et al. MR RESCUE Investigators. A trial of imaging selection and endovascular treatment for ischemic stroke. N Engl J Med. 2013; 368(10):914–923

[9] Adams HP Jr, Bendixen BH, Kappelle LJ, et al. Classification of subtype of acute ischemic stroke: definition for use in a multicenter clinical trial. Trial of Org 10172 in Acute Stroke Treatment. Stroke. 1993; 24:35–41

[10] Jovin TG, Chamorro A, Cobo E, et al. REVASCAT Trial Investigators. Thrombectomy within 8 hours after symptom onset in ischemic stroke. N Engl J Med. 2015; 372(24):2296–2306

[11] Nogueira RG, Jadhav AP, Haussen DC, et al. DAWN Trial Investigators. Thrombectomy 6 to 24 hours after stroke with a mismatch between deficit and infarct. N Engl J Med. 2018; 378(1):11–21

[12] Albers GW, Marks MP, Kemp S, et al. DEFUSE 3 Investigators. Thrombectomy for stroke at 6 to 16 hours with selection by perfusion imaging. N Engl J Med. 2018; 378(8):708–718

[13] Fiorelli M, Bastianello S, von Kummer R, et al. Hemorrhagic transformation within 36 hours of a cerebral infarct: relationships with early clinical deterioration and 3-month outcome in the European Cooperative Acute Stroke Study I (ECASS I) cohort. Stroke. 1999; 30(11):2280–2284

[14] Wu S, Yuan R, Wang Y, et al. Early prediction of malignant brain edema after ischemic stroke: a systematic review and meta-analysis. Stroke. 2018; 49(12):2918–2927

[15] Simard JM, Sahuquillo J, Sheth KN, Kahle KT, Walcott BP. Managing malignant cerebral infarction. Curr Treat Options Neurol. 2011; 13(2):217–229

[16] Togha M, Sharifpour A, Ashraf H, Moghadam M, Sahraian MA. Electrocardiographic abnormalities in acute cerebrovascular events in patients with/without cardiovascular disease. Ann Indian Acad Neurol. 2013; 16(1):66–71

[17] Kallmünzer B, Breuer L, Kahl N, et al. Serious cardiac arrhythmias after stroke: incidence, time course, and predictors—a systematic, prospective analysis. Stroke. 2012; 43(11):2892–2897

[18] Jensen JK, Atar D, Mickley H. Mechanism of troponin elevations in patients with acute ischemic stroke. Am J Cardiol. 2007; 99(6):867–870

[19] Yaghi S, Chang AD, Ricci BA, et al. Early elevated troponin levels after ischemic stroke suggests a cardioembolic source. Stroke. 2018; 49(1):121–126

[20] Alexander P, Heels-Ansdell D, Siemieniuk R, et al. Hemicraniectomy versus medical treatment with large MCA infarct: a review and meta-analysis. BMJ Open. 2016; 6(11):e014390

[21] Jüttler E, Unterberg A, Woitzik J, et al. DESTINY II Investigators. Hemicraniectomy in older patients with extensive middle-cerebral-artery stroke. N Engl J Med. 2014; 370(12):1091–1100

[22] Tanious A, Pothof AB, Boi, tano LT, et al. Timing of carotid endarterectomy after stroke: retrospective review of prospectively collected national database. Ann Surg. 2018; 268(3):449–456

3 Cerebrovascular Emergency: Spontaneous Intracerebral Hemorrhage (ICH)

Syed Omar Shah

Abstract

Spontaneous ICH remains a significant cause of morbidity and mortality throughout the world. The aim of this chapter is to provide the etiology, presentation, and treatment of this disease.

Keywords: ICH, hemorrhage, hypertension, amyloid, reversal

3.1 Epidemiology

- About 40 to 80% of ICH patients die within the first 30 days and half of all deaths occur within the first 48 hours.[1]
- Incidence is 12 to 31 per 100,000 people and increases with age, doubling every 10 years after age 35.[2,3]
- Occurs most in Asians followed by African Americans followed by Caucasians.[4]
- Risk factors include hypertension, age, alcohol intake, very low low-density lipoprotein (LDL) and cholesterol levels.[5]

3.2 Etiologies/Differential Diagnosis

- Hypertension is the most common cause
- Cerebral amyloid angiopathy (in elderly, age > 60 years)
- Vascular malformations
- Trauma
- Coagulopathy
- Aneurysm
- Hemorrhagic transformation of infarction
- Tumors
- Neoplasm
- Venous sinus thrombosis
- Drugs—cocaine and appetite suppressants

3.3 Common Clinical Presentations

- Headache, seizures, vomiting, worsening Glasgow coma score (GCS)
- Neurologic deterioration can be gradual or rapid, depending on location and size of hemorrhage
- Hypertensive hemorrhage tends to occur in the following locations (▶ Fig. 3.1)
  - Basal ganglia/thalamus > lobar > cerebellum > pons
  - Localizing symptoms
    - **Basal ganglia/thalamus:** hemisensory loss, hemiplegia, aphasia, homonymous hemianopsia, eye deviation toward the lesion but in rare cases have eye deviation away from lesion ("wrong way eyes"), upgaze palsy
    - **Lobar:** seizures, homonymous hemianopsia, plegia or paresis more commonly in the leg than arm
    - **Cerebellum:** ataxia, nystagmus, intractable vomiting, hydrocephalus
    - **Pons:** pinpoint pupils, quadraparesis, coma, locked-in syndrome
- Amyloid bleed is mostly lobar
- Vascular malformations (cavernous malformation, arteriovenous malformation [AVM], dural arteriovenous fistula [dAVF]) can occur anywhere

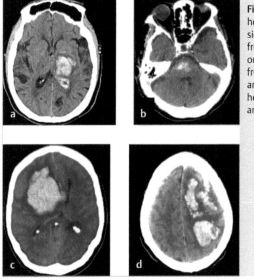

Fig. 3.1 (a) Basal ganglia hemorrhage due to hypertension. (b) Pontine hemorrhage from hypertension or cavernous malformation. (c) Right frontal hemorrhage due to amyloid angiopathy. (d) Left hemispheric hemorrhage from anticoagulation.

3.4 Neuroimaging

- Computed tomography (CT) of the head without contrast as soon as possible and then 24 hours after admission. If the patient is on anticoagulation more frequent imaging may be warranted (at 12 and 24 hours) while reversal of coagulopathy is in process.
- CT angiography (CTA) of the head and neck is usually not indicated. However, in the following circumstances, a CTA may be helpful to rule out
  - Subarachnoid hemorrhage
  - AVM/Cavernous malformation
  - Hemorrhagic brain tumor
- Fluid levels seen on CT scan indicate a coagulopathy
- **Volume assessment:** ABC/2 estimate

$$\frac{\text{A (largest diameter in cm on largest hemorrhage CT slice)} \times \text{B (largest diameter 90 degrees to A)} \times \text{C (number of 10 cm CT slices))}}{2}$$

- Can use ABC/3 for hemorrhages secondary to warfarin
- Magnetic resonance imaging (MRI) of brain with and without contrast to evaluate for underlying mass if no etiology is found (4–6 weeks post hemorrhage)
- Appearance of hemorrhages on MRI (see ▶ Table 3.1)

3.5 Treatment

- Blood pressure (BP) (see ▶ Fig. 3.2).
  - Elevated BP is associated with hematoma expansion, neurologic deterioration, and death and dependency.[6] Early control is essential.

Table 3.1 Appearance of blood on MRI

Phase	Time	T1	T2
Hyperacute	<12 hours	Isodense	Bright
Acute	12 hours to 3 days	Isodense	Dark
Early Subacute	3–7 days	Bright	Dark
Late Subactute	7–14 days	Bright	Bright
Chronic	>14 days	Dark	Dark

Mnemonic: "I Bring itty bitty baby doo doo" (I-B, I-D, B-D, B-B, D-D)
Abbreviation: MRI: magnetic resonance imaging.

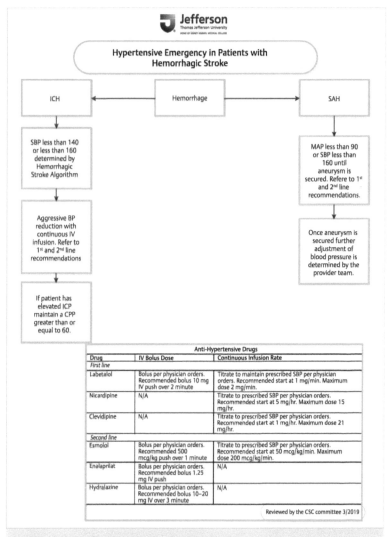

Fig. 3.2 Thomas Jefferson University algorithm for the management of hypertensive emergency in patients with hemorrhagic stroke.

- Antihypertensive Treatment of Acute Cerebral Hemorrhage (ATACH) and Intensive Blood Pressure Reduction in Acute Cerebral Hemorrhage (INTERACT) found reduction of systolic blood pressure (SBP) < 140 to be safe.[7,8]
- INTERACT2 showed no increase in death or serious adverse events from early intensive BP lowering.[9]
- For ICH patients presenting with SBP between 150 and 220 mm Hg and without contraindication to acute BP treatment, acute lowering of SBP to 140 mm Hg is safe and can be effective for improving functional outcome.[6]

3.5.1 Aggressive Reduction in SBP to Goal of 140

- Place arterial line and peripheral intravenous (IV) medications
- Use continuous IV medications
  - Clevidipine, 4 to 6 mg/hour (start 1–2 mg/hour)
  - Labetalol, 2 mg/min (max 300 mg per day)
  - Nicardipine, 5 to 15 mg/hour (start 5 mg/hour)

3.5.2 Seizures

- Frequency of clinical seizures within 1 week of ICH is 16%, with majority occurring at onset.[10]
- Clinical seizures should be treated with IV antiepileptics.
- Continuous electroencephalography (EEG) monitoring for those with depressed mental status that is out of proportion to injury.
- Prophylactic antiepileptic medication is not recommended.[6]

3.5.3 Intracranial Pressure

See Chapter 6.

3.5.4 Medical Issues

- Hypoglycemia and hyperglycemia should be avoided.
- Goal normothermia should be achieved.
- After documentation of cessation of bleeding, **subcutaneous heparin should be considered for prevention of venous thromboembolism** in patients with lack of mobility after 1 to 4 days from onset.[6]
  - At Thomas Jefferson University we routinely start subcutaneous heparin 24 to 48 hours after onset of hemorrhage after a repeat stable CT scan.

3.5.5 Coagulopathies

Reversing anticoagulant or antiplatelet agents is often necessary to minimize rebleeding or prevent bleeding when surgical procedures are required emergently. See ▶ Table 3.2 and ▶ Fig. 3.3 for details of specific reversal agents.

3.5.6 Surgical Options

- Intraventricular tPA
- **Clot Lysis:** Evaluating Accelerated Resolution of IVH (CLEAR-IVH) trial demonstrated that intraventricular administration of tPA reduced intracranial pressure (ICP), lowered external ventricular drain (EVD) obstructions, and shortened duration of EVD but mortality and mRS (modified Rankin Scale) were not different.[11]
- Phase 3 randomized CLEAR III trial is in progress.
- Efficacy and safety of this treatment remains uncertain.[6]

3.5.7 Craniotomy

- The International Surgical Trial in Intracerebral Hemorrhage (STICH) found no overall statistically significant difference in mortality or functional outcome for patients who underwent early surgery.[12]
  - Subgroup analysis suggested that patients with lobar hemorrhages within 1 cm of the cortex might benefit from surgery.
- STICH II trial showed no benefit for patients with superficial lobar hemorrhages within 1 cm of the cortex and without IVH.[13]
- An updated analysis showed advantage for surgery when all patients were considered, but there was significant heterogeneity in the data.
- Patients with cerebellar ICH who deteriorate neurologically or have brainstem compression and/or hydrocephalus should undergo surgical removal of the hemorrhage as soon as possible.[6]
  - Initial treatment of these patients with ventricular drainage rather than surgical evacuation is not recommended.
- For most patients with supratentorial ICH, the usefulness of surgery is not well established.[6]
  - Consider in deteriorating patients for life-saving measures.

3.5.8 Craniectomy

- No large randomized controlled trials
- Might reduce mortality for patients who are in a coma, have large hematomas with significant midline shift, or have elevated ICP refractory to medical management[6]

Table 3.2 List of anticoagulant and antiplatelet agents with current reversal

Drug	Reversal agent	Dose	Max infusion rate
Warfarin	Vitamin K	10 mg IVP (intravenous push)	N/A
	Prothrombin Complex Concentrates (PCC)	25–50 IU/kg IV	2 mL/min
	Recombinant activated Factor Seven (rFVIIa)	Not recommended	
Unfractionated heparin Or Low-molecular-weight heparin	Protamine Sulfate	• If the dose was given 8 hours or less, 1 mg/ 100 units of heparin IV (Max dose 50 mg) • 8–12 hours, administer 0.5 mg protamine/100 units of heparin • >12 hours, administer 0.25 mg protamine/100 units heparin	5 mg/min
Dabigatran	Activated charcoal (if < 2 hours)		
	Idarucizumab (Praxbind)	2.5 GM/50 mL slow IVP over 5 min, total of 2 doses	2 mL/min
Apixaban, Rivaroxaban	Activated charcoal (if < 2 hours)		
	PCC K-Centra (4PCC)	25–50 IU/kg IVP 50 units/kg IVP (max dose 5,000 units)	2 mL/min
	Andexxa (Xa inhibitor antidote)	Dose and agent dependent Dose based on timing of last oral dose taken; contact pharmacy for specific dosing	
Argatroban	None		
Bivalirudin	Consider rFVIIa	90 mcg/kg	

(*Continued*)

Table 3.2 (*Continued*) List of anticoagulant and antiplatelet agents with current reversal

Drug	Reversal agent	Dose	Max infusion rate
Alteplase (tPA)	Cryoprecipitate Tranexamic Acid E-Aminocaproic Acid	10 units over 10–30 min can re-dose if fibrinogen is < 200 1,000 mg IV infused over 10 min 5 gm IV over 1 hour followed by 1 gm IV until bleeding is controlled	
Antiplatelets	Platelets	One donor apheresis unit (equivalent to five pooled units) for patients undergoing a neurosurgical procedure	

Abbreviations: IU, international unit; IV, intravenous; IVP.

3.5.9 Minimally Invasive Surgical Evacuation

- Minimally invasive aspiration of hemorrhage
- The Minimally Invasive Surgery Plus Recombinant Tissue-Type Plasminogen Activator for ICH Evacuation Trial II (MISTIE II) demonstrated a significant reduction in perihematomal edema and a trend to a trend toward improved outcomes in patients who received minimally invasive surgery plus tPA.[14]
- MISTIE III is currently in progress.
- The effectiveness of this procedure is still uncertain.

3.6 Prognosis

- There continues to be no change in mortality for patients with ICH even with the abovementioned treatments.[1]
- ICH Score
  - Simple clinical grading scale that allows prognostication at presentation (▶ Table 3.3)[15]
  - Final score represents 30-day mortality risk (▶ Table 3.4)

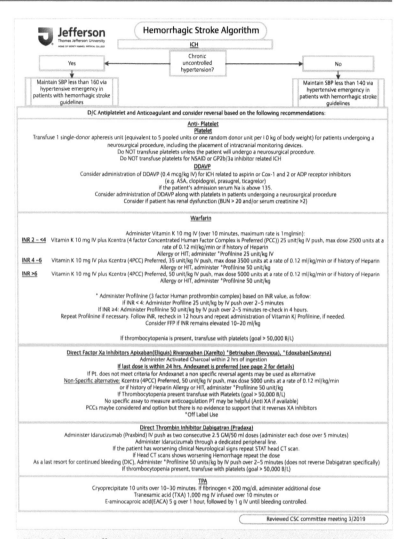

Fig. 3.3 Thomas Jefferson University algorithm for the reversing anticoagulants or antiplatelet agents with acute hemorrhagic stroke.

Table 3.3 ICH score

	Points
GCS	
3–4	2
5–12	1
13–15	0
ICH Volume	
≥ 30 cm^3	1
< 30 cm^3	0
Intraventricular Hemorrhage	
Yes	1
No	0
Location	
Infratentorial	1
Supratentorial	0
Age	
Age ≥ 80 years	1
Age < 80 years	0
Total Points	

Abbreviations: GCS, Glasgow coma score; ICH, intracerebral hemorrhage.

Table 3.4 Risk of mortality based on ICH score

ICH score	Mortality (%)
0	0
1	13
2	26
3	72
4	97
5	100
6	100

Abbreviation: ICH, intracerebral hemorrhage.

References

[1] Rincon F, Mayer SA. The epidemiology of intracerebral hemorrhage in the United States from 1979 to 2008. Neurocrit Care. 2013; 19(1):95–102

[2] Stein M, Misselwitz B, Hamann GF, Scharbrodt W, Schummer DI, Oertel MF. Intracerebral hemorrhage in the very old: future demographic trends of an aging population. Stroke. 2012; 43 (4):1126–1128

[3] van Asch CJ, Luitse MJ, Rinkel GJ, van der Tweel I, Algra A, Klijn CJ. Incidence, case fatality, and functional outcome of intracerebral haemorrhage over time, according to age, sex, and ethnic origin: a systematic review and meta-analysis. Lancet Neurol. 2010; 9(2):167–176

[4] Labovitz DL, Halim A, Boden-Albala B, Hauser WA, Sacco RL. The incidence of deep and lobar intracerebral hemorrhage in whites, blacks, and Hispanics. Neurology. 2005; 65(4):518–522

[5] Ariesen MJ, Claus SP, Rinkel GJ, Algra A. Risk factors for intracerebral hemorrhage in the general population: a systematic review. Stroke. 2003; 34(8):2060–2065

[6] Hemphill JC, III, Greenberg SM, Anderson CS, et al. American Heart Association Stroke Council, Council on Cardiovascular and Stroke Nursing, Council on Clinical Cardiology. Guidelines for the management of spontaneous intracerebral hemorrhage: a guideline for healthcare professionals from the American Heart Association/American Stroke Association. Stroke. 2015; 46(7):2032–2060

[7] Qureshi AI, Palesch YY, Martin R, et al. Antihypertensive Treatment of Acute Cerebral Hemorrhage Study Investigators. Effect of systolic blood pressure reduction on hematoma expansion, perihematomal edema, and 3-month outcome among patients with intracerebral hemorrhage: results from the antihypertensive treatment of acute cerebral hemorrhage study. Arch Neurol. 2010; 67 (5):570–576

[8] Arima H, Huang Y, Wang JG, et al. INTERACT1 Investigators. Earlier blood pressure-lowering and greater attenuation of hematoma growth in acute intracerebral hemorrhage: INTERACT pilot phase. Stroke. 2012; 43(8):2236–2238

[9] Anderson CS, Heeley E, Huang Y, et al. INTERACT2 Investigators. Rapid blood-pressure lowering in patients with acute intracerebral hemorrhage. N Engl J Med. 2013; 368(25):2355–2365

[10] De Herdt V, Dumont F, Hénon H, et al. Early seizures in intracerebral hemorrhage: incidence, associated factors, and outcome. Neurology. 2011; 77(20):1794–1800

[11] Naff N, Williams MA, Keyl PM, et al. Low-dose recombinant tissue-type plasminogen activator enhances clot resolution in brain hemorrhage: the intraventricular hemorrhage thrombolysis trial. Stroke. 2011; 42(11):3009–3016

[12] Mendelow AD, Gregson BA, Fernandes HM, et al. STICH investigators. Early surgery versus initial conservative treatment in patients with spontaneous supratentorial intracerebral haematomas in the International Surgical Trial in Intracerebral Haemorrhage (STICH): a randomised trial. Lancet. 2005; 365(9457):387–397

[13] Mendelow AD, Gregson BA, Rowan EN, Murray GD, Gholkar A, Mitchell PM, STICH II Investigators. Early surgery versus initial conservative treatment in patients with spontaneous supratentorial lobar intracerebral haematomas (STICH II): a randomised trial. Lancet. 2013; 382(9890):397–408

[14] Mould WA, Carhuapoma JR, Muschelli J, et al. MISTIE Investigators. Minimally invasive surgery plus recombinant tissue-type plasminogen activator for intracerebral hemorrhage evacuation decreases perihematomal edema. Stroke. 2013; 44(3):627–634

[15] Hemphill JC, III, Bonovich DC, Besmertis L, Manley GT, Johnston SC. The ICH score: a simple, reliable grading scale for intracerebral hemorrhage. Stroke. 2001; 32(4):891–897

4 Cerebrovascular Emergencies: Aneurysmal Subarachnoid Hemorrhage (SAH)

Norman Ajiboye, Yu Kan Au, and Syed Omar Shah

Abstract

Aneurysmal subarachnoid hemorrhage (SAH) is a devastating neurologic disorder which requires early recognition for optimal patient management. It is associated with a very high mortality if it is not recognized early and treated appropriately. This chapter provides a quick guide to the early diagnosis and proper management of patients with SAH. It reveals the barriers to early diagnosis and it provides the tools needed to manage such patients. Furthermore, it provides the treatments of frequently encountered medical complications of SAH. Finally, it provides a synoptic algorithm that may be used for the evaluation and management of patients with SAH.

Keywords: subarachnoid hemorrhage, rebleeding, hydrocephalus, delayed cerebral ischemia, vasospasm

4.1 Epidemiology[1,2,3]

- **Incidence:** 10 to 15 per 100,000 in USA.
- Average age of onset is 50 years old.
- It affects up to 30,000 persons annually in the Unites States of America.
- In-hospital mortality rates range between 18 and 21.5%.
- Overall mortality rates continue to decline but still remain high between 40 and 70%.

4.2 Risk Factors[1,4]

See ► Table 4.1.

4.3 Diagnosis[1,4,5]

- A high level of suspicion is warranted when a patient presents with the worst headache of life (thunderclap headache). It is described in 80% of patients with SAH. A sentinel headache, which is a less severe headache and could precede the aneurysm rupture, occurs in approximately 20%.

Table 4.1 Risk factors for aneurysm formation

Nonmodifiable	Modifiable
Prior SAH	HTN
Family history of aneurysms	Tobacco use
Genetic syndrome (PCKD, Ehlers-Danlos)	Alcohol use
Female	Sympathomimetic drug use
Black or Hispanic ethnicity	

Abbreviations: HTN, hypertension; PCKD, polycystic kidney disease; SAH, subarachnoid hemorrhage.
Note: Autosomal Dominant Polycystic kidney disease, Fibromuscular dysplasia, Ehlers-Danlos Type IV, Sickle Cell Disease, Osler-Weber-Rendu Syndrome, Arteriovenous Malformations.

- Nausea and/or vomiting, stiff neck, loss of consciousness, or focal neurologic deficits may occur.
- The diagnostic sensitivity of computed tomography (CT) of the head is about 95% within the first 12 hours. Therefore, if the initial CT of head is negative and clinical suspicion is high a lumbar puncture (LP) is warranted.
- LP findings of xanthochromia (yellow discoloration of cerebrospinal fluid [CSF]) can be seen around 12 hours after rupture.
- CT angiography (CTA) should be considered in the workup of aneurysmal SAH. If the CTA is negative, digital subtraction angiography (DSA) is recommended.
- Misdiagnosis or delay in diagnosis carries a fourfold increased risk of death or disability.

4.4 Grading System

There are two main grading scales that are primarily commonly used to describe the severity of the hemorrhage. The scale can be used to help in prognosis; however, it should not be used as an absolute. Hemorrhage is graded based on either the presenting symptoms or Glasgow Coma Scale with the presence or absence of motor deficit.

4.4.1 Hunt and Hess Grade[6]

See ▶ Table 4.2.

4.4.2 World Federation of Neurological Surgeons Grade[7]

See ▶ Table 4.3.

4.4.3 Modified Fischer Scores[8,9]

The Modified Fisher Score first published in 2001 serves to predict the risk of symptomatic vasospasm that can develop after aneurysm rupture.

See ▶ Table 4.4.

4.5 Management of Subarachnoid Hemorrhage

There are two phases to the management of aneurysmal subarachnoid hemorrhage[10]:

1. Early phase comprises preventing rebleeding, securing the aneurysm, and managing immediate complications.

Table 4.2 Hunt and Hess Grade

Grade 1	Asymptomatic or mild headache and slight nuchal rigidity
Grade 2	Moderate to severe headache, nuchal rigidity, no neurologic deficit other than cranial nerve palsy
Grade 3	Drowsiness, confusion, or mild focal deficit
Grade 4	Stupor, moderate to severe hemiparesis
Grade 5	Deep coma, decerebrate rigidity, moribund appearance

Table 4.3 World Federation of Neurological Surgeons Grade

WFNS Grade	GCS Score	Motor Deficit
I	15	Absent
II	13–14	Absent
III	13–14	Present
IV	7–12	Present or absent
V	3–6	Present or absent

Abbreviations: GCS, Glasgow Coma Scale; WFNS, World Federation of Neurological Surgeons Grade.

Table 4.4 Modified Fisher Score

Scale	Findings	Percentage with symptomatic vasospasm
1	Focal or diffuse thin SAH, no IVH	24
2	Focal or diffuse thin SAH, with IVH	33
3	Thick SAH present, no IVH	33
4	Thick SAH present, with IVH	40

Abbreviations: IVH, intraventricular hemorrhage; SAH, subarachnoid hemorrhage.

2. Late phase comprises maintenance of metabolic homeostasis as well as monitoring and prevention of delayed cerebral ischemia.

▶ Fig. 4.1 details Thomas Jefferson University protocol for subarachnoid hemorrhage.

4.5.1 Early Phase
Rebleeding[10]

- Suspect if early deterioration occurs. Mortality is reported to be as high as 80%.
- There is higher risk if patient has a poor-grade SAH, previous sentinel headache, or a large aneurysm.
- Rebleeding is at its highest risk within 12 to 24 hours, with rates of rebleeding estimated to occur at 30% within 3 hours, 50% within 6 hours, and 4 to 13% in first 24 hours. Time to treatment is crucial.
- To minimize the risk of rebleeding prior to securing the aneurysm, current recommendations include[11]:
  - Early repair (> 6 hours post rupture) when appropriate
  - Blood pressure control with systolic blood pressure (SBP) < 160 mm Hg or mean arterial pressure (MAP) < 110 mm Hg; care should be taken to avoid extremes in either direction
  - Early use of anti-fibrinolytics can be considered from admission until time of aneurysm securing. Anti-fibrinolytics should not be started > 48 hours or used longer than 72 hours due to risk of rebleeding.[4,10,11]
  - Anyone treated with anti-fibrinolytics should be screened for deep vein thrombosis.
- No current consensus on blood pressure management prior to securing the aneurysm. Current recommendation for SBP < 160 mm Hg or MAP < 110 mm Hg.

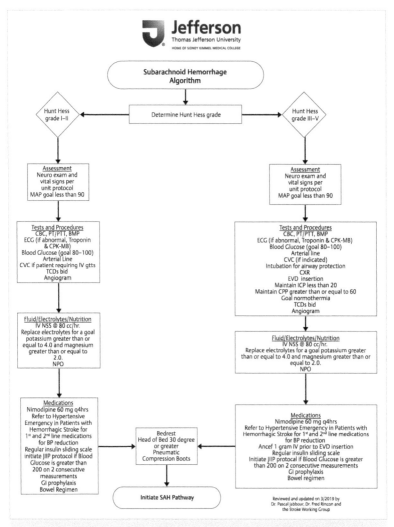

Fig. 4.1 Thomas Jefferson University early management of acute aneurysmal subarachnoid hemorrhage protocol.

Aneurysm Treatment

There are two current methods for securing aneurysms: surgical clipping or endovascular coiling/embolization. The details regarding aneurysm treatment are outside the scope of this book.

Hydrocephalus[4,5,12]

1. Acute hydrocephalus occurs in about 30% of patients but can vary widely from 15 to 87%. Drainage with external ventricular drainage (EVD) is associated with improved neurologic status.
2. In a recent study comparing management of EVDs, the majority of institutions preferred to keep the EVD continuously open in both the unsecured and secured aneurysm (81 and 94%, respectively).[13]
3. Most institutions favor a gradual wean (96 hours) over a rapid wean (< 24 hours). Shunt placement has not been clearly associated with either weaning method.[5,12]

Seizures and Prophylactic Anticonvulsant Use[11,14]

- Up to 26% of SAH patients have seizure-like episodes.
- Risk factors include age > 65 years old, thick SAH clot, intraparenchymal hemorrhage, rebleeding, and cerebral infarct.
- There is no randomized controlled trial on prophylactic antiepileptic drug (AED) in SAH.
- Nonconvulsive seizures are detected in 10 to 20% of comatose SAH patients.
- Current recommendations include:
  - Phenytoin should **NOT** be used for routine prophylaxis as it has been associated with worse outcome. Other anticonvulsant agents may be considered for prophylaxis.
  - A short course of anticonvulsant (3–7 days) may be considered for patients without a history of seizure. Long-term use of anticonvulsant is NOT recommended.
  - For patients with a seizure on admission, anticonvulsant agents should be continued at the discretion of the management team.
  - Continuous electroencephalography (EEG) monitoring should be considered for high-grade SAH patients in coma and patients with acute neurologic decline.

Cardiopulmonary Complications[11,14,15]

- Sympathetic stimulation and catecholamine surge mediate myocardial injury.
  - 35% elevated troponins, 35% arrhythmias, and 25% wall motion abnormalities

- "Neurogenic Stress Cardiomyopathy" or "Stunned Myocardium"
  - Syndrome of chest pain, dyspnea, hypoxemia, and cardiogenic shock
  - Occurs within hours of aneurysm rupture
  - Risk of sudden death in approximately 12% of the patients
  - Symptoms are transient and can resolved within 1 to 3 days
  - Supportive management
- Cardiac abnormalities in patients who develop delayed cerebral ischemia have worse outcomes.
- Symptomatic pulmonary complications can occur in approximately 20% of the patients while up to 80% may have impaired oxygenation.
  - Neurogenic or cardiogenic pulmonary edema
  - Acute lung injury
  - Acute respiratory distress syndrome (ARDS)
- Pulmonary complications are associated with higher clinical grade SAH and higher mortality.
- Current recommendations include:
  - Baseline electrocardiogram (ECG), transthoracic echocardiogram (TTE), and cardiac enzymes must be obtained on admission.
  - Target euvolemia: If pulmonary edema is present then avoiding increased fluids and careful use of diuretics should be considered.
  - Standard management of heart failure is indicated although tempered by the BP/cerebral perfusion pressure (CPP) goals needed to maintain neurologic stability.

4.5.2 Late Phase

Volume Assessment and Management[11,15,16]

- Target fluid balance of **euvolemia**.
- Avoid hypovolemia. It is associated with cerebral infarcts and worse outcome.
- Isotonic fluids are recommended for volume replacement.
- Avoid hypotonic fluids.
- Regular assessment of volume status with both clinical data and physical examination can be supplemented by the use of noninvasive or invasive monitoring technologies when needed.
- Routine use of pulmonary artery catheter is NOT recommended and central venous pressure (CVP) monitoring is NOT recommended as the sole measurement for volume status.
- Fludrocortisone or hydrocortisone can be considered in patients who persistently maintain a negative fluids balance.

Glucose Management[11,17]

- No randomized control trial of strict versus liberal glucose control in SAH.
- Both hypoglycemia and hyperglycemia have been associated with vasospasm.
- Hyperglycemia is seen as marker of SAH severity and risk for infection.
- Recommendation is to maintain serum glucose of 80 to 200 mg/dL.

Temperature Management[11,18]

- Fever occurs in 40 and 70% of the SAH patients.
- Fever is defined as temperature ≥ 38.3 °C (101 °F) and has been associated with secondary brain injury including infarct.
- Fever occurs more frequently in patients with high-grade SAH, large hemorrhage burden, and/or intraventricular hemorrhage.
- Treatment with ice packs, fans, cold saline infusion, and cooling blanket have not been shown to be effective.
- Surface and intravascular cooling devices have been shown to be more effective at controlling fever.
- Recommendations for fevers are as follows:
  - Temperature elevation can be due to infectious and noninfectious etiologies. Infection must be ruled out and/or treated.
  - Acetaminophen (intravenous [IV] or oral) or ibuprofen (IV or oral) should be used as first-line therapies.
  - Surface or intravascular cooling devices can be implemented when antipyretic agents fail with targeted temperature of 37 °C.
  - When surface or intravascular cooling devices are used, monitoring using the bedside shivering assessment scale (BSAS)[19] and implementing a preemptive treatment algorithm are critical.
  - When surface cooling devices are employed regular skin assessments should be completed every 2 to 4 hours to avoid potential burn injury.
  - Surface cooling or intravascular cooling should be avoided in patients with a pre-existing skin condition or who are in vasodilatory shock requiring multiple vasopressors.

Deep Venous Thrombosis Prophylaxis[10,11]

- SAH increases a patient's risk of deep vein thrombosis (DVT) by inducing a prothrombotic state.
- The incidence of DVT varies widely between 1.5 and 18%, with poor-grade SAH patients having the highest rate.
- DVT prevention should be initiated in all SAH patients.
- Initial prevention includes the use of sequential compression devices.

- Chemoprophylaxis should be withheld until 24 hours after the aneurysm has been secured.
- Despite low-molecular-weight heparin being associated with higher risk of intracerebral and noncerebral minor hemorrhage, it showed similar effectiveness to SCDs (sequential compression devices) and unfractionated heparin in preventing DVTs.

Magnesium and Statins[10,16]

- Magnesium acts as noncompetitive calcium antagonist. It has multiple vascular roles which potentially carry a neuroprotective effect by:
  - Promoting vasodilation by blocking voltage gated calcium channels
  - Decreasing glutamate release and decreasing calcium entry into cells
  - Attenuating the effect of endothelin 1
  - Blocking the formation of reactive O_2 species
- Normomagnesemia recommended
- No definitive evidence to support the initiation of a statin to reduce vasospasm and delayed cerebral ischemia (DCI)
- STASH trial[20] did not show long- or short-term benefits
- Patients on statins prior to admission with an SAH should be continued
- Routine use of statin in statin naïve patients should be avoided

4.6 Vasospasm, Delayed Neurologic Deterioration (DND), and Delayed Cerebral Ischemia (DCI)[4,11,16]

- Vasospasm refers to the narrowing of an artery following SAH. It can be seen radiographically (on CTA) or sonographically (transcranial Doppler [TCD]).
- Vasospasm can cause cerebral ischemia or infarction by decreasing blood flow and oxygen delivery. It occurs generally between post-bleed day 3 and 7.
- Vasospasm can begin post-bleed day 3 and peak between days 7 and 10, generally resolving by day 21.
- Delayed neurologic deterioration (DND) is a clinical decline in neurologic function after initial stabilization (excluding rebleeding). Common causes for DND include: hydrocephalus, cerebral edema, seizures, fever, metabolic derangement, and vasospasm or DCI.
- DCI refers to any neurologic deterioration related to ischemia from cerebral vasospasm with symptoms lasting > 1 hour without another explanation (fever, seizure, etc.).
- Both DCI and vasospasm can be symptomatic or asymptomatic.

- DCI when secondary to vasospasm is a major cause of death and disability and occurs in 15 to 20% of patients.

4.6.1 Detection and Management of Vasospasm and DCI[10,11,14,15,16]

Vasospasm Detection

- DSA is considered the gold standard in detecting large vessel spasm.
- CTA has a high specificity of 87 to 95% and can be used to screen prior to obtaining a DSA.
- TCDs also have a high sensitivity of 90% with a specificity of 71% when evaluating the middle cerebral vessels.
- TCD follows mean blood flow and Lindegaard ratio to categorize severity of vasospasm. See ▶ Table 4.5.
- TCD has a high specificity with a moderate sensitivity. Velocities > 200 cm/s or rapidly increasing as well as Lindegaard ratio (middle cerebral artery [MCA]/internal carotid artery [ICA]) > 6 are concerning for vasospasm.
- EEG shows reduced alpha variability.

Vasospasm Treatment

- Oral nimodipine should be given to all SAH patients unless contraindicated starting on the day of admission. Recommended dose of 60 mg every 4 hours for 21 days has been shown to improve neurologic outcome but NOT cerebral vasospasm. Dose can be decreased to 30 mg every 2 hours if unable to tolerate due to hypotension.
- For radiographic vasospasm (CTA, TCD, or DSA) with or without DCI, initial management is a trial of induced hypertension to increase cerebral blood

Table 4.5 Transcranial Doppler velocities and Lindegaard ratio

Criteria and Severity of Cerebral Vasospasm		
Severity of vasospasm	Mean flow velocity of MCA cm/s	Lindegaard Ratio (MCA/ICA)
Normal	< 90	< 3
Mild-Hyperemia	< 120	< 3
Moderate	120–150	3–4.5
Severe	150–200	4.5–6
Critical	> 200	> 6

Abbreviations: ICA, internal carotid artery; MCA, middle cerebral artery.

flow and oxygen delivery. Although there is no current guideline on the optimal target blood pressure, it is generally agreed upon that using a stepwise approach of increasing the blood pressure while monitoring the physical examination to see the response is appropriate.

- Phenylephrine and norepinephrine are first-line agents for induced hypertension. Caution in patients who may have underlying cardiac disease.
- Inotropic agents (milrinone or dobutamine) can be considered in certain circumstances with careful monitoring of cardiac index and cardiac output.
- Hypervolemia is NOT recommended although a fluid bolus while initiating induced hypertension is not unreasonable.
- Endovascular intra-arterial vasodilation and/or angioplasty should be considered if no response to, or in conjunction with, medical therapy.
- Asymptomatic infarcts can be detected in 10 to 20% of CT scans and 23% of magnetic resonance imaging (MRI) images.

DCI Treatment

- Initiation of medical therapy should be implemented in any patient who: (1) has radiographic vasospasm or DCI demonstrated on CTA or DSA or (2) is considered high risk with strong clinical picture to suggest DCI.
- Endovascular treatment with intra-arterial calcium channel blocker, intra-arterial vasodilator, or balloon angioplasty can be considered if no response to, or in addition with, medical therapy.
- High-grade SAH patients may not show clinical deterioration. Vasospasm and DCI can be monitored with multiple neuro-monitoring modalities (CTA, TCD, EEG, PbtO2, cerebral microdialysis), either individually or simultaneously.

Anemia and Transfusion[4,11,21]

- Anemia is common in SAH patients, occurs in around 50% of patients. It usually occurs 3 to 4 days post-ictus.
- Maintain hemoglobin concentration above 8 to 10 g/dL to improve cerebral oxygen delivery.
- In patients with symptomatic vasospasm/DCI, it is not unreasonable to transfuse to a hemoglobin of ≥ 10 g/dL.
- Weigh risks versus benefit of transfusion if patient is low-grade SAH, with no evidence of vasospasm or DCI.
- Some strategies to employ to prevent iatrogenic anemia include:
  ○ Minimizing unnecessary blood draws
  ○ Use pediatric tubes
  ○ Use point of care testing if serial labs are needed

○ Use of VAMP system, Edwards LifeSciences (Venous Arterial Blood Management and Protection) to decrease blood loss during sampling

4.7 Hyponatremia and Endocrine Dysfunction[4,10,11]

4.7.1 Hyponatremia

- Hyponatremia is the most common electrolyte abnormality in SAH and can be found in 30 to 50% of patients.
- Trigger for initiating treatment is a serum $[Na^+] < 135$ mEq/L or if there is a neurologic change with the decrease in Na^+.
- Assessment of volume status is important in distinguishing the etiology of hyponatremia.
  ○ SIADH (syndrome of inappropriate antidiuretic hormone secretion) is associated with euvolemia or hypervolemia
  ○ Cerebral salt wasting is associated with hypovolemia
- Treatment can involve:
  ○ Setting a goal of normonatremia with serum sodium between 135 and 145 mEq/dL
  ○ Free water restriction
  ○ Hypertonic saline
  ○ Early use of fludrocortisone or hydrocortisone may help limit natriuresis and hyponatremia, paying special attention to serum glucose and potassium levels
  ○ Salt tablets
  ○ Vasopressin-receptor antagonists (tolvaptan or conivaptan)

4.7.2 Endocrine Dysfunction

- In the hyperacute phase of SAH, elevation of cortisol levels is normal.
- Adrenal insufficiency can occur but continues to be a difficult diagnosis in the intensive care unit (ICU) due to confounders.
- Stress-dose steroids may be useful in patients with symptomatic vasospasm who are not responsive to vasopressors.
- High-dose steroids are **NOT** recommended for routine use.

References

[1] Lantigua H, Ortega-Gutierrez S, Schmidt JM, et al. Subarachnoid hemorrhage: who dies, and why? Crit Care. 2015; 19:309

[2] Chan V, Lindsay P, McQuiggan J, Zagorski B, Hill M, O'Kelly C. Declining admission and mortality rates for subarachnoid hemorrhage in Canada between 2004 and 2015. Stroke. 2019; 50(1):181–184

[3] Grasso G, Alafaci C, Macdonald RL. Management of aneurysmal subarachnoid hemorrhage: state of the art and future perspectives. Surg Neurol Int. 2017; 8:11

[4] Connolly ES, Jr, Rabinstein AA, Carhuapoma JR, et al. American Heart Association Stroke Council, Council on Cardiovascular Radiology and Intervention, Council on Cardiovascular Nursing, Council on Cardiovascular Surgery and Anesthesia, Council on Clinical Cardiology. Guidelines for the management of aneurysmal subarachnoid hemorrhage: a guideline for healthcare professionals from the American Heart Association/American Stroke Association. Stroke. 2012; 43(6):1711–1737

[5] Edlow JA, Figaji A, Samuels O. Emergency neurological life support: subarachnoid hemorrhage. Neurocrit Care. 2015; 23:S103–S109

[6] Hunt WE, Hess RM. Surgical risk as related to time of intervention in the repair of intracranial aneurysms. J Neurosurg. 1968; 28(1):14–20

[7] Drake CG, Hunt WE, Sano K, et al. Report of World Federation of Neurological Surgeons Committee on a Universal Subarachnoid Hemorrhage Grading Scale. J Neurosurg. 1988; 68(6):985–986

[8] Frontera JA, Claassen J, Schmidt JM, et al. Prediction of symptomatic vasospasm after subarachnoid hemorrhage: the modified fisher scale. Neurosurgery. 2006; 59(1):21–27, discussion 21–27

[9] Fisher CM, Kistler JP, Davis JM. Relation of cerebral vasospasm to subarachnoid hemorrhage visualized by computerized tomographic scanning. Neurosurgery. 1980; 6(1):1–9

[10] Seder DB, Mayer SA. Critical care management of subarachnoid hemorrhage and ischemic stroke. Clin Chest Med. 2009; 30(1):103–122, viii–ix

[11] Diringer MN, Bleck TP, Claude Hemphill J, III, et al. Neurocritical Care Society. Critical care management of patients following aneurysmal subarachnoid hemorrhage: recommendations from the Neurocritical Care Society's Multidisciplinary Consensus Conference. Neurocrit Care. 2011; 15 (2):211–240

[12] Klopfenstein JD, Kim LJ, Feiz-Erfan I, et al. Comparison of rapid and gradual weaning from external ventricular drainage in patients with aneurysmal subarachnoid hemorrhage: a prospective randomized trial. J Neurosurg. 2004; 100(2):225–229

[13] Chung DY, Leslie-Mazwi TM, Patel AB, Rordorf GA. Management of external ventricular drains after subarachnoid hemorrhage: a multi-institutional survey. Neurocrit Care. 2017; 26(3):356–361

[14] Muench E, Horn P, Bauhuf C, et al. Effects of hypervolemia and hypertension on regional cerebral blood flow, intracranial pressure, and brain tissue oxygenation after subarachnoid hemorrhage. Crit Care Med. 2007; 35(8):1844–1851, quiz 1852

[15] Lennihan L, Mayer SA, Fink ME, et al. Effect of hypervolemic therapy on cerebral blood flow after subarachnoid hemorrhage: a randomized controlled trial. Stroke. 2000; 31(2):383–391

[16] Egge A, Waterloo K, Sjøholm H, Solberg T, Ingebrigtsen T, Romner B. Prophylactic hyperdynamic postoperative fluid therapy after aneurysmal subarachnoid hemorrhage: a clinical, prospective, randomized, controlled study. Neurosurgery. 2001; 49(3):593–605, discussion 605–606

[17] Schlenk F, Graetz D, Nagel A, Schmidt M, Sarrafzadeh AS. Insulin-related decrease in cerebral glucose despite normoglycemia in aneurysmal subarachnoid hemorrhage. Crit Care. 2008; 12(1):R9

[18] Fernandez A, Schmidt JM, Claassen J, et al. Fever after subarachnoid hemorrhage: risk factors and impact on outcome. Neurology. 2007; 68(13):1013–1019

[19] Badjatia N, Strongilis E, Gordon E, et al. Metabolic impact of shivering during therapeutic temperature modulation: the Bedside Shivering Assessment Scale. Stroke. 2008; 39(12):3242–3247

[20] Kirkpatrick PJ, Turner CL, Smith C, Hutchinson PJ, Murray GD, STASH Collaborators. Simvastatin in aneurysmal subarachnoid haemorrhage (STASH): a multicentre randomised phase 3 trial. Lancet Neurol. 2014; 13(7):666–675

[21] Oddo M, Milby A, Chen I, et al. Hemoglobin concentration and cerebral metabolism in patients with aneurysmal subarachnoid hemorrhage. Stroke. 2009; 40(4):1275–1281

5 Transfusion Medicine and Anticoagulation

Bhuvanesh Govind and Matthew Vibbert

Abstract

Anemia of critical illness, thromboses, and coagulopathies are common complications in the neurologic intensive care unit (ICU). A judicious approach that considers risks of therapy while optimizing tissue oxygen delivery, restoring homeostatic balance in coagulopathy, and treating arterial or venous thromboses should be pursued to improve outcomes. The chapter will discuss high-yield points in pertinent transfusion topics in the neurocritical care unit, including a review of the pharmacology and reversal of commonly encountered anticoagulant medications.

Keywords: transfusion, coagulopathy, anticoagulation, deep vein thrombosis, venous thromboembolism

5.1 Introduction

Anemia in critically ill patients is not uncommon. It has been estimated to occur in up to 95% of patients within 3 days of hospitalization.[1] Studies estimate that patients can lose between 40 and 60 mL/day through phlebotomy in the intensive care unit (ICU).[1] The etiology behind anemia is varied with some of the most common causes listed below. The decision to transfuse packed red blood cells (RBCs) in neurologically injured patients is often based on the underlying brain injury, indication for surgery, and optimization for cerebral metabolic demands.

5.2 Anemia in the ICU

- Defined as a reduction in RBC mass
- Mechanism of anemia is beyond the scope of this chapter, but etiology could be related to RBC production, survival, or destruction
- Common finding in many ICU patients is that it is often from a multifactorial etiology[2]
  - Bleeding
  - Frequent phlebotomy
  - Hemodilution secondary to fluid resuscitation
  - Anemia of critical illness

– Reduced red cell production and survival
– Iron sequestration due to increased ferritin in acute inflammatory states

5.3 Red Cell Transfusion

One unit of packed red blood cell (PRBC) raises hemoglobin by 1 g/dL and hematocrit by 3% approximately. Most of the plasma component is removed and RBC component is mixed with about 100 mL of nutrient solution for extended storage life. Additional modifications considered include the following.

5.3.1 Leukocyte Reduction Indications

Reduction of febrile nonhemolytic transfusion reaction after multiple transfusions or in multiparous females, human leukocyte antigen (HLA) alloimmunization, or transfusion-related immunomodulation (TRIM) especially in postoperative patients.

5.3.2 Washed RBC

Reduction of severe allergic reactions, anaphylaxis in IgA deficiency.

5.3.3 Irradiation

Reduction of rare and fatal risk of transfusion-associated graft-versus-host disease (TA-GVHD) in certain at-risk populations such as neonates, patients with hematologic malignancies or stem cell transplants, or patients with congenital immune deficiency.

5.3.4 Complications of Red Blood Cell Transfusion

• Minor allergic reaction
• Acute or delayed hemolytic reaction
• Fever
• Transfusion-related acute lung injury (TRALI)
• Transfusion-associated circulatory overload (TACO)
• Transmission of viruses (hepatitis B virus [HBV], hepatitis B virus [HCV], human immunodeficiency virus [HIV])
• Increased risk of infection, pneumonia, and sepsis

Table 5.1 Hemorrhagic Shock Classification[7]

	1 (Compensated)	2 (Mild)	3 (Moderate)	4 (Severe)
Blood Loss (cc)	<750	750 – 1500	1500 – 2000	>2000
Pulse (bpm)	<100	>100	>120	>140
Blood Pressure	Normal	Decrease	Marked decrease	Profound decrease
Urine Output	>30	20–30	5–15	Negligible
Respiratory Rate	Normal	Mild Increase	Moderate increase	Severe tachypnea
CNS Symptoms	Alert	Anxious	Confusion	Lethargy, obtundation

5.3.5 Benefits to Transfusion

• Rapid volume expansion which is needed with acute blood loss. Symptoms of shock from blood loss do not usually manifest until a patient has lost approximately 1,500 mL of blood. ▶ Table 5.1 highlights the symptoms which can be found with acute blood loss.
• Increasing hemoglobin

5.4 Hemoglobin "Triggers"

• RBC transfusion in a dose-dependent manner is an *independent predictor of mortality* in critically ill adult trauma and surgical patients, despite premorbid level of anemia.[14,15,16]
• Trial of Transfusion Requirements in Critical Care (TRICC) defined universal hemoglobin goal of *at least 7 mg/dL* in critically ill patient.[3]
• Given that patients with primary neurologic injury were a small portion of the TRICC study population, concern exists that restrictive transfusion practices may not be generalizable in patients suffering severe brain injury, where signs and symptoms of tissue hypoxia may be difficult to detect.
• Moderate evidence exists to individualize hemoglobin goals based on specific disease states. Although there is no strong evidence toward suggesting significant improvement in outcomes, may consider transfusing for a liberalized goal of *8 to 10 mg/dL* in[4,5,6]:
  ○ Poor-grade subarachnoid hemorrhage (SAH)
  ○ Large ischemic stroke (more than two-third of middle cerebral artery [MCA] territory)
  ○ Severe traumatic brain injury

• Except in situations where a massive transfusion protocol is implemented, all transfusions should occur 1 unit at a time along with reassessment.

5.5 Thrombocytopenia

Thrombocytopenia is another major concern in the hospitalized patients and has been estimated to occur in upwards of 60% of ICU patients. In the critically ill patient, thrombocytopenia has been associated with a wide variety of causes. Trending the platelet count during the hospitalization is important and can lead to early recognition of life-threatening conditions such as heparin-induced thrombocytopenia (HIT). Common causes of thrombocytopenia include:

• Medications: ▶ Table 5.2 shows examples of specific medications
• Sepsis
• Disseminated intravascular coagulation (DIC)
• Acute respiratory distress syndrome
• Cardiopulmonary resuscitation (CPR)
• Massive bleeding
• Multifactorial

Either prophylactic transfusion for prevention of bleeding or treatment of active bleeding in specific scenarios must be utilized with fair consideration of the risks of transfusion.

• Risks are similar to those associated with red cell transfusion.
• Transfusion is not indicated in HIT, thrombotic thrombocytopenic purpura (TTP), or autoimmune thrombocytopenic purpura (ATP), unless significant bleeding occurs.

Table 5.2 Medications associated with thrombocytopenia

Antibiotics	Vancomycin, penicillin, trimethoprim-sulfamethoxazole, piperacillin
Anticonvulsants	Carbamazepine, phenytoin, valproic acid, levetiracetam
Anti-inflammatory	NSAIDs, naproxen, acetaminophen
Cardiovascular	Amiodarone, quinidine, furosemide, digoxin
H2 blockers	Famotidine, ranitidine, cimetidine
Other	Simvastatin, haloperidol, heparin, Lovenox, lithium

Abbreviation: NSAIDs, nonsteroidal anti-inflammatory drugs.

Table 5.3 Platelet transfusion goals for common procedures

Planned invasive procedure (lumbar puncture, CVC)	>50,000/mm³ New limited data suggest thresholds for CVC placement can be as low as 20,000 mm;³ may be targeted if placement can be done safely with low risk of arterial puncture performed by an experienced operator[19,22]
Bronchoscopy with lavage (without biopsy)	>20,000/mm³
Major surgery goals vary by situation and type of procedure (**neurosurgical procedures may require higher goals**):	>50,000/mm³

Abbreviation: CVC, central venous catheter.

5.6 Prophylaxis Thresholds[2,20,21,22]

See ▶ Table 5.3.

5.6.1 Treatment of Bleeding

- Intracerebral hemorrhage with anticoagulant use (warfarin, oral Xa inhibitor, direct thrombin inhibitor): >50,000/mm³ (*institutional threshold*)
- Current American Heart Association (AHA)/American Stroke Association (ASA) guidelines (2015) on spontaneous intracerebral hemorrhage (ICH) recommend that patients with severe thrombocytopenia should receive platelet replacement (Class IC recommendation),[18] but it does not recommend at what threshold the platelets should be given or to what target.

5.7 Antiplatelet Reversal in Intracranial Hemorrhage

- Our institutional practice is to consider location and severity of bleeding, prior single versus dual antiplatelet use, and/or signs of early hematoma expansion and to target a goal of >50,000/mm³ if transfusion is considered in this setting (see ▶ Fig. 5.1).
  - Consider goal of >80,000 to 100,000/mm³ if undergoing neurosurgical procedures[20,21]
- No specific replacement strategy is recommended. Our institutional practice varies by antiplatelet agent:
  - **Aspirin**: 10 units of platelets, once

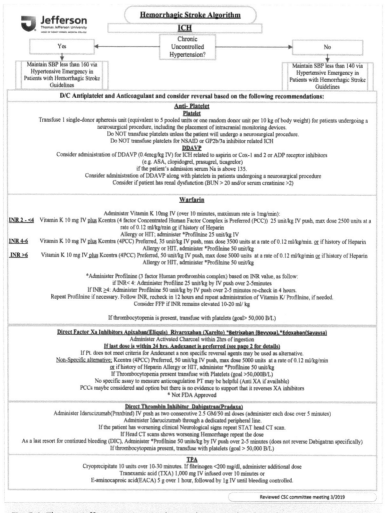

Fig. 5.1 Thomas Jefferson University hemorrhagic stroke algorithm.

○ **Clopidogrel, prasugrel, ticagrelor, ticlopidine**: 10 units of platelets once but can be repeated every 8 hours until demonstration of radiographic stability of the hemorrhage for up to 48 hours

There is lack of strong evidence to support aggressive platelet transfusion.[18] Evidence from PATCH trial and other studies examined in the Neurocritical Care Society guidelines statement calls into question historical practice of transfusing platelets solely for prior antiplatelet use in the setting of spontaneous ICH and suggests that platelet transfusion for any antiplatelet agent or hemorrhage volume provides no clear benefit in those patients *not* undergoing neurosurgical procedure.[17,18,19,20,21,22]

5.8 Coagulation Cascade (▶ Fig. 5.2) and Anticoagulants

- Arterial and venous thromboses are important causes of morbidity and mortality following brain injury.
- Prevention and treatment of thrombosis is an important consideration in the management of the neurocritical care patient.
- Indications may include ischemic stroke, carotid occlusion, cardiac thrombus, and pulmonary embolism (PE).

5.9 Anticoagulants

5.9.1 Warfarin

Indications

Wide range of thromboembolic, valvular, and cardiac disease states.

Dosing

Dosing is individualized and depends on:
- Hepatic impairment, nutritional state, age, cardiac function, risk for bleeding, genetic variants of CYP2C9 or VKORC1 enzymes, and concomitant use of enzyme-inducing medications
- Therapeutic international normalized ratio (INR) level generally is 2.0 to 3.0. Exceptions include 2.5 to 3.5 for mechanical mitral valve, mechanical aortic valve PLUS risk factors, and mechanical valve in aortic and mitral locations.

Mechanism

Inhibits vitamin-K dependent coagulation factor synthesis (II, VII, IX, X, Protein C, Protein S).

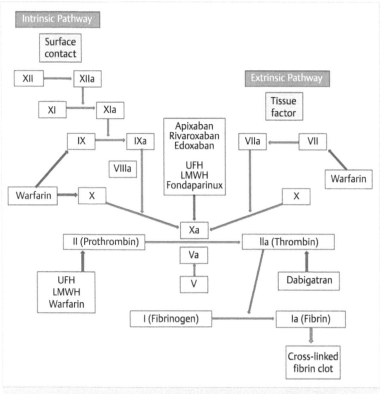

Fig. 5.2 Mechanisms of Pharmacologic Anticoagulation.

Metabolism

CYP system, $t_{1/2} = 20 - 60$ hours, rapid absorption, time to peak = 4 hours, time to full therapeutic effect may take days.

Pros

Established reversal agents, very low financial costs of long-term therapy.

Cons

Multiple drug–drug interactions, difficulty in maintaining therapeutic INR, long-term monitoring.

Adverse Drug Effects

- **Bleeding is rare:** Anaphylaxis, calciphylaxis, atheromatous plaque or cholesterol microemboli, skin necrosis or gangrene
- Contraindicated in active state of HIT as it inhibits Protein C, which can worsen thrombotic process

Reversal

- Vitamin K 10 mg IV *PLUS*
- Three- or four-factor Prothrombin Complex Concentrate (PCC) IV 25 to 50 unit/kg IVP over 2 to 5 minutes (dosing dependent on INR, PCC type)

Or
- Fresh frozen plasma (FFP) 10 to 15 cc/kg. This carries a risk of causing volume overload depending on the number of units needed.
- INR should be checked 2 to 4 hours after administering PCC and IV vitamin K. Repeat PCC dose can be given if there is no improvement. Recheck INR after 6 to 12 hours.

5.10 Oral Factor Xa Inhibitors

5.10.1 Apixaban, Rivaroxaban, Edoxaban

Indications

Nonvalvular atrial fibrillation stroke prevention (primary or secondary prophylaxis), deep vein thrombosis (DVT) and PE treatment (apixaban, edoxaban), hip/knee surgery postoperative thromboprophylaxis (apixiban, rivaroxaban)

Mechanism

Factor Xa inhibition

Metabolism (By Agent)

- **Apixiban:** CYP3A4/5 system, $t_{1/2}$ = 12 hours, rapid absorption, time to peak = 3–4 hours

- **Rivaroxaban:** CYPA4/5 and CYP2J2, $t_{1/2}$ = 5–9 hours, rapid absorption, time to peak = 2–4 hours
- **Edoxaban:** minimal CYP3A4, $t_{1/2}$ = 10–14 hours, rapid absorption, time to peak = 1–2 hours
- Renal clearance; reduced dosing for CrCl 15–50 mL/min. Not recommended for CrCl < 15 mL/min. Poorly removed with dialysis

Pros

No long-term blood tests, noninferior to warfarin in treatment of DVT or PE.

Cons

Use and half-life affected by impaired renal clearance, moderate-severe hepatic impairment (Child-Pugh class B and C), extremes of BMI, and medication costs.

Reversal

- Andexanet indication and dosing listed in ▶ Fig. 5.3.
- Transfuse for concomitant thrombocytopenia of > 50,000/mm^3
- If ingestion within 2 hours, activated charcoal 50 g by mouth
- Three- or four-factor PCC 50 units/kg IV can be considered to reverse anticoagulation activity

5.11 Thrombin Inhibitors

5.11.1 Oral

Dabigatran

Indications

Nonvalvular atrial fibrillation stroke prevention (primary or secondary prophylaxis), DVT and PE treatment, and hip/knee surgery postoperative thromboprophylaxis.

Mechanism

Thrombin (IIa) inhibition

Metabolism

Hepatic esterases, not a substrate of the P450 system, $t_{1/2}$ = 12–17 hours; elderly = 14–17 hours; hepatic metabolism; rapid absorption; time to peak is 1 hour.

Andexanet Use for Apixaban or Rivaroxaban Associated ICH
Alternative to PCC (Kcentra, Profilnine) when last dose of apixaban/rivaroxaban was ≤ 24 hours

<u>Inclusion Crtieria for Use</u>

The following inclusion criteria were developed as a tool to assist the clinician in determining potential eligibility for the use of andexanet.
The use of andexanet versus concentrated prothrombin complex concentrate should be determined on an individualized basis with recommendations from the attending physician.

- Restricted to life threatening, salvageable apixaban or rivaroxaban associated CNS bleeding (intracranial or intraspinal)
- No history of prior exposure to andexanet
- No sepsis or septic shock

<u>Alternative treatment options if patient does not meet criteria</u>

Use 4 factor PCC (Kcentra) if last dose administered >24 hrs ago, or for other non CNS serious/life threatening hemorrhages (if 4 factor PCC is not available, alternative treatment is a 3 factor PCC (Profilnine) +/- fresh frozen plasma. FFP). Please refer to ICH algorithm and ICH order set for additional details.

<u>Exclusion Criteria</u>

Patient must have undergone a head CT or MRI scan demonstrating evidence of new or expanding intracranial bleeding, based on clinical trial criteria, patients excluded if any of the following are present:

- Baseline modified rankin score of >4 prior to ICH
- Glasgow coma score <7
- Intracerebral hematoma volume >60 cc as assessed by the CT volumetric formula ABC/2 (see below*)
- For subdural hematomas: maximum thickness >10 mm and midline shift >5 mm
- For subarachnoid hematomas, any evidence of hydrocephalus
- Hemorrhagic conversion of an ischemic CVA for patients initiated on apixaban or rivaroxaban
- Infratentorial ICH location
- Epidural hematomas
- Intraventricular extension of hemorrhage
*ABC/2 Formula: A is the greatest hemorrhage diameter by CT, B is the diameter 90° to A, and C

<u>Determination of Andexanet Dose</u>

Last DOAC dose administered <8 hrs: use High dose protocol
Last DOAC dose administered >8 but <24 hrs: use Low dose protocol
If DOAC administered <2 hrs ago, consider concomitant administration of activated charcoal
Concomtiant Antiplatelet Therapy: refer to antiplatelet therapy reversal guideline in ICH algorithm in addition to direct factor Xa reversal algorithm

FXa Inhibitor	FXa Inhibitor Last Dose	Timing of FXa Inhibitor Last Dose Before Andexanet alfa Initiation	
		< 8 Hours or Unknown	≥ 8 Hours
Rivaroxaban	≤ 10 mg	Low Dose	Low Dose
	> 10 mg / Unknown	High Dose	
Apixaban	≤ 5 mg	Low Dose	
	> 5 mg / Unknown	High Dose	

<u>Administration</u>

Total infusion time 2 ¼ - 2 ½ hours, use 0.22 micron filter
Andexanet Bolus and Infusion Rates

Dose*	Initial IV Bolus	Follow-On IV Infusion
Low dose	400 mg at a target rate of 30 mg/min	4 mg/min for 120 minutes 480 mg
High dose	800 mg at a target rate of 30 mg/min	8 mg/min for 120 minutes 960 mg

- Repeat Head CT recommended at 6 and 24 hours after administration of andexanet for reevaluation. There is no indication for redosing of andexanet after initial dose.

Please refer to andexanet checklist / fact sheet for additional information

Fig. 5.3 Andexanet Use for Apixaban or Riveroxaban Associated ICH.

Reversal

Idarucizumab 5 g IV (administered in 2.5 g doses)
- Activated charcoal 50 g by mouth if ingestion within 2 hours

• Three- or four-factor PCC 50 units/kg IV and hemodialysis are other options to consider to help reverse anticoagulation activity if bleeding is severe

Pros

No long-term monitoring, noninferior to warfarin

Cons

Caution in impaired renal clearance, severe hepatic impairment, and body mass index (BMI) > 40. Adverse reactions reported include bleeding and gastrointestinal (dyspepsia and gastroesophageal reflux disease [GERD]-like symptoms).

5.11.2 Intravenous

Argatroban

Indication

Prophylaxis or treatment for patient with HIT.

Mechanism

Inhibits fibrin formation, V/VIII/XIII/Protein C activation, and platelet and aggregation.

Metabolism

Hepatic hydroxylation and aromatization; $t_{1/2}$ = 39–51 minutes (181 minutes in moderate-severe hepatic impairment), time to peak = 1–3 hours.

Pros

Discontinuation of infusion should reverse effects quickly given short half-life (unless moderate-severe hepatic impairment).

Cons

• Can be difficult to titrate to therapeutic window
• Wide spectrum of cardiovascular effects: Chest pain, hypotension, bradycardia, ventricular tachycardia, and coronary thrombosis
• Headache, pain, rash, nausea/vomiting/diarrhea, dyspnea, cough, abdominal pain
• Falsely elevates INR on plasma testing
• Conversion from argatroban to warfarin involves consideration of current INR and rate of argatroban infusion

Reversal

No specific direct reversal agent

5.12 The Heparins

5.12.1 Unfractionated Heparin

- **Indication:** Venous thromboembolism (DVT, PE, cerebral venous sinus thrombosis), non-ST elevation myocardial infarction (non-STEMI), cardiac thrombus, and in certain situations with mobile thrombus (cardiac or arterial) on a case by case basis
- Subcutaneous heparin (SQH) used as chemoprophylactic agent for venous thromboembolism (VTE) (see DVT prophylaxis for dosing)
- **Mechanism:** Very large molecular weight heparin (3,000 to 30,000 Daltons) that acts via thrombin inhibition and factors IIa, Xa, IXa, and XIIa inactivation via serine protease antithrombin III (ATIII) activation
- **Metabolism:** Via reticuloendothelial system; $t_{1/2}$ = 1.5 hours
- Dose adjustment may be needed for low body weight
- **Pros:** Ideal in the brain injured patient where there may be need for anticoagulation but with elevated adverse risk of major bleeding or worsening given short half-life allows for relatively fast reversal of anticoagulant effect
- **Cons:** Hemorrhage, thrombocytopenia or HIT, hypersensitivity reactions, drug fever, rigors
- Reversal
  - In most cases, discontinuation of infusion is sufficient given short half-life (waiting at least four half-lives equates to approximately 6 hours prior to near-complete reversal of heparin effect by partial thromboplastin time [PTT] parameter)
  - For severe bleeding, reversal agent is protamine sulfate (1 mg IV for every 100 units heparin administered in previous 2 to 3 hours with maximum of 50 mg dose)

5.12.2 Low-Molecular-Weight Heparin (LMWH)

Indication

Venous thromboembolism (DVT or PE), knee or hip replacement prophylaxis, and acute coronary syndromes including unstable angina and acute STEMI.

Mechanism

2,000 to 9,000 Daltons heparin primarily inactivates factor Xa and less so thrombin inhibition (most of the pentasaccharide chains are not long enough to induce thrombin inhibition but does have some effect).

Dose Adjustment

Needed for low body weight.

Metabolism

Hepatic metabolism (CYP450), urine excretion (40%)
$t_{1/2} = 4.5 - 7$ hours

Pros

Predictable pharmacokinetics compared to unfractionated heparins; activity can be measured via anti-Xa assay if necessary; no serum testing needed to monitor anticoagulant effect.

Cons

Hemorrhage, spinal/epidural hematoma, prosthetic heart valve thrombosis, thrombocytopenia, HIT, hypersensitivity reactions, skin necrosis, hyperkalemia, hepatotoxicity, injection site reaction, osteoporosis (with long-term use), nausea, diarrhea, and drug fever

Reversal

- No specific direct reversal agent
- Protamine sulfate 1 mg for every 1 mg of enoxaparin given in previous 8 hours or 0.5 mg for every 1 mg enoxaparin given prior to 8 hours and up to preceding 12 hours (maximum 50 mg of protamine sulfate)
- Ratio for other agents is protamine sulfate 1 mg for every 100 units of either dalteparin or tinzaparin in previous 8 hours

5.12.3 Fondaparinux

- **Indication:** Prophylaxis or treatment for patient with HIT
- Subcutaneous option, compare to argatroban (IV option and a direct thrombin inhibitor)
- **Mechanism:** Inactivation of Xa

- **Metabolism:** Metabolism is not clearly well established; urine excretion; $t_{1/2}$ = 17 – 21 hours
- **Pros:** Subcutaneous option for prophylaxis or treatment with history of HIT, no monitoring required (generally does not increase the PTT)
- **Cons:** Hemorrhage, epidural/spinal hematoma, thrombocytopenia, hypersensitivity reactions, injection site reactions (rash), anemia, and drug fever
- Can be used in patients weighing < 50 kg in dose-adjusted manner but contraindicated if concomitantly undergoing hip fracture, hip replacement, knee replacement, or abdominal surgeries
- **Reversal:** If severe bleeding occurs, use recombinant factor VIIa 90 mcg/kg

5.13 Deep Vein Thrombosis (DVT) Prophylaxis

- Venous thromboembolism occurs as a result of venous stasis, endothelial injury, and/or hypercoagulable state. Increased incidence of venous thromboembolic events specifically occurs in critically ill patient with brain injury compared to medical or surgical ICU patients.[8,9]
  - ○ Endothelial injury and dysfunction secondary to primary brain injury leads to release of excess tissue factor, compromising homeostatic mechanisms toward prothrombotic state.[9,11,12,13]
- Screening versus symptomatic assessment varies by institution. Given the propensity of neurocritical care patients to experience VTE relative to medical or surgical ICU patients, it is routine practice at our institution to perform *screening* of lower extremity Doppler studies to rule out DVT.
- Several risk factors for VTE development have been studied. Significant factors that have been associated with an increased risk include[8,9]:
  - ○ Timing of chemoprophylaxis initiation: Patients with severe acute brain injury are at high risk for VTE; VTE incidence increases during the initial days of hospitalization (3 to 6 days).[9] Timing of initiation of chemoprophylaxis depends on type of primary insult and individualized injury pattern but earlier prophylaxis with SQH and interpneumatic compression (IPC) devices is generally advised. Summary of a recent statement from the Neurocritical Care Society[11]:
    - – **ICH:** As soon as hemorrhagic progression risk of a brain injury is determined clinically or radiographically stable within 48 hours.[12] Our institutional practice is to start chemoprophylaxis at 24 hours if radiographically stable.
    - – **Ischemic stroke:** Delayed by 24 hours if IV tPA is given or as soon as feasible if no tPA.
    - – **Aneurysmal SAH:** As soon as aneurysm is secured and SAH is deemed radiographically stable on 24-hour follow-up.

- **Spinal cord injury:** Within 72 hours of injury and after control of any source of bleeding.
  - **Brain tumor:** As soon as feasible if risk for major bleeding is low and there are no signs of hemorrhagic conversion.
  - Neuromuscular disease: As soon as feasible.
  - BMI > 30 kg/m^2
  - Increasing severity of brain injury[12,13]
- No strong recommendation exists toward any one specific agent, dosing, and timing,[12,13] our institutional practice is to initiate subcutaneous unfractionated heparin 5000 units every 8 hours for patients > 50 kg and every 12 hours for patients < 50 kg.

References

[1] Pendem S, Rana S, Manno EM, Gajic O. A review of red cell transfusion in the neurological intensive care unit. Neurocrit Care. 2006; 4(1):63–67

[2] Hoffman R. Hematology: Basic Principles and Practice. 6th ed. Philadelphia (PA): Churchill Livingstone;

[3] Hébert PC, Wells G, Blajchman MA, et al. A multicenter, randomized, controlled clinical trial of transfusion requirements in critical care. Transfusion requirements in critical care investigators, Canadian Critical Care Trials Group. N Engl J Med. 1999; 340(6):409–417

[4] Oddo M, Milby A, Chen I, et al. Hemoglobin concentration and cerebral metabolism in patients with aneurysmal subarachnoid hemorrhage. Stroke. 2009; 40(4):1275–1281

[5] Naidech AM, Jovanovic B, Wartenberg KE, et al. Higher hemoglobin is associated with improved outcome after subarachnoid hemorrhage. Crit Care Med. 2007; 35(10):2383–2389

[6] Lelubre C, Bouzat P, Crippa IA, Taccone FS. Anemia management after acute brain injury. Crit Care. 2016; 20(1):152

[7] Gutierrez G, Reines HD, Wulf-Gutierrez ME. Clinical review: hemorrhagic shock. Crit Care. 2004; 8(5):373–381

[8] Skrifvars M, Bailey M, Presneill J, et al. Venous thromboembolic events in critically ill traumatic brain injury patients. Intensive Care Med. 2017; 43(3):419–428

[9] Tracy BM, Dunne JR, O'Neal CM, Clayton E. Venous thromboembolism prophylaxis in neurosurgical trauma patients. J Surg Res. 2016; 205(1):221–227

[10] Abdel-Aziz H, Dunham CM, Malik RJ, Hileman BM. Timing for deep vein thrombosis chemoprophylaxis in traumatic brain injury: an evidence-based review. Crit Care. 2015; 19:96–105

[11] Nyquist P, Bautista C, Jichici D, et al. Prophylaxis of venous thrombosis in neurocritical care patients: an evidence-based guideline: a statement for healthcare professionals from the neurocritical care society. Neurocrit Care. 2016; 24(1):47–60

[12] Carney N, Totten A, O'Reilly C, et al. Guidelines for the Management of Severe Traumatic Brain Injury. 4th ed. Brain Trauma Foundation TBI Guidelines. Neurosurgery 2016;0:1–10

[13] McCully SP, Schreiber MA. Traumatic brain injury and its effect on coagulopathy. Semin Thromb Hemost. 2013; 39(8):896–901

[14] Vincent JL, Baron JF, Reinhart K, et al. ABC (Anemia and Blood Transfusion in Critical Care) Investigators. Anemia and blood transfusion in critically ill patients. JAMA. 2002; 288(12):1499–1507

[15] Marik PE, Corwin HL. Efficacy of red blood cell transfusion in the critically ill: a systematic review of the literature. Crit Care Med. 2008; 36(9):2667–2674

[16] Kumar MA. Red blood cell transfusion in the neurological ICU. Neurotherapeutics. 2012; 9(1):56–64

[17] Baharoglu MI, Cordonnier C, Al-Shahi Salman R, et al. PATCH Investigators. Platelet transfusion versus standard care after acute stroke due to spontaneous cerebral haemorrhage associated with antiplatelet therapy (PATCH): a randomised, open-label, phase 3 trial. Lancet. 2016; 387 (10038):2605–2613

[18] Hemphill JC, III, Greenberg SM, Anderson CS, et al. American Heart Association Stroke Council, Council on Cardiovascular and Stroke Nursing, Council on Clinical Cardiology. Guidelines for the management of spontaneous intracerebral hemorrhage: a guideline for healthcare professionals from the American Heart Association/American Stroke Association. Stroke. 2015; 46 (7):2032–2060

[19] Frontera JA, Lewin JJ, III, Rabinstein AA, et al. Guideline for reversal of antithrombotics in intracranial hemorrhage: a statement for healthcare professionals from the Neurocritical Care Society and Society of Critical Care Medicine. Neurocrit Care. 2016; 24(1):6–46

[20] Kaufman RM, Djulbegovic B, Gernsheimer T, et al. AABB. Platelet transfusion: a clinical practice guideline from the AABB. Ann Intern Med. 2015; 162(3):205–213

[21] Reddy GD, Gopinath S, Robertson CS. Transfusion in traumatic brain injury. Curr Treat Options Neurol. 2015; 17(11):46

[22] Kumar A, Mhaskar R, Grossman BJ, et al. AABB Platelet Transfusion Guidelines Panel. Platelet transfusion: a systematic review of the clinical evidence. Transfusion. 2015; 55(5):1116–1127, quiz 1115

[23] Zeidler K, Arn K, Senn O, Schanz U, Stussi G. Optimal preprocedural platelet transfusion threshold for central venous catheter insertions in patients with thrombocytopenia. Transfusion. 2011; 51 (11):2269–2276

6 Cerebral Edema and Elevated Intracranial Pressure

Anna Karpenko and Michelle Ghobrial

Abstract

Elevated intracranial pressure (ICP) is a medical condition commonly encountered in the intensive care unit (ICU) and can be seen in association with several highly morbid processes including traumatic brain injury, global hypoxic injury, large territory strokes, intracranial hemorrhage, brain tumor, and hepatic encephalopathy among other etiologies. In this chapter, we will discuss the stepwise management of elevated ICP.

Keywords: cerebral edema, intracranial pressure, cerebral perfusion pressure, management, therapeutic temperature management, hyperosmolar therapy

6.1 The Basics

6.1.1 Monro-Kellie Doctrine (▶ Fig. 6.1)

- There is a fixed volume within the cranial vault consisting of:
  - Blood (arterial and venous), 10%
  - Cerebrospinal fluid (CSF), 10%
  - Brain parenchyma, 80%
- An increase in any one will lead to a decrease in the other two
  - Example: intracranial tumor will take up space at the expense of CSF and blood volume which can lead to elevated intracranial pressure (ICP) and decreased blood flow

6.1.2 ICP and Cerebral Perfusion Pressure (CPP)

- Normal ICP in adults is 5 to 15 mm Hg
- CSF is produced and reabsorbed in a continuous fashion. The body produces approximately 500 mL/day.
- CPP = MAP – ICP
- Normal CPP is 50 to 90 mm Hg
- Cerebral autoregulation (▶ Fig. 6.2) allows cerebral blood flow to be maintained across a range of cerebral perfusion pressures (50–150 mm Hg)
- Intracranial hypertension is defined as sustained ICP > 20 mm Hg
  - ICP elevation is independent risk factor for poor outcome in brain trauma[5]
  - ▶ Table 6.1 lists some of the more common causes of elevated ICP

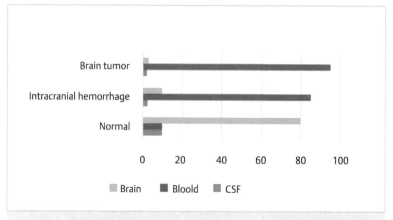

Fig. 6.1 Monro-Kellie doctrine states that the sum of the components within the cranial vault is constant (normal). When intracranial hemorrhage occurs, it increases the volume of the parenchyma and decreases the volume of the cerebrospinal fluid (CSF) without compromising the total blood volume. With a brain tumor, the mass adds volume to the parenchyma at the expense of both the CSF volume and blood volume.

- Indications for ICP monitoring
  - Obstructive hydrocephalus
  - Communicating hydrocephalus with early signs of high ICP
  - Severe traumatic brain injury (TBI) patients
  - ICP monitors are addressed within Chapter 17

6.1.3 Intracranial Compliance (▶ Fig. 6.3)

- Intracranial compliance is defined as the change in volume over the change in pressure ($\Delta V/\Delta P$)[1]
- With increase in intracranial volume
  - ICP slowly increases
  - CSF displaces into the thecal sac
  - Decrease in venous return from compression of the cerebral veins
  - Without intervention ICP becomes malignant and deadly

6.1.4 ICP Waveforms and Herniation Syndromes

- With ICP monitoring, it is common to review the waveform at the bedside
- Three components to the ICP waveform (▶ Fig. 6.4)

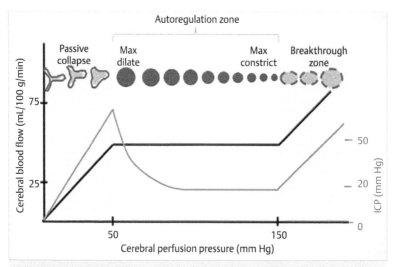

Fig. 6.2 Cerebral autoregulation curve. In a normal brain, varying the size of the blood vessel allows the brain to maintain a constant cerebral blood flow over a range of cerebral perfusion pressures (50–150 mm Hg). When the cerebral perfusion pressure (CPP) is > 150 mm Hg (hyperemic state), blood vessels become "leaky." There is blood–brain barrier breakdown and endothelial injury causing cerebral edema. On the other end, when the CPP is < 50 mm Hg (reactive vasodilation), the vessels are maximally dilated and blood flow continues to fall causing hypoperfusion and ischemia. On both ends there is an increase in intracranial pressure (ICP) when autoregulation is disrupted. (Reproduced with permission from Rose J.C. et al. Optimizing blood pressure in neurological emergencies. Springer Nature Jan 1, 2004.)

Table 6.1 Conditions associated with elevated intracranial pressure

Brain tumor	Meningitis/Encephalitis
Traumatic brain injury	Fulminant hepatic failure
Hemispheric stroke	Eclampsia
Subarachnoid hemorrhage	Hypertensive encephalopathy
Anoxic brain injury	Subdural, epidural, or intracranial hemorrhage

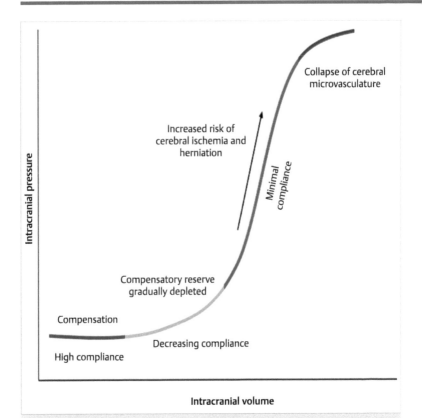

Fig. 6.3 Intracranial compliance curve. Pressure volume curve has four zones: Zone 1: Baseline intracranial volume with good compensatory reserve and high compliance (blue). Zone 2: Gradual depletion of compensatory reserve as intracranial volume increases (yellow). Zone 3: Poor compensatory reserve and increased risk of cerebral ischemia and herniation (red). Zone 4: Critically high intracranial pressure (ICP) causing collapse of cerebral microvasculature and disturbed cerebrovascular reactivity (grey) (From Hagay M. Intracranial pressure monitoring-review and avenues for development. Sensors 2018;18;465:1–15.)

- ○ P1: percussive wave represents arterial pulsation transmitted through the choroid plexus to the CSF
- ○ P2: tidal wave represents cerebral compliance
- ○ P3: dicrotic wave represents closure of aortic valve (venous outflow)
- When P2 is elevated above P1 it is a sign of poor intracranial compliance (▶ Fig. 6.5) and that management is needed

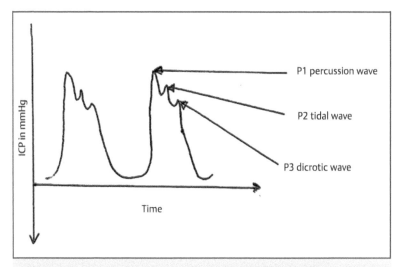

Fig. 6.4 Normal intracranial pressure waveforms. (Adapted from Abraham M and Singhal V. Intracranial Pressure Monitoring. Journal of Neuroanaesthesiology and Critical Care. Thieme 2015.)

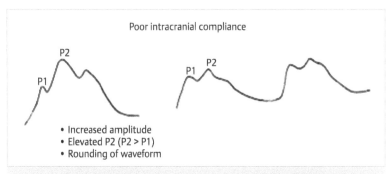

Fig. 6.5 Pathologic waveforms indicating poor compliance. (Adapted from Abraham M and Singhal V. Intracranial Pressure Monitoring. Journal of Neuroanaesthesiology and Critical Care. Thieme 2015.)

- Pathologic ICP waveforms[4,5,6] (Lundberg waves) (▶ Fig. 6.6)
  - Occur when ICP is increased and intracranial compliance is decrease
  - Three waveforms that occur
    - **Lundberg A:** sustained elevated ICP that needs immediate treatment
    - **Lundberg B:** unstable ICP and should be aggressively managed
    - **Lundberg C:** clinically insignificant

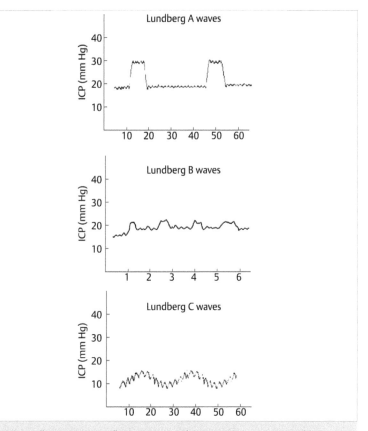

Fig. 6.6 Lundberg waves. Lundberg A waves, "Plateau waves," represent sudden increased in intracranial pressure (ICP) > 20 mm Hg for > 5 minutes; sign of impending herniation. Lundberg B waves, "Pressure Waves," are smaller increases in ICP for shorter period of time; self-limited associated with vasomotor changes and unstable ICP. Lundberg C waves are low amplitude period waves. They occur every 4 to 8 minutes and are of unknown significance. (From Hirzallah MO, Choi HA. The Monitoring of Brain Edema and Intracranial Hypertension. J Neurocit Care 2016;9:92–104.)

- Herniation syndromes[7,8] (► Table 6.2; ► Fig. 6.7)
  - Brain herniation occurs when pressure gradients cause the brain parenchyma to shift displacing and compressing surrounding tissues, cranial nerves, and blood vessels
  - Note that herniation occurs in approximately one-third of patients without elevated ICP

Table 6.2 Herniation syndromes

Syndrome	Clinical finding
Uncal herniation	Ipsilateral fixed and dilated pupil due to 3rd nerve palsy Can be signs of confusion or agitation prior to pupil change Motor posturing contralateral or bilateral
Subfalcine (Cingulate) herniation	Can be asymptomatic until the anterior cerebral artery is compressed Decreased mental status Contralateral leg weakness
Central (Transtentorial) herniation • There are stages of herniation • Diencephalic • Midbrain-upper pons • Power pons-upper medullary • Medullary (terminal)	Diabetes insipidus due to shearing of the pituitary stalk Cortical blindness from entrapment of the posterior cerebral arteries Altered consciousness → coma Bilateral pupil dilation Extensor motor posturing Respiratory changes (not normally seen on mechanically ventilated patients)
Upward herniation	Bilateral pupillary dilation Extensor posturing Altered consciousness → coma
Cerebellar (Tonsillar) downward herniation	Altered consciousness → coma Respiratory arrest Cardiac arrhythmias
External or transcalvarial herniation • Post decompressive surgery • Due to skull fracture	Symptoms depend on area affected

6.2 Cerebral Edema

- Common complication for patients in the neurologic intensive care unit (ICU)
- Approximately half of the patients will develop increase in ICP or cerebral edema requiring intervention
- There are two types of cerebral edema:
  - Vasogenic edema
    - Breakdown of blood–brain barrier
    - Increased fluid within the extracellular space
    - Commonly associated with:
      - ►Brain tumor
      - ►Infection: Meningitis, encephalitis, abscess
      - ►Cerebral contusion

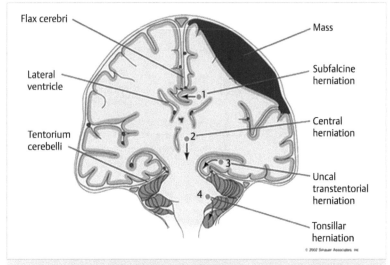

Fig. 6.7 Brain herniation subtypes: (**a**) Subfalcine, (**b**) Central, (**c**) Uncal, (**d**) Upward/ Tonsillar. (Reproduced with permission from ICP management. In Jallo G, Kothbauer K, Recinos V. ed, Handbook of Pediatric Neurosurgery. 1st edition. Thieme; 2018.)

- Affects white matter rather than grey matter within the brain. On imaging there is preservation of the grey–white junction.
- Managed mostly with glucocorticoids and mannitol
- Cytotoxic edema
- Intracellular accumulation of fluid; metabolic changes within the cell
- Swelling of cells
- Commonly associated with
  ► Stroke
  ► Liver failure
  ► Water intoxication
- Affects grey and white matter within the brain with loss of the grey–white junction on imaging
- Managed primarily with hyperosmolar medications, not responsive to glucocorticoids

6.3 Stepwise Approach to the Management of Elevated ICP

Refer to ► Fig. 6.8.

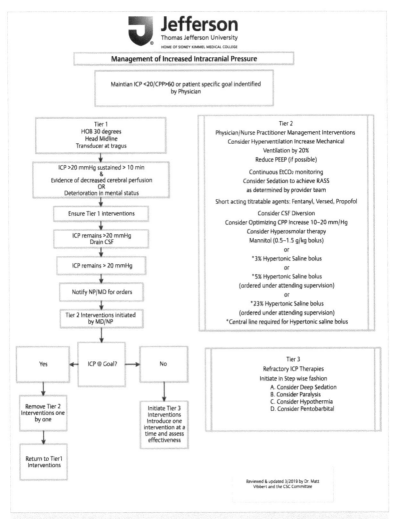

Fig. 6.8 Thomas Jefferson University management of increased intracranial pressure.

6.4 Management of Increased Intracranial Pressure

6.4.1 Tier 1

- Conservative measures
  - Head of bed is elevated 30 degrees
  - Head midline
  - Ensure ICP transducer is at the level of the tragus
  - Treat fever
  - Ensure normovolemia
  - Treat seizure if witnessed (can connect to electroencephalography [EEG] if nonconvulsive seizures are suspected)
- Reevaluate ICP if it remains > 20 mm Hg and CPP < 60 mm Hg OR there is decreased mental status
  - Drain CSF to keep ICP < 20 mm Hg
  - If no improvement in ICP or CPP with these measures proceed to Tier 2

6.4.2 Tier 2

- Add or increase sedation using short-acting agents with goal of decreasing the ICP (note: may need to add or increase vasopressors to maintain CPP)
  - Propofol
  - Fentanyl
  - Versed
- Consider hyperventilation by increasing minute ventilation by 20% to achieve a PaCO2 of 28 to 30 mm Hg
  - Should be used as temporizing measure while hyperosmolar medications or glucocorticoids are being ordered
    - Causes vasoconstriction
    - For every 1 mm Hg decrease in PaCO2 there is a 3% decrease in cerebral blood flow
    - Prolonged hyperventilation increases the risk of ischemia
    - The goal of these practices is to manage edema, lower ICP while maintaining mean arterial pressure[9]
- Optimize CPP by increasing MAP by 10 to 20 mm Hg
- Consider adding hyperosmolar therapy
  - Hyperosmolar therapy
    - Mannitol[10]
      - ►Osmotic diuretic, increases CPP through plasma expansion and reduced viscosity of blood by altering the rheology of RBCs, and therefore promotes CBF (cerebral blood flow)
      - ►20% solution given in 0.25 to 1 g/kg bolus; repeat every 6 hours

- ► Monitor serum osmolality (SOsm) and hold for SOsm > 320 or osmolal gap > 20
- ► Can cause hypovolemia from diuretic effect
- ► Cautious use with renal failure
- ► Replace fluid loss cc per cc with isotonic solution
- ► Can get rebound intracranial hypertension with prolonged use
- ► Increased risk for rebound edema with abrupt discontinuation after prolonged use
- – Hypertonic saline 3%
  - ► As efficacious as mannitol,[11,12] also supports intravascular volume, blood pressure, and thus CPP
  - ► Dosing
    - - Can be started peripherally with 18 G IV or larger at no more than 30 mL/hour; cannot bolus peripherally
    - - With central access: Bolus 250 mL for over 30 minutes
    - - After bolus begin infusion at 30 mL/hour
    - - Check Serum Na and serum Osm every six hours
    - - Goal Na$^+$ 150–155
    - - Can rebolus and increase infusion every 6 hours if not at goal. See
      - ▶ Table 6.3 for infusion adjustment.
    - - Maximum rate is 100 mL/hour

Table 6.3 Na goal-based titration schedule for 3% normal saline infusion

Serum Na$^+$ (mmol/L)	Rate (mL/hr)	Expected Δ Na$^+$ (mmol/L/ 6 hours)	Recheck Na$^+$
≤ 135	Increased rate by 40 mL/hr	6	6 hours
136–137	Increased rate by 35 mL/hr	6	6 hours
138–139	Increased rate by 30 mL/hr	5	6 hours
140–141	Increased rate by 25 mL/hr	5	6 hours
142–143	Increased rate by 20 mL/hr	4	6 hours
144–145	Increased rate by 15 mL/hr	4	6 hours
146–147	Increased rate by 10 mL/hr	3	6 hours
148–149	Increased rate by 5 mL/hr	3	6 hours
150–155	Continue current rate		6 hours
≥ 156	Stop infusing and call ordering physician		6 hours

- ► De-escalation
  - Wean slowly over 24 to 48 hours to avoid rebound intracranial hypertension
  - Continue to follow serum Na+ every 6 hours
  - Avoid dropping Na by more than 8 mmol/L/day (can restart at higher dose with significant drop)
- ► Precautions
  - Can precipitate decompensated heart failure
  - Can cause tissue necrosis if extravasates
  - Can cause hypotension with rapid infusion
  - Can induce platelet dysfunction, monitor platelets
  - Avoid increasing Na+ by more than 10 mmol/L/day
  - Monitor electrolytes
  - Can cause hyperchloremic metabolic acidosis
  - Cautious use in patient with renal failure or on hemodialysis
  - Cautious use in patients with Na+ < 130 mmol/L due to risk of osmotic myelinolysis
  - Can cause thrombophlebitis
- – Hypertonic saline alternative dosing
  - ► **5% NaCl:** Bolus 3 mL/kg over 10 to 20 minutes
  - ► **7.5% NaCl:** Bolus 2 mL/kg over 10 to 20 minutes
  - ► 23.4% NaCl should be reserved for herniation syndrome only. Bolus 30 mL over 3 to 5 minutes via central line only
- ○ Reevaluate ICP and clinical examination: If no improvement in ICP, refer to Tier 3 for refractory management

6.4.3 Tier 3

Deep Sedation

- Increase sedation to induce coma Richmond Agitation Sedation Scale (RASS) Score of −4
- If there is no improvement of ICP, add paralytics
- Used to prevent coughing, shivering, spontaneous posturing, or other reflexive movements or to offset effects of abdominal hypertension which may contribute to elevation of ICP
- Commonly used:
  - ○ Rocuronium 0.6 mg/kg IVP bolus followed by 0.3 mg/kg/hour continuous infusion
  - ○ Cisatracurium 0.1 mg/kg IVP bolus followed by 0.15 mg/kg/hour continuous infusion
- Monitoring with train of four (sequential electrical stimulation to facial, ulnar, or posterior tibial nerves), target one to two twitches

- Long-term neuromuscular blockade (NMB) associated with ICU acquired weakness, DVT, corneal abrasions, anaphylaxis, and awareness during paralysis if sedation is insufficient
- Guidelines recommend against routine use of paralytics for ICP

Therapeutic Temperature Management for Refractory ICP

Mechanism

Reduces ICP by lowering metabolic rate of O_2 consumption and thus cerebral blood volume (CBV).

Contraindications (*Relative Contraindications)

- Do-not-resuscitate (DNR)/do-not-intubate (DNI) status
- Brain death
- Skin condition that would preclude use of cooling pads
- Patients with vasodilatory shock requiring multiple vasoactive agents
- Chronic renal failure
- Severely impaired pre-arrest cognitive status (modified Rankin Scale [mRS] > 4 or Glasgow Outcome Scale [GOS] < 3)
- Follows commands
- Uncontrolled arrhythmias
- Other obvious reasons for coma, trauma, intoxication, etc.
- Multi-organ dysfunction syndrome
- Evident sepsis
- *Bleeding or coagulopathy (international normalized ratio [INR] > 2.0, DIC, platelet < 50,000)
- *Shock
- *Pregnancy

Protocol

- Obtain baseline basic metabolic panel (BMP), partial thromboplastin time (PTT), prothrombin time (PT), platelet, and arterial blood gas (ABG)
- Consider continuous EEG monitoring and cardiac monitoring (if not already on)
- Surface or endovascular cooling methods can be used
- Rectal, esophageal, pulmonary artery, or bladder thermometer
- Every 1 hour for vital signs every one hour while on protocol, need A-line for BP monitoring, I/Os, patient and water temperature
- Target temperature
  - Normothermia (37 °C) if febrile and unable to control with medications or
  - Mild-moderate hypothermia (33–36 °C) within 3 hours

- Assess for signs of shivering every 1 hour using the bedside shivering assessment scale[13] (▸ Table 6.4)
- Implement anti-shivering protocol[14] (▸ Table 6.5)

Other Medications

Pentobarbital

- Acts by reducing the metabolic rate of the brain
- Continuous EEG, target burst suppression with two to three bursts/screen
- Loading dose of 3 to 5 mg/kg with repeat boluses every 15 to 30 minutes as needed to reach ICP < 20 mm Hg
- Maintenance dose of 1 to 4 mg/kg/hour
- Complications: Hypotension, ileus

Table 6.4 Bedside shivering assessment score

Score	Type of shivering	Location
0	None	No shivering noted on palpation of masseter, neck, or chest wall
1	Mild	Localized shivering of neck and thorax (may only be seen on ECG monitor)
2	Moderate	Intermittent visible shivering of upper extremities in addition to the neck and thorax
3	Severe	Generalized shivering or sustained shivering in the upper extremities

Abbreviation: ECG, electrocardiogram.

Table 6.5 Anti-shivering protocol

Goal	Intervention	Dosing	Additional concerns
Peripheral vasoconstriction			
	Warming blanket at max temp (42 °C)		Apply hand and foot warmer if available
	Magnesium sulfate infusion	0.5–1 mg/hour IV Goal mag level 3–4 mg/dL Follow every 6 hours	Monitor daily ECG Daily K$^+$ and Ca^{++} Monitor for toxicity
	Acetaminophen	650–1,000 mg by mouth or IV every 4–6 hours standing	

(Continued)

Table 6.5 (*Continued*) Bedside shivering assessment score

Goal	Intervention	Dosing	Additional concerns
Central alpha receptors			
	Buspirone	30 mg by mouth every 8 hours	
	Dexmedetomi-dine infusion	0.2–1.5 mcg/kg/hour	
	or		
	Fentanyl infusion	25 mcg/hour titrate up	
	or		
	Meperidine	25–50 mg IV or IM every 4 hours as needed (max dose 600 mg/24 hours)	Contraindicated • Renal insufficiency (SCr > 1.2) • CVVHD and HD • MOAI use in prior 14d • Active or ongoing seizures
Skeletal muscle activity			
For refractory shivering, not for routine use	Rocuronium	0.6 mg/kg IVP bolus followed by 0.3 mg/kg/hour infusion	Follow train of four Goal 1–2 twitches
	Or		
	Cisatracurium	0.1 mg/kg IVP bolus followed by 0.15 mg/kg/hour infusion	Follow train of four Goal 1–2 twitches
	Or		
	Dantrolene	2.5 mg/kg IV every 6 hours	• Cannot be used for more than three consecutive days • Follow liver function panel daily while medication is being given

Abbreviations: CVVHD, continuous veno-venous hemodialysis; ECG, electrocardiogram; HD, hemodialysis; IM, intramuscular; IV, intravenous; MOAI, monoamine oxidase inhibitor; SCr, serum creatinine.

References

[1] Harary M, Dolmans RGF, Gormley WB. Intracranial pressure monitoring-review and avenues for development. Sensors (Basel). 2018; 18(2):1–15

[2] Abraham M, Singhal V. Intracranial pressure monitoring. J Neuroanaesth Crit Care. 2015; 2 (3):193–203

[3] Balestreri M, Czosnyka M, Hutchinson P, et al. Impact of intracranial pressure and cerebral perfusion pressure on severe disability and mortality after head injury. Neurocrit Care. 2006; 4(1):8–13

[4] Wijdicks EFM. Lundberg and his waves. Neurocrit Care. 2019; 31(3):546–549

[5] Hirzallah MI, Choi HA. The monitoring of brain edema and intracranial hypertension. J Neurocrit Care.. 2016; 9(2):92–104

[6] Greenberg M. Handbook of Neurosurgery. 6th ed. Thieme Medicial Publishers; 2006

[7] Stevens RD, Shoykhet M, Cadena R. Emergency neurological life support: intracranial hypertension and herniation. Neurocrit Care. 2015; 23 Suppl 2:S76–S82

[8] Bhardwaj A, Mirski M. Handbook of Neurocritical Care. 2nd ed. Springer Publishing; 2011

[9] Tyagi R, Donaldson K, Loftus CM, Jallo J. Hypertonic saline: a clinical review. Neurosurg Rev. 2007; 30(4):277–289, discussion 289–290

[10] Battison C, Andrews PJ, Graham C, Petty T. Randomized, controlled trial on the effect of a 20% mannitol solution and a 7.5% saline/6% dextran solution on increased intracranial pressure after brain injury. Crit Care Med. 2005; 33(1):196–202, discussion 257–258

[11] Carney N, Totten AM, O'Reilly C, et al. Guidelines for the management of severe traumatic brain injury, Fourth Edition. Neurosurgery. 2017; 80(1):6–15

[12] Francony G, Fauvage B, Falcon D, et al. Equimolar doses of mannitol and hypertonic saline in the treatment of increased intracranial pressure. Crit Care Med. 2008; 36(3):795–800

[13] Choi HA, Ko S-B, Presciutti M, et al. Prevention of shivering during therapeutic temperature modulation: the Columbia anti-shivering protocol. Neurocrit Care. 2011; 14(3):389–394

[14] Badjatia N, Strongilis E, Gordon E, et al. Metabolic impact of shivering during therapeutic temperature modulation: the bedside shivering assessment scale. Stroke. 2008; 39(12):3242–3247

7 Fevers and Infections in the Neuro-ICU

Deena M. Athas, Amna Sheikh, and Jacqueline S. Urtecho

Abstract
Fever, both infectious and noninfectious, is a common occurrence in neuro-critical care unit (neuro-ICU). This chapter will discuss key components in diagnosis and management of some of the most common infectious and noninfectious causes of fever in the neuro-ICU.

Keywords: meningitis, HIV, toxoplasmosis, fevers, infection and central fevers

7.1 Brain

7.1.1 Meningitis

Meningitis is inflammation of the leptomeninges which consist of three layers (dura, arachnoid, and pia mater) which surround the brain and spinal cord. There are various causes of meningitis (▶ Table 7.1).

Signs/Symptoms

Most patients present with one or more of the following symptoms:
- Headache
- Fever
- Stiff neck
- Nausea/Vomiting
- Rash (petechial or vesicular)
- Altered mental status
- Sensitivity to light or sound
- Physical examination findings of:
  ○ Brudzinski's sign—flexion of the knees and hips upon neck flexion
  ○ Kernig's sign—flexion of the knees and hips to 90 degrees, and then extension of knees causes pain and resistance

Risk Factors

- Age
- Living conditions
- Medical conditions/diseases
- Exposure
- Travel

Table 7.1 Various causes of meningitis

Bacteria	Viral	Fungal	Tubercular	Noninfectious
S. pneumoniae	HSV	Cryptococcus	Mycobacteria	Malignancy
N. meningitidis	VZV	Coccidioides		Medications/
H. Flu	Enterovirus	Histoplasma		drugs (NSAIDs,
L. monocytogenes	HIV	Aspergillosis		IVIG, antibiotics,
Aerobic gram (−)	Arboviruses			antiepileptic
bacilli	(West Nile)			medications)
	Lymphocytic			Autoimmune
	choriomeningitis			diseases

Abbreviations: HIV, human immunodeficiency virus; HSV, herpes simplex virus; IVIG, intravenous immunoglobulin; NSAIDs, nonsteroidal anti-inflammatory drugs; VZV, varicella-zoster virus.

Workup

Laboratory Studies

- Complete blood count (CBC), chemistry, coagulation panel, blood cultures, and liver function
- Human immunodeficiency virus (HIV), Lyme, Lupus Ab, Purified protein derivative (PPD), Rapid Plasma Reagin (RPR) or Fluorescent treponemal antibody absorption (FTA-ABS)
- Lumbar puncture (LP) sending cell count and culture can help to narrow the diagnosis (▶ Table 7.2). For patients on anticoagulants or antiplatelet agents other than aspirin, a hematology consultation can be considered prior to reversal recommendations. Do not delay antibiotics if the LP is delayed.

Imaging

Computed tomography (CT) scan of brain is not recommended routinely prior to the LP. According to the Infectious Disease Society of America, a CT scan should be performed prior to performing the LP when any of the following conditions apply (▶ Table 7.3).

7.1.2 Acute Bacterial Meningitis

Epidemiology

According to Centers for Disease Control and Prevention (CDC), bacterial meningitis affects 4,000 people every year worldwide. Common causative organisms include: *Streptococcus pneumoniae* (61%) and *Neisseria meningitidis* (16%).

Table 7.2 CSF profiles by cause

Test			Viral	Fungal	Tubercular
Appearance	Clear	Purulent or clear	Clear	Clear to fibrous	Opaque, cob-web formation
Opening pressure	Normal <20 mm Hg	Elevated	Normal	Normal to elevated	Normal to elevated
WBC	0–8/mm³	>1,000/mm³	<100 to 1,000/mm³	100–500/mm³	Variable
Cell differential	Lymphocyte and monocytes	Predominance of PMN	Lymphocytes	Lymphocytes	Lymphocytes
Protein	15–45 mg/dL	100–500 mg/dL	Normal to elevated 50–250 mg/dL	Elevated 100–500 mg/dL	Elevated 100–500 mg/dL
Glucose	50–80 mg/dL	<40 mg/dL	50–80 mg/dL	30–45 mg/dL	<50 mg/dL
CSF:serum glucose	0.6	<0.4	>0.6	<0.4	<0.4
Organisms	None	S. pneumoniae, Neisseria, H. Flu, Listeria, S. aureus, Gram (–) bacilli	HSV-2, VZV, Enterovirus, HIV, West-Nile	Crypto, Coccidioides, Histoplasma, Aspergillosis	Mycobacteria

Abbreviations: CSF, cerebrospinal fluid; HIV, human immunodeficiency virus; HSV-2, herpes simplex virus 2; VZV, varicella-zoster virus.

Group B streptococcus (14%), *Haemophilus influenzae* (7%), and *Listeria mono-cytogenes* (2%).

Diagnosis

All patients with suspicion of bacterial meningitis should get immediate blood cultures and LP (lumbar puncture) and antibiotics started without significant delay. ► Fig. 7.1 details the algorithm for suspected bacterial meningitis.

Table 7.3 Conditions when patients should obtain CT of head prior to performing lumbar puncture. (Adapted from Tunkel et al.[3])

Conditions	Details
Abnormal neurologic exam	Nonreactive pupils, arm/leg drift, gaze deviation, cranial nerve palsy, aphasia
Altered mental status	Inability to follow commands or answer questions
Papilledema	Presence of papilledema suggests increased ICP
Seizure	Within 1 week
Immunocompromised state	HIV/AIDS, cancer, any immunosuppressive therapy, post-transplantation
History of prior CNS disease	Mass lesion (tumor/abscess), large stroke, etc.

Abbreviations: AIDS, acquired immunodeficiency syndrome; CNS, central nervous system; CT, computed tomography; HIV, human immunodeficiency virus; ICP, intracranial pressure.

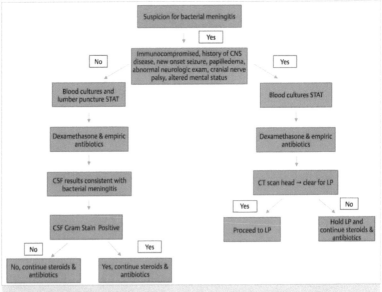

Fig. 7.1 Management algorithm for adults with suspected bacterial meningitis.[3] (Adapted from Tunkel A, et al. Practice guidelines for the management of bacterial meningitis.)

Table 7.4 Antibiotic therapy for meningitis based on predisposing factors. (Adapted Practice Guidelines for bacterial meningitis.[3])

Predispos- ing factor	Common bacteria	First-line antibiotic therapy	Alternative antibi- otic therapy
Age: 2–50 years	N. meningitidis S. pneumoniae	Third-generation cephalosporin Vancomycin plus third-generation cephalospo-rin (ceftriaxone or cefotaxime)	Penicillin G, ampicil-lin, chloramphenicol, fluoroquinolone or aztreonam meropenem, fluoroquinolone
Age: > 50 years	S. pneumoniae, N. meningitidis, L. monocytogenes, aerobic gram-negative bacilli	Vancomycin + ampicillin + third-generation cephalospo-rin (ceftriaxone or cefotaxime)	
Basilar skull fracture Penetrating trauma	S. pneumoniae, H. influen-zae, Group A β-hemolytic streptococci S. aureus, coagulase-negative staphylococci, aerobic gram-negative bacilli (including P. aeruginosa)	Vancomycin + third-generation cephalosporin Vancomycin + cefepime or Vancomycin + ceftazidime or Vanco-mycin + meropenem	
Post-neuro-surgical procedure	Aerobic gram-negative bacilli (including P. aerugi-nosa), S. aureus, coagu-lase-negative staphylo-cocci (especially S. epidermidis)	Vancomycin + cefepime or Vancomycin + ceftazidime or Vanco-mycin + meropenem	
CSF shunt	Coagulase-negative staphylococci (especially S. epidermidis), S. aureus, aerobic gram-negative bacilli (including P. aeruginosa), Propionibacterium acnes	Vancomycin + cefepime or Vancomycin + ceftazidime or Vancomycin + meropenem	

Abbreviation: CSF, cerebrospinal fluid.

Treatment

Empiric antibiotics should be started as soon as possible. Broad-spectrum antibiotics are chosen initially based on risk factors or age (▶ Table 7.4). As specific pathogens are identified, the antibiotic of choice should be narrowed.

Dexamethasone (10 mg IV every 6 hours) should be started 10 to 20 minutes prior to first dose of antibiotics whenever pneumococcal meningitis is suspected.[27] Steroids should be continued for 2 to 4 days when pneumococcal meningitis is confirmed. If LP results are not consistent with bacterial meningitis then steroids should be discontinued. Antibiotics can be continued until cultures are finalized.

7.1.3 Aseptic Meningitis

Meningitis with clinical symptoms but negative bacterial cultures is called aseptic meningitis. Some of the more common causes of aseptic meningitis include:

- **Viruses:** Enterovirus, HIV, herpes simplex virus (HSV), mumps, Epstein-Barr virus (EBV), cytomegalovirus (CMV), human herpesvirus 6 (HHV-6), and adenovirus
- **Fungal infections:** Cryptococcal infection and coccidioidal infection
- **Spirochetes:** Lyme and syphilis
- Leptomeningeal neoplasm
- **Drug-induced meningitis:** Nonsteroidal anti-inflammatory drugs (NSAIDs), intravenous immunoglobulin (IVIG), antibiotics, and antiepileptic drugs

Diagnosis

LP should be done in all patients with suspected meningitis (▶ Fig. 7.1).

Treatment

All patients with suspected meningitis should be started on antibiotics until bacterial causes are ruled out.

7.1.4 Viral Meningitis

It is the most common form of meningitis but less severe than bacterial meningitis. Enteroviruses (coxsackievirus, echovirus, non-polio enteroviruses) which occur in the summer and fall are the most common cause of viral meningitis.

Treatment

Most cases are self-limited and resolve within 7 to 10 days. Generally, most patients can be managed with supportive treatment (antipyretics, IV fluids, pain medications, etc.). Antiviral treatment is required for some viruses such as HSV-2 and varicella-zoster virus (VZV) which are treated with acyclovir and HIV which is treated with anti-retrovirals.

Table 7.5 Common fungal infections and treatment

Fungi	Transmission	Treatment
Cryptococcus	Soil Bird droppings Decaying wood	IV Amphotericin B + 5-Flucytosine x 2 weeks then oral fluconazole
Coccidioides	Soil in the southwest United States, Central and South America	Oral fluconazole induction IV fluconazole with IT Amphotericin B for patients who fail oral therapy
Histoplasma	Bird/bat droppings Central and Eastern USA	IV Amphotericin B with transition to oral itraconazole or fluconazole
Aspergillosis	From sinusitis, IVDA	IV Voriconazole or Amphotericin B
Blastomyces	Moist soil Decaying wood/leaves Midwest, Southcentral, and Southeast USA	IV Amphotericin B
Candida	Colonized on body, hematogenous spread	Amphotericin B + 5-Flucytosine

7.1.5 Fungal Meningitis

Although relatively rare in the United States, they can occur in patients who are immunocompromised. Risk factors include organ transplantation, chemotherapy, or chronic steroid use. They present in a subacute or chronic fashion. Fungal meningitis does not spread person to person but rather patients inhale the spores which then spread from the lungs to the brain or spinal cord. Special attention should be paid to patients who have recently moved and may have been exposed based on their prior geographic location. ▶ Table 7.5 notes some of the more common fungal infections according to the CDC.

7.1.6 Ventriculitis

Inflammation of ependymal lining of cerebral ventricles due to infection is called ventriculitis.

Etiology

- Causes include meningitis, cerebral abscess, trauma, external ventricular drains, intraventricular shunts, and intrathecal chemotherapy[31]
- Common causative organisms include staphylococcus species, gram-positive skin flora, gram-negative rods, and *S. pneumoniae*

Incidence

Ventriculitis rates ranges from 0 to 45% in the setting of intraventricular catheter.[25]

Clinical Features

Fever, seizures, nuchal rigidity, new headache,[1] photophobia, nausea, lethargy, altered mental status, erythema, and tenderness over the tubing in patients with ventriculoperitoneal shunt (VPS). Pleuritis in cases of ventriculopleural shunt infection, peritonitis, abdominal pain, abdominal fluid collections in cases of ventriculoperitoneal shunt infection,[2,3] and blood stream infection and endocarditis in cases of ventriculoatrial shunt infection.

Diagnosis

- According to Infectious Diseases Society of America (IDSA) guidelines[1] diagnosis of a cerebrospinal fluid (CSF) drain infection
  - Single or multiple positive CSF culture with pleocytosis, hypoglycorrhachia, and increasing cell count and clinical symptoms are ventriculitis and meningitis.
- However, abnormalities in CSF cell count and glucose/protein may not be reliable indicators of infection, and normal CSF does not exclude infection.
- If cultures are negative initially, they should be held for at least 10 days for slow growing organisms.
- If a CSF device (including shunt, intrathecal pump, deep brain stimulatory, vagal nerve stimulator or associated hardware) is infected then current recommendations are to remove the infected device. Any device/shunt that is removed should be sent for culture.
- In addition to CSF cultures, blood cultures should be obtained for any patient with a ventriculoatrial shunt and should be considered for patients with a ventriculoperitoneal or ventriculopleural shunt.

Imaging

- Magnetic resonance imaging (MRI) with gadolinium is recommended for anyone with suspected CSF device infection.
- CT of head with contrast can be considered an alternative if MRI is unavailable or contraindicated.
- Abdominal imaging with CT of chest/abdomen or ultrasound of the abdomen should be completed in patients with peritoneal or pleural shunts and abdominal or pleuritic chest pain.

Table 7.6 Empiric antibiotic coverage in patients with suspected healthcare-associated ventriculitis/meningitis

No beta-lactam allergy or carbapenem allergy	With serious beta-lactam or carbapenem allergy
Vancomycin + antipseudomonal beta-lactam agent (cefepime, ceftazidime, or meropenem)	Vancomycin + Aztreonam or Ciprofloxacin

Treatment

- Includes antibiotic therapy and removal of infected shunt or device (▶ Table 7.6).
- Once a specific pathogen is identified, antibiotics should be narrowed (▶ Table 7.7).
- Duration of antibiotic is between 10 and 14 days depending on the pathogen, can extend to 21 days for some gram-negative bacilli. Duration should be determined after the last positive CSF culture.

7.1.7 HIV-Related Infections

Cerebral Toxoplasmosis

Central nervous system (CNS) opportunistic infections caused by the parasite *Toxoplasma gondii*.[4] It is one of the major causes of mortality and morbidity in patients with HIV. Toxoplasmosis is the most common of these infections. Patients with HIV are at risk for toxoplasmosis reactivation when CD4 cell count drops to < 200.[4] Its manifestations in CNS infections range from focal brain lesions to diffuse encephalitis.[4,5]

Diagnosis

- Clinical presentation:
  - Fever, headache, seizures, altered mental status, and focal neurologic deficit
- Laboratory studies:
  - HIV
  - CD4
  - Anti-toxoplasma IgG antibodies[23]
  - Blood cultures
- LP: Should be performed in all patients suspected unless contraindicated. Opening pressure should be noted and CSF should be sent for:
  - Cell count

Table 7.7 Antimicrobial selection based on organism and sensitivity

Specific antimicrobial agents based on pathogen	
Pathogen	**Antimicrobial agent**
Methicillin-susceptible *S. aureus*	Nafcillin or oxacillin (unless beta-lactam allergy then vancomycin can be alternative)
Methicillin-resistant *S. aureus*	Vancomycin Second-line therapy would be linezolid, daptomycin, or trimethoprim-sulfamethoxazole if unable to use vancomycin
Coagulase-negative staphylococci	Vancomycin Rifampin: this agent should be added in combination, if sensitivities allow Linezolid or daptomycin or trimethoprim-sulfamethoxazole can be used for patients unable to use beta-lactams or vancomycin
P. acnes	Penicillin G
Gram negative bacilli (non-pseudomonal) Enterobacter Klebsiella Citrobacter Serratia *H. influenzae* Proteus Neisseria	Based on sensitives and CNS penetration Ceftriaxone or cefotaxime
Pseudomonas	Cefepime, ceftazidime, or meropenem Alternative would be aztreonam or a fluroquinolone
Acinetobacter	Meropenem If carbapenem resistant, can use colistimethate sodium or polymyxin B
Candida	Liposomal Amphotericin B with 5-flucytosine
Aspergillus or Exserohilum	Voriconazole

- Protein, glucose
- Cytology
- Culture
- Cryptococcal antigen
- Toxoplasma polymerase chain reaction (PCR)[23]

- History of immunocompromised state (T-cell deficiency) due to HIV, cancer, or immunosuppressive therapy
- **Positive imaging:** MRI with gadolinium is preferred to CT[6]
  - Ring enhancing lesions with surrounding edema
  - Lesions tend to be in the deeper grey matter (basal ganglia, thalamus)
  - Can use MR spectroscopy or positron emission tomography to differentiate from cerebral lymphoma[7,8]

Treatment

- Consists of induction then maintenance therapy (▶ Table 7.8)
- Corticosteroids can be used to treat cerebral edema
- Anticonvulsant agents should be used for all patients who present with seizure. Seizure prophylaxis should be based on location of lesion.
- Antiretroviral therapy (ART) initiation: Patients with HIV not receiving ART should be evaluated regarding timely initiation of ART since suppression of HIV viral load and reconstitution of the immune system by increasing CD^4 count following diagnosis of an opportunistic infection such as toxoplasmosis has been shown to decrease AIDS progression and mortality.

Cryptococcus

Cryptococcus neoformans is a fungus that can cause meningitis in patients with immunosuppression or advanced HIV disease, often with CD count < 100.[4]

Table 7.8 Treatment of cerebral toxoplasmosis[28,29]

	Medication	Duration
Induction Dose	Pyrimethamine 200 mg PO	1 dose
Maintenance Dose < 60 kg	Pyrimethamine 50 mg PO daily + Sulfadiazine 1,000 mg PO every 6 hours + Leucovorin 10–25 mg PO daily (can be increased to 50 mg daily or two times per day if needed)	Minimum 6 weeks—longer therapy may be needed for extensive disease or partial response
Maintenance Dose > 60 kg	Pyrimethamine 50 mg PO daily + Sulfadiazine 1,000 mg PO every 6 hours + Leucovorin 10–25 mg PO daily (can be increased to 50 mg daily or two times per day if needed)	Minimum 6 weeks—longer therapy may be needed for extensive disease or partial response

Symptoms: Malaise, fever, headache, nausea, photosensitivity, visual disturbances, altered mental status, and cranial nerve palsies in cases of high intracranial pressure.[9]

Diagnosis

- LP should be done in all cases with suspicion of cryptococcal meningitis.
  - It may show elevated opening pressures > 25 cm H_2O.
  - CSF profile usually shows low white blood cell (WBC) of < 50 cells/microL, low to normal glucose, and mild protein elevation.
  - Positive cryptococcal antigen in CSF establishes the diagnosis.
- In patients who cannot undergo LP, serum antigen should be tested. It has been shown to be comparable to CSF antigen.[10] CT of head or MRI of brain with gadolinium should be performed to rule out other causes.

Treatment

- **Consists of three phases:** Induction, consolidation, and maintenance[8] (▶ Table 7.9)
- Induction with amphotericin and 5-flucytosine has shown a decrease in early mortality (within the first 2 weeks) when compared to amphotericin and fluconazole combination.[11]
- May require serial LPs for patients with elevated opening pressure or persistent intracranial symptoms suggestive of high intracranial pressure. Lumbar drain or ventriculoperitoneal shunt can be considered but should not be routine.

Table 7.9 Treatment guidelines for cryptococcal meningitis

Phase	Duration	Treatment
Induction Phase	2 weeks	Liposomal amphotericin B 3–4 mg/kg IV daily AND 5-flucytosine 25 mg/kg PO four times a day[11]
Consolidation Phase: Follows successful induction phase defined as clinical improvement and negative CSF cultures on repeat LP	8 weeks	Fluconazole 400 mg PO daily
Maintenance Phase	Minimum 1 year	Fluconazole 200 mg PO daily

Abbreviations: CSF, cerebrospinal fluid; IV, intravenous; LP, lumbar puncture.

- In contrast to toxoplasmosis, initiation of ART should be delayed in the setting of acute cryptococcal infection.

7.1.8 Empyema

An infected fluid collection inside a body cavity is referred to as an empyema. Empyemas can occur intracranially or in the spinal canal. When the collection occurs between the dura and the arachnoid it is called a subdural empyema,[26] likewise a collection located between the skull and dura is referred to as an epidural empyema. Subdural empyemas still carry a high morbidity and mortality with rates estimated as high as 55% and 48% respectively.

Risk Factors

Sinusitis (commonly), dental and ear infections, cranial surgery, trauma, and bacteremia.[12]

Microbiology

S. pneumoniae, H. influenzae, aerobic streptococci, Staphylococcus aureus, anaerobes, Pseudomonas aeruginosa, and Staphylococcus epidermidis

Clinical Presentation

Fever,[13] headache, nausea vomiting, altered mental status, earache, seizures,[13] meningismus, and focal neurologic signs.[12,13]

Diagnosis

- Laboratory studies
  - CBC, erythrocyte sedimentation rate (ESR), C-reactive protein (CRP), and blood cultures
- Imaging: All patients with suspected intracranial empyema should undergo brain imaging
  - MRI with gadolinium[14] preferred choice
  - CT of head with contrast can be performed if MRI is unavailable or contraindicated
  - MRV should be performed if there is a suspicion for infected sinus venous thrombosis
- LP: can be performed based on clinical suspicion but imaging should be completed first to avoid potential risk of herniation
- Operative cultures

Treatment

- Early diagnosis, early empiric antibiotic therapy, and surgical evacuation are the main stay of treatment.
- Empiric antibiotics include vancomycin, metronidazole, and ceftriaxone or cefepime or ceftazidime (pseudomonal coverage).
- Conservative treatment with antibiotics alone can be considered provided that the is no focal neurologic deficit, the collection is limited and localized (not in the posterior fossa) and there is rapid improvement with the initiation of antibiotic therapy. The drawbacks to conservative treatment are the patient will require frequent imaging to evaluate resolution and will require long-term broad-spectrum antibiotics, which carry risk of adverse effect.[26]

Complications

Cerebritis, venous sinus thrombosis, septic thrombophlebitis, venous infarction, cerebral edema, and cranial osteomyelitis.[12,14]

7.2 Spine

7.2.1 Epidural Abscess

Presence of purulent material between the dura and vertebral bodies is called spinal epidural abscess.[15] It can cause injury to the spinal cord by direct compression, or by causing septic thrombophlebitis causing vascular occlusion. This can lead to permanent loss of neurologic function.

Epidemiology

The incidence of spinal abscess is about 0.2 to 1.2 cases per 10,000.[15] The incidence has increased over the past 25 years. It is more common in men than women.

Risk Factors

- Diabetes
- Spinal surgery/procedure/instrumentation
- Spinal deformity
- Immunosuppression
- Alcoholism
- Trauma
- Intravenous drug abuse (IVDA)
- Bacteremia

Microbiology

S. aureus accounts for two-thirds of the cases, and MRSA accounts for about 15% of cases. Other organisms include: Coagulase-negative staphylococci (*S. epidermidis*), *Escherichia coli*, *P. aeruginosa*, anaerobic bacteria (rare), and mycobacteria including tuberculosis (rare). Approximately one-third of patients have no identifiable cause.

Clinical Presentation

- Neurologic deficits are the most common feature: Motor weakness, numbness, and bladder or bowel dysfunction
- Pain: Back pain, radicular pain, and shooting pain, electric shock like. On physical examination, palpation along the spinal axis can help to localize the suspected area of injury
- Fever

Diagnosis

Laboratory studies: CBC, ESR, CRP, and blood cultures

Imaging

- MRI spinal access (gold standard),
- CT of spine with intravenous contrast, or
- CT myelogram if MRI is unavailable or contraindicated

Treatment (▶ Table 7.10)

- Surgical decompression should be performed as early as possible to avoid permanent neurologic injury.
- Empiric systemic antibiotics should be initiated upon presentation.

Table 7.10 Treatment for spinal epidural abscess

	Medication	Duration
Empiric treatment	Vancomycin + cefotaxime, ceftriaxone, cefepime, or ceftazidime OR Meropenem	Minimum 6 weeks[16]
If high suspicion for pseudomonas	Vancomycin + cefepime or ceftazidime or meropenem	

- Antibiotic therapy
  - Vancomycin + ceftriaxone (ceftazidime or cefepime); narrow based on culture results; duration of treatment at least 6 weeks[16]
- Patients with high-risk perioperative risk, panspinal infection, irreversible paralysis, or those who decline surgery may be treated with antibiotics alone.
- CT-guided aspiration of the abscess for organism identification should be done if surgical decompression is not an option.
- If unable to obtain direct cultures, antibiotics can be tapered based on blood culture results.

7.2.2 Osteomyelitis

Vertebral osteomyelitis is usually an indolent disease with chronic symptoms that can lead to misdiagnosis.[30] It is usually the result of hematogenous spread but can also be from contiguous spread from surrounding soft tissues.

Risk Factors

- IVDA
- Diabetes
- Degenerative joint disease
- Endocarditis
- Spinal surgery/procedure or instrumentation
- Immunocompromised state

It occurs twice as often in men than women.

Microbiology

Most common organism: *S. aureus*[17]

   Foreign-body-associated infection: Coagulase-negative staphylococci or *Propionibacterium* spp.

   Common in nosocomial infections: Enterobacteriaceae, *P. aeruginosa*, *Candida* spp.

   TB prevalent areas: *Mycobacterium tuberculosis*

   Endemic pathogens: *Brucella* spp., *Coxiella burnetti*, fungi[17]

Clinical Presentation

- Pain over the affected vertebra is the most common presenting feature. Patients can have pain for days to weeks. Pain can be elicited on physical examination by palpation along the spinal axis.

- Fever is not always present.
- Lumbar vertebra is more commonly involved than thoracic and cervical.

Diagnosis

- Laboratory studies
  - CBC, ESR, CRP, and blood cultures
- Imaging
  - Echocardiogram should be performed in all patients with positive blood cultures.
  - **X-ray:** Low sensitivity and low specificity. Can take up to 2 weeks before imaging is abnormal:
    - Soft tissues swelling
    - Bone destruction
    - Periosteal reaction
    - Widening or narrowing of joint spaces
  - MRI with and without gadolinium
  - CT has limited use except in cases when MRI is unavailable or contraindicated. Poor resolution of soft tissue and inability to show bone marrow edema. A normal CT scan does not exclude the diagnosis of osteomyelitis.
- **Tissue culture:** Image-guided needle aspiration should be performed when blood cultures are negative. Tissue cultures should be sent for bacteria, fungus, mycobacteria, and brucella (when appropriate).

Treatment

If patients are hemodynamically stable and without evidence of epidural abscess, antibiotics can be held until the microbiologic diagnosis is established. Antibiotic therapy can be tailored to the specific pathogen as shown in ▶ Table 7.11. Total treatment duration is generally a minimum of 6 weeks.

Monitoring

Assess clinical improvement and trend ESR and CRP after 4 weeks of antimicrobial therapy. In patients who do not improve, repeat MRI is warranted; additional tissue specimen should be obtained if there is evidence of clinical and radiographic failure of therapy.[18]

Surgical Intervention

Surgery is recommended for patients who have progressive neurologic deficits, or epidural or paravertebral abscesses, cord compression due to vertebral

Table 7.11 Antimicrobial selection for osteomyelitis without abscess. (Adapted from IDSA guidelines 2015[18])

Micro-organisms	First choice
Empiric therapy	Vancomycin plus cefotaxime or ceftazidime or ceftriaxone or cefepime
MSSA	Nafcillin or oxacillin or cefazolin
MRSA	Vancomycin
Enterococcus species, penicillin susceptible	Penicillin G or ampicillin
Enterococcus species, penicillin resistant	Vancomycin IV
P. aeruginosa	Cefepime/Meropenem/Doripenem
Enterobacteriaceae	Cefepime/Ertapenem
Propionibacterium acnes	Penicillin G/ceftriaxone

Abbreviations: MRSA, methicillin-resistant Staphylococcus aureus; MSSA, methicillin-susceptible Staphylococcus aureus.

collapse, or persistent or recurrence of disease in spite of antimicrobial therapy.[17,18]

7.3 Central Fever

Central fevers are fevers without any identifiable cause (infectious or noninfectious) in the setting of acute neurologic injury. Fever has been defined as a body temperature $\geq 38.3\,°C$ daily for 2 consecutive days.[19] Fever has been associated with increased mortality rate, worse neurologic outcome, longer ICU stay, and higher cost of care.[19,20]

- Predictors of central fevers include
  - Early onset within 72 hours of admission to ICU[19,20]
  - Persistent fevers lasting for more than 6 hours for 2 or more days[20,21,22]
  - Recent blood transfusion
  - Diagnosis of traumatic brain injury, subarachnoid hemorrhage, intraventricular hemorrhage, or tumor

Central fever is also a diagnosis of exclusion. Infectious and noninfectious causes need to be ruled out before a diagnosis of central fever can be made.

- Other noninfectious causes of fever include the following:
  - Drug induced
  - Superficial thrombophlebitis

- Acute deep vein thrombosis
- Pancreatitis
- Acalculous cholecystitis

Aggressive management of all fevers is recommended. Acetaminophen and surface cooling agents are the recommended treatment. Details on methods for temperature management can be found in Chapter 6.

References

[1] Tunkel AR, Hasbun R, Bhimraj A, et al. 2017 Infectious Diseases Society of America's Clinical Practice Guidelines for Healthcare-Associated Ventriculitis and Meningitis. Clin Infect Dis. 2017; 64 (6):e34–e65

[2] Fukui MB, Williams RL, Mudigonda S. CT and MR imaging features of pyogenic ventriculitis. AJNR Am J Neuroradiol. 2001; 22(8):1510–1516

[3] Tunkel AR, Hartman BJ, Kaplan SL, et al. Practice guidelines for the management of bacterial meningitis. Clin Infect Dis. 2004; 39(9):1267–1284

[4] Basavaraju A. Toxoplasmosis in HIV infection: an overview. Trop Parasitol. 2016; 6(2):129–135

[5] Gray F, Gherardi R, Wingate E, et al. Diffuse "encephalitic" cerebral toxoplasmosis in AIDS. Report of four cases. J Neurol. 1989; 236:273–277

[6] Levy RM, Mills CM, Posin JP, Moore SG, Rosenblum ML, Bredesen DE. The efficacy and clinical impact of brain imaging in neurologically symptomatic AIDS patients: a prospective CT/MRI study. J Acquir Immune Defic Syndr (1988). 1990; 3(5):461–471

[7] Ernst TM, Chang L, Witt MD, et al. Cerebral toxoplasmosis and lymphoma in AIDS: perfusion MR imaging experience in 13 patients. Radiology. 1998; 208(3):663–669

[8] Panel on Opportunistic Infections in HIV-infected Adults and Adolescents. Guidelines for the prevention and treatment of opportunistic infections in HIV-infected adults and adolescents: recommendations from the Center of Disease Control and Prevention, the National Institutes of Health, and the HIV Medical Association of the Infectious Disease Society of America. Available at http://aidsinfo.nih.gov/contentfiles/ivguidelines/adult_oi.odf. Accessed January 17, 2017. C1–8

[9] Jarvis JN, Harrison TS. HIV-associated cryptococcal meningitis. AIDS. 2007; 21(16):2119–2129

[10] Asawavichienjinda T, Sitthi-Amorn C, Tanyanont V. Serum cyrptococcal antigen: diagnostic value in the diagnosis of AIDS-related cryptococcal meningitis. J Med Assoc Thai. 1999; 82(1):65–71

[11] Larsen RA, Leal MA, Chan LS. Fluconazole compared with amphotericin B plus flucytosine for cryptococcal meningitis in AIDS: a randomized trial. Ann Intern Med. 1990; 113(3):183–187

[12] Agrawal A, Timothy J, Pandit L, Shetty L, Shetty JP. A review of subdural empyema and its management. Infect Dis Clin Pract. 2007; 15(3):149–153

[13] Bruner DI, Littlejohn L, Pritchard A. Subdural empyema presenting with seizure, confusion, and focal weakness. West J Emerg Med. 2012; 13(6):509–511

[14] Weingarten K, Zimmerman RD, Becker RD, Heier LA, Haimes AB, Deck MD. Subdural and epidural empyemas: MR imaging. AJR Am J Roentgenol. 1989; 152(3):615–621

[15] Tompkins M, Panuncialman I, Lucas P, Palumbo M. Spinal epidural abscess. J Emerg Med. 2010; 39 (3):384–390

[16] Darouiche RO. Spinal epidural abscess. N Engl J Med. 2006; 355(19):2012–2020

[17] Lew DP, Waldvogel FA. Osteomyelitis. Lancet. 2004; 364(9431):369–379

[18] Berbari EF, Kanj SS, Kowalski TJ, et al. Infectious Diseases Society of America. 2015 Infectious Disease Society of America (IDSA) clinical practice guidelines for the diagnosis and treatment of native vertebral osteomyelitis in adults. Clin Infect Dis. 2015; 61(6):e26–e46

[19] Rabinstein AA, Sandhu K. Non-infectious fever in the neurological intensive care unit: incidence, causes and predictors. J Neurol Neurosurg Psychiatry. 2007; 78(11):1278–1280

[20] Hocker SE, Tian L, Li G, Steckelberg JM, Mandrekar JN, Rabinstein AA. Indicators of central fever in the neurologic intensive care unit. JAMA Neurol. 2013; 70(12):1499–1504

[21] Kamel H. Fever without infection in the neurological intensive care unit. JAMA Neurol. 2013; 7:4354

[22] Honig A, Michael S, Eliahou R, Leker RR. Central fever in patients with spontaneous intracerebral hemorrhage: predicting factors and impact on outcome. BMC Neurol. 2015; 15(6):6

[23] Colombo FA, Vidal JE, Penalva de Oliveira AC, et al. Diagnosis of cerebral toxoplasmosis in AIDS patients in Brazil: importance of molecular and immunological methods using peripheral blood samples. J Clin Microbiol. 2005; 43(10):5044–5047

[24] Navia BA, Petito CK, Gold JW, Cho ES, Jordan BD, Price RW. Cerebral toxoplasmosis complicating the acquired immune deficiency syndrome: clinical and neuropathological findings in 27 patients. Ann Neurol. 1986; 19(3):224–238

[25] Lyke KE, Obasanjo OO, Williams MA, O'Brien M, Chotani R, Perl TM. Ventriculitis complicating use of intraventricular catheters in adult neurosurgical patients. Clin Infect Dis. 2001; 33(12):2028–2033

[26] de Bonis P, Anile A, Pompucci A, Labonia M, Lucantoni C, Mangiola A. Cranial and spinal subdural empyema. Journal of Neurosurgery 2009; 23(3):335–340.

[27] de Gans J, van de Beek D, European Dexamethasone in Adulthood Bacterial Meningitis Study Investigators. Dexamethasone in adults with bacterial meningitis. N Engl J Med. 2002; 347 (20):1549–1556

[28] Katlama C, De Wit S, O'Doherty E, Van Glabeke M, Clumeck N. Pyrimethamine-clindamycin vs. pyrimethamine-sulfadiazine as acute and long-term therapy for toxoplasmic encephalitis in patients with AIDS. Clin Infect Dis. 1996; 22(2):268–275

[29] Nath A, Sinai AP. Cerebral toxoplasmosis. Curr Treat Options Neurol. 2003; 5(1):3–12

[30] Sapico FL, Montgomerie JZ. Vertebral osteomyelitis. Infect Dis Clin North Am. 1990; 4(3):539–550

[31] Agrawal A, Cincu R, Timothy J. Current concepts and approach to ventriculitis. Infect Dis Clin Pract. 2008; 16(2):100–104

8 Treatment of Status Epilepticus in Adults

James Park, Alan Wang, Andres Fernandez, and Sara Hefton

Abstract

Status epilepticus is a neurologic emergency that requires immediate evaluation and treatment in order to prevent significant morbidity and mortality. Seizures can present in many different ways, and therefore status epilepticus can be varied in its presentation, as well (i.e. convulsive, nonconvulsive, focal motor, myoclonic). Status epilepticus can become refractory; timely recognition and treatment is necessary to avoid the refractory state/neurologic damage that can occur with prolonged status epilepticus. Here, we will define status epilepticus and detail its management.

Keywords: status epilepticus, status, seizure(s), convulsive, nonconvulsive, refractory status

8.1 Overview and Definitions

Status epilepticus (SE) is a neurologic emergency. This chapter will address the evaluation and management of a seizing patient.

- Seizures may be focal (starting in one part of the brain) or generalized (starting in the whole brain at once)
  - Focal seizures may impair consciousness or may occur without impaired consciousness
  - Generalized seizures will always cause impaired consciousness
- Seizures may consist of tonic (stiffening) and clonic (rhythmic jerking) phases, but may also consist of staring, nonresponsiveness, and automatisms (unconscious movements)

There are two types of SE: convulsive SE (CSE) and nonconvulsive SE (NCSE)
- Clinical presentation:
  - **CSE:** Rhythmic jerking of the extremities, impairment in mental status, and may have postictal focal neurologic deficits[1]
  - **NCSE:** Subtle and variable semiology (may have positive or negative symptoms)[1,2]
- SE definitions were applied generally to CSE and NCSE in the past (refer to the points below). But now the definition of NCSE is evolving as continuous

EEG monitoring has become more readily available and we can learn more about it (see below in NCSE section for definitions).

- SE is defined by the Neurocritical Care Society Status Epilepticus guidelines as:
  - Continuous clinical and/or electrographic seizure activity of 5 minutes or more[1]
  - Recurrent seizure activity without a return to baseline between seizures[1]
- Epidemiology:
  - 50,000 to 150,000 SE cases per year are reported in the United States[3]
  - Up to 30% mortality in adults[3]
- Pathophysiology
  - SE occurs due to the failure of mechanisms that terminate seizures or initiation of mechanisms that lead to prolonged seizures[4]
  - There is a decrease in inhibitory receptors and an increase in excitatory receptors[5,6]
  - Key timepoints as per the ILAE Task Force on Classification of Status Epilepticus[4]:
    - t_1: when seizures are likely to be prolonged and become continuous
      - ► Tonic-clonic: 5 minutes
      - ► Focal SE with impaired consciousness: 10 minutes
      - ► Absence: 10 to 15 minutes
    - t_2: when seizures can cause long-term consequences
      - ► Tonic-clonic: 30 minutes
      - ► Focal SE with impaired consciousness: > 60 minutes
      - ► Absence: unknown

8.2 Convulsive Status Epilepticus Management

- Two main CSE treatment guidelines
  - Neurocritical Care Society[1]
  - American Epilepsy Society[3]
  - See ► Fig. 8.1 for timeline and medication doses[3]
- Initial SE management (the below management is based on the NCS and AES guidelines in addition to our local institutional practice) [1,2,3]
  - Evaluate and secure adequate airway, breathing, and circulation (ABCs)
  - Obtain intravenous (IV) access
  - Check finger-stick glucose
    - If glucose < 60 mg/dL, give thiamine 100 mg IV × 1, then 50 mg D50 IV
  - Monitor SpO2, blood pressure, heart rate, and rhythm as vital signs may become unstable
  - Treat hyperthermia
  - Obtain labs: CBC, CMP, ABG, PT, INR, aPTT, Ca^{2+}, Mg^{2+}, $PO4^{-2}$, troponin, HCG (if appropriate), ammonia (if appropriate)
  - Check toxicology screen

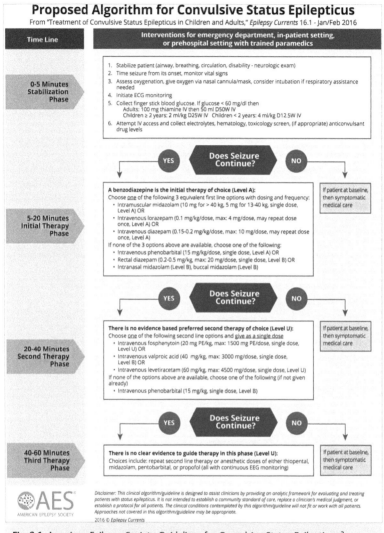

Fig. 8.1 American Epilepsy Society Guidelines for Convulsive Status Epilepticus.[3]

- ○ Check antiepileptic drug (AED) levels (if appropriate)
- ○ Obtain computed tomography (CT) of the head to evaluate for structural lesion if no history of seizures

- May consider magnetic resonance imaging (MRI) of brain with and without contrast after seizures are controlled
  - Consider lumbar puncture and/or antibiotics if there is clinical suspicion of infection
  - Begin continuous electroencephalography (cEEG) if appropriate; considering the indications outlined by the consensus statement by American Clinical Neurophysiology Society (ACNS)[2]
    - Electroencephalography (EEG) is required for the diagnosis of nonconvulsive seizures and NCSE
      - ►CSE may transition to NCSE; cEEG should be used in patients who do not return to baseline despite therapy
    - EEG is required for the assessment of efficacy of continuous IV therapy in SE
    - cEEG should be continued until patient is seizure free for at least 24 hours
- Initial medical therapy
  - Benzodiazepines[1,3] should be administered in parallel with the initial management steps listed above
    - IV Lorazepam 2 to 4 mg at a time for up to 0.1 mg/kg total dose
    - IM Midazolam (especially in prehospital[8] setting) 10 mg × 1 (if the patient weighs more than 40 kg)
    - IV Diazepam 0.15 to 0.2 mg/kg/dose for up to 10 mg/dose
- Second medical therapy
  - Administered if benzodiazepines fail, but often concurrently ordered
  - No definitive evidence for a preferred AED[3]
  - AED options include:
    - IV Fosphenytoin/Phenytoin (20 PE/kg or 20 mg/kg load, max 1,500 mg/dose)
      - ►Fosphenytoin may be administered more rapidly than phenytoin and does not have risk of purple glove syndrome
      - ►Patients must be monitored on telemetry, given risk of cardiac arrhythmias
      - ►Post-load phenytoin level 2 hours after administration, goal 15 to 20 µg/mL
    - IV Valproic Acid (40 mg/kg load, max 3,000 mg/dose)
      - ►May cause hepatotoxicity, hyperammonemia, and thrombocytopenia
      - ►Post-load level 1 hour after administration, target level 70 to 100 µg/mL
    - IV Levetiracetam (60 mg/kg load, max 4,500 mg/dose)
      - ►Renal clearance; dose must be adjusted for creatinine clearance
    - IV Phenobarbital (if the above options are not available, 15 mg/kg load)
      - ►May cause hypotension, metabolic acidosis, and respiratory depression
    - While more research needs to be done lacosamide is commonly used in the clinical setting for the treatment of SE. As it is more recent it is not part of the guidelines. IV lacosamide is typically given as a 300 or 400 mg load.

- ►A systematic review of the available evidence showed most clinicians using anywhere from 200 to 400 mg.[11]
- ►However, another study using weight-adjusted dosing showed better efficacy when a loading dose of 5.3 mg/kg was administered (for the average 60-70 kg person this would equate to 300-400 mg).[11]
- ►May cause PR prolongation and AV block. Hypotension and arrhythmias have also been occasionally reported.
  - ○ Individual patient scenario may play a role in the choice of AED[1]
    - – Consider patient comorbidities and potential side effects of AEDs noted above
  - ○ In patients with known epilepsy and on an AED, it is reasonable to give an IV bolus of that AED if IV formulation is available[1]
- The Established Status Epilepticus Treatment Trial (ESETT)[12,13]
  - ○ No statistically significant difference was seen in terms of efficacy and safety outcome between the three drugs (fosphenytoin, valproic acid, and levetiracetam) for the treatment of benzodiazepine-refractory SE

8.3 Nonconvulsive Status Epilepticus (NCSE)

- Variable definitions have been used in the past such as:
  - ○ Nonconvulsive status lasting more than 30 minutes or recurrent over 30 minutes without return to normal consciousness[2]
  - ○ Continuous nonconvulsive seizure lasting more than 5 minutes[1]
  - ○ Electrographic seizures seen on more than 50% of an EEG epoch[2]
- There are upcoming new definitions for nonconvulsive status epilepticus based on the American Clinical Neurophysiology Society's Standardized Critical Care EEG Terminology: 2021 version
  - ○ This document is currently in "public comment format" after which the revision and publication process will occur; see the public comment link.[26]
  - ○ Based on this upcoming publication:
    - – The definition should change from NCS ≥30 minutes to electrographic seizure for ≥10 continuous minutes
    - – The required seizure burden to diagnose NCSE will also decrease from 50% to 20% or more of a 60-minute epoch
- Must be monitored on EEG[2]
  - ○ EEG recording lasting less than 1 hour only identifies 45 to 58% of patients who eventually have seizures
  - ○ Recording for at least 24 hours is recommended
- Often occurs after CSE
- Worse prognosis,[7] especially if no history of seizures[14]
- Treatment typically extrapolated from the guidelines for the treatment of CSE and practice is variable
- Determining and treating the underlying etiology is important

8.4 Refractory Status Epilepticus (RSE)

- Defined as failure of benzodiazepines (initial medical therapy) and standard AED (second medical therapy)[1]
- No definitive evidence for a preferred AED agent[3]
  - One randomized controlled trial could not be completed due to poor enrollment[15]
- Management
  - Must be monitored on EEG[16,17]
  - Identify and treat the underlying etiology where possible
  - Ensure AEDs are at therapeutic levels
  - Intubate for airway protection and admit to intensive care unit (ICU)
- Third medical therapy:
  - Continuous infusion of anesthestics[18,19]
    - Midazolam, propofol, or pentobarbital may be used[1]
    - Case reports and series have shown ketamine to be effective, but clinical trials are ongoing to prove its efficacy and safety in the treatment of RSE. There are some questions about using ketamine earlier in SE because of neuroprotective effects seen in rodent models[27,28,29]
  - No standard approach and practice is variable
  - May target burst suppression or seizure suppression on cEEG; no clear superiority for effective seizure control.[1,18]
  - Maintain adequate dosing of second medical therapy medications
  - Wean infusion gradually after targeted EEG pattern (burst suppression or seizure suppression) has been maintained for 24 hours and monitor for recurrence of seizures
- Focal motor seizures without loss of awareness (epilepsia partialis continua)
  - Often difficult to control
  - Risk of escalation of care with intubation and anesthetics must be weighed against benefits
  - Often treated with nonsedating medications requiring polypharmacy

8.5 Super Refractory Status Epilepticus (SRSE)

- Defined as SE that continues for ≥ 24 hours after the onset of anesthesia, including when SE recurs with the reduction or withdrawal of anesthesia[18]
- Anywhere from 4 to 26% of SE cases have been reported as becoming super refractory[20,21,22,23,24]
- Treatment
  - There is no consensus on treatment.

- Anesthetics: Typically IV anesthesia is weaned every 24 to 48 hours. If seizures recur, anesthesia is restarted and the duration of each cycle can be gradually increased. Slower weaning of anesthetics should also be considered.[18]
- In select cases based on the clinical picture, immunotherapy (steroids, intravenous immunoglobulin [IVIG], and/or plasma exchange) is considered to treat possible autoimmune etiologies.
- Consider neurosurgical evaluation if a structural lesion is present.
- Other potential therapies include: inhaled anesthetics, ketamine[25], hypothermia, ketogenic diet, and electroconvulsive therapy.[25]

References

[1] Brophy GM, Bell R, Claassen J, et al. Neurocritical Care Society Status Epilepticus Guideline Writing Committee. Guidelines for the evaluation and management of status epilepticus. Neurocrit Care. 2012; 17(1):3–23

[2] Herman ST, Abend NS, Bleck TP, et al. Critical Care Continuous EEG Task Force of the American Clinical Neurophysiology Society. Consensus statement on continuous EEG in critically ill adults and children, part I: indications. J Clin Neurophysiol. 2015; 32(2):87–95

[3] Glauser T, Shinnar S, Gloss D, et al. Evidence-based guideline: treatment of convulsive status epilepticus in children and adults: Report of the Guideline Committee of the American Epilepsy Society. Epilepsy Curr. 2016; 16(1):48–61

[4] Trinka, E, Cock, H, Hesdorffer, D, et al. A definition and classification of status epilepticus-Report of the ILAE Task Force on Classification of Status Epilepticus. Epilepsia. 2015; 56: 1515–1523.

[5] Foreman B, Hirsch LJ. Epilepsy emergencies: diagnosis and management. Neurol Clin. 2012; 30 (1):11–41, vii

[6] Betjemann JP, Lowenstein DH. Status epilepticus in adults. Lancet Neurol. 2015; 14(6):615–624

[7] Treiman DM, Meyers PD, Walton NY, et al. Veterans Affairs Status Epilepticus Cooperative Study Group. A comparison of four treatments for generalized convulsive status epilepticus. N Engl J Med. 1998; 339(12):792–798

[8] Silbergleit R, Durkalski V, Lowenstein D, et al. NETT Investigators. Intramuscular versus intravenous therapy for prehospital status epilepticus. N Engl J Med. 2012; 366(7):591–600

[9] Alldredge BK, Gelb AM, Isaacs SM, et al. A comparison of lorazepam, diazepam, and placebo for the treatment of out-of-hospital status epilepticus. N Engl J Med. 2001; 345(9):631–637

[10] Strzelczyk A, Zollner JP, et al. Lacosamide is status epilepticus: Systematic review of current evidence. Epilepsia. 2017; 58(6): 933–950.

[11] Santamarina E, et al. Intravenous lacosamide (LCM) in status epilepticus (SE): Weight-adjusted dose and efficacy. Epilepsy and Behavior. 2018; 84:93–98.

[12] Kapur J, et al. Randomized trial of three anticonvulsant medications for status epilepticus. N Engl J Med. 2019; 381(22):2103–2113.

[13] Chamberlain JM, et al. Efficacy of levetiracetam, fosphenytoin, and valproate for established status epilepticus by age group (ESETT): A double-blind, responsive-adaptive, randomised controlled trial. Lancet. 2020; 395:1217–1224.

[14] Power KN, Gramstad A, Gilhus NE, Engelsen BA. Adult nonconvulsive status epilepticus in a clinical setting: semiology, aetiology, treatment and outcome. Seizure. 2015; 24:102–106

[15] Rossetti AO, Milligan TA, Vulliémoz S, Michaelides C, Bertschi M, Lee JW. A randomized trial for the treatment of refractory status epilepticus. Neurocrit Care. 2011; 14(1):4–10

[16] Abend NS, Dlugos DJ, Hahn CD, Hirsch LJ, Herman ST. Use of EEG monitoring and management of non-convulsive seizures in critically ill patients: a survey of neurologists. Neurocrit Care. 2010; 12(3):382–389

[17] Claassen J, Mayer SA, Kowalski RG, Emerson RG, Hirsch LJ. Detection of electrographic seizures with continuous EEG monitoring in critically ill patients. Neurology. 2004; 62(10):1743–1748

[18] Shorvon S and Ferlisi M. The treatment of super-refractory status epilepticus: a critical review of available therapies and a clinical treatment protocol. Brain. 2011; 134(10):2802–2818

[19] Fernandez A, Lantigua H, Lesch C, et al. High-dose midazolam infusion for refractory status epilepticus. Neurology. 2014; 82(4):359–365

[20] Delaj L, Novy J, Ryvlin P, Marchi NA, Rossetti AO. Refractory and super-refractory status epilepticus in adults: a 9-year cohort study. Acta Neurol Scand. 2017; 135(1):92–99

[21] Jayalakshmi S, Ruikar D, Vooturi S, et al. Determinants and predictors of outcome in super refractory status epilepticus—a developing country perspective. Epilepsy Res. 2014; 108(9):1609–1617

[22] Tian L, Li Y, Xue X, et al. Super-refractory status epilepticus in West China. Acta Neurol Scand. 2015; 132(1):1–6

[23] Kantanen A-M, Reinikainen M, Parviainen I, et al. Incidence and mortality of super-refractory status epilepticus in adults. Epilepsy Behav. 2015; 49:131–134

[24] Mayer SA, Claassen J, Lokin J, Mendelsohn F, Dennis LJ, Fitzsimmons BF. (2002) Refractory status epilepticus: frequency, risk factors, and impact on outcome. Arch Neurol 59:205–210.

[25] Alkhachroum A, Caroline A. Der-Nigoghossian C.A, Elizabeth Mathews E. et al. Ketamine to treat super-refractory status epilepticus. Neurology Sep 2020. https://n.neurology.org/content/early/2020/09/01/WNL.0000000000010611

[26] Hirsch LJ, Fong MWK et al, https://www.acns.org/UserFiles/file/ACNSNomenclature2021_MAIN-TEXT_2020_08-22ForPublicComment.pdf

[27] Rosati A, De Masi S, Guerrini R. Ketamine for Refractory Status Epilepticus: A Systematic Review. CNS Drugs. 2018;32(11):997-1009.

[28] Höfler J, Trinka E. Intravenous ketamine in status epilepticus. Epilepsia, 2018. https://onlinelibrary.wiley.com/doi/full/10.1111/epi.14480

[29] G Fujikawa D. Starting ketamine for neuroprotection earlier than its current use as an anesthetic/antiepileptic drug late in refractory status epilepticus. Epilepsia 2019. https://onlinelibrary.wiley.com/doi/full/10.1111/epi.14676

9 Trauma

Ravichandra Madineni and Christian Hoelscher

Abstract

Traumatic brain injury (TBI) and traumatic spinal cord injury (SCI) are serious neurologic injuries with potentially devastating impact on patients, caregivers, and society. The pathophysiologic mechanisms of these injuries are complex. While the primary injury is likely associated with irreversible deficit, increasing research and better treatment protocols aimed at mitigating secondary injury cascades has led to consistent progress in taking care of this critically ill patient population.

Keywords: traumatic brain injury, spinal cord injury, primary injury, secondary injury, dysautonomia

9.1 Acute Spinal Cord Injury

9.1.1 Introduction

Spinal cord injury (SCI) is an increasingly common problem posed to both neurosurgeons and neuro-intensivists, with an estimated incidence of up to 0.05%, with about 10,000 to 15,000 SCI occurring each year in the United States alone.[1,2,3] The consequences can be devastating, with long-term clinical, functional, and financial burdens imposed on providers, care-takers, and, of course, the patient. Managing SCI patients requires a general understanding of the involved physiology, which includes:

- **Primary injury:** The result of direct tissue damage to the spinal cord, either from penetrating or blunt trauma, that causes irreversible tissue damage via direct compression, distraction, or laceration of the spinal cord.[4]
- **Secondary injury:** Damage to potentially salvageable tissue caused by inflammation, hypoperfusion, thrombosis, edema, and accumulation of toxic metabolites and reactive oxygen species.[5]

Given that the underlying primary insult causes irreparable tissue damage, the bulk of research in the field of SCI has been directed toward modulating and reducing secondary injury cascades. This can be accomplished via medical and surgical interventions.

9.1.2 Medical Treatment of Acute SCI

Medical management of SCI begins at the scene with strict spine precautions, immobilization on a hard backboard, and placement of a hard cervical collar.

Acute SCI is often caused by high-energy mechanisms with potentially unstable injuries, and particular attention must be provided to avoid causing or worsening a SCI during patient transfer and transport. Upon arrival at an appropriate trauma center, standard Advanced Trauma Life Support (ATLS) protocols should be followed to identify all injuries. Particular attention should be paid to maintenance of the airway and adequate respiration/ventilation. This is especially true in cases of cervical SCI, as such patients may have significant neck soft-tissue edema that places their airway at high risk for progressive compromise in a manner that may make urgent intubation increasingly difficult. Injuries above the C5 level are additionally at high risk for respiratory failure given the impaired or absent innervation to the diaphragm. As such, there should be a very low threshold for intubation to ensure adequate respiratory function.[6,7]

The next most important consideration in acute SCI patients is aggressively supporting the systemic circulation. The traumatized central nervous system often displays significantly dysfunctional vascular autoregulation, and tissue perfusion is often directly dependent on mean arterial pressure (MAP). Avoidance of hypotension is critical, with many centers pursuing a prolonged (e.g., 5–7 days) course of artificially elevated MAP (> 85–90 mm Hg) in an effort to ensure adequate perfusion of any potentially salvageable ischemic penumbra in the traumatized spinal cord. This often requires the administration of pressors to achieve this goal, especially in patients with neurogenic shock due to loss of sympathetic tone to the vasculature. This is common after cervical and high thoracic injuries, and often manifests as hypotension without an appropriate tachycardic response (i.e., bradycardia or an inappropriately normal heart rate). The data in the literature in support of this protocol is unfortunately of low quality, but the available data from two prospective studies support this elevated MAP goal in an effort to maximize neurologic recovery.[8]

The spine is stabilized, a detailed neurologic examination is critical. This is often performed according to the standards of the American Spinal Injury Association (ASIA) scale. This takes into account strength in 10 core myotomes, as well as light touch and pinprick sensation in all dermatomes including sacral, and is graded A–E (▶ Table 9.1). Accurate ASIA classification is essential as there is prognostic significance and it forms the baseline for monitoring future recovery.

Use of steroids in the setting of blunt trauma to the spinal cord has been a topic of debate in the literature. The NASCIS[9,10,11] trials attempted to establish the role of steroids, specifically methylprednisolone, in SCI with the results suggesting benefit when used within 8 hours of injury, for a duration of up to 48 hours. However, neurologic recovery gained in follow-up periods was modest at best, and the use of high-dose steroids in this setting is maintained cautiously as an option but with the caveat that the evidence is more convincing for adverse effects, including death, than it is for significant clinical benefit.

Table 9.1 American Spinal Injury Association impairment scale

A   No motor or sensory function below the level of injury, including sacral segments. Complete injury.

B   Preservation of at least partial sensory function below the level of injury, without motor preservation. Incomplete injury.

C   Preservation of partial motor function below the level of injury, with fewer than 50% of key myotomes showing < 3/5 strength grade. Incomplete injury.

D   Preservation of partial motor function below the level of injury, with fewer than 50% of key myotomes showing ≥ 3/5 strength grade. Incomplete injury.

E   Normal sensory and motor function in a patient with a previously documented spinal cord injury.

There are a variety of other pharmacologic agents being studied in myriad clinical trials, but these are used only in carefully constructed research protocols and none have reached standard clinical practice as yet.

9.1.3 Surgical Management of Acute SCI

Many patients with SCI require surgical intervention for stabilization of unstable spinal column injuries and/or decompression of neural elements, with an added benefit being early mobilization and avoidance of prolonged periods of bedrest that are associated with complications such as pneumonia, deep venous thrombosis, pulmonary embolism, and general deconditioning. The exact timing of surgery for SCI has been an area of debate. Several animal studies have shown that earlier decompression of the spinal cord leads to improved neurologic outcomes, presumably as a result of improved tissue perfusion and reduced secondary injury cascades.[12,13] This bench research led to optimism that early decompression would clearly benefit actual SCI patients, and led many surgeons to support earlier (originally defined as < 72 hours after injury) rather than later surgery for decompression and stabilization. However, early studies did not necessarily support this hypothesis, with one review of incomplete cervical SCI showing no direct correlation between early surgery and functional recovery,[14] and another review of about 800 patients who underwent early, late, or no surgery showing no difference in recovery or functional improvement between the early and late surgical groups, and in fact at 1-year follow-up noted motor improvements were more likely in the nonsurgical cohort.[15] A high degree of variability in defining "early" versus "late" surgery was thought to be a factor in this lack of clinical benefit. A follow-up systematic review, using < 24 hours as the cutoff for "early surgery" found significant benefit for early surgery, which led the Spine Trauma Study Group to adopt this threshold in its clinical guidelines. However, the quality of the evidence remained relatively poor. Several small studies have noted better neurologic recovery in those operated on early (< 24 hours after injury), as well as fewer complications related to reduced length of stay and bedrest.[16,17,18,19] In 2012, the first multicenter, prospective cohort study evaluated early versus late surgery for acute cervical SCI, with 19.8% in the early surgery group versus 8.8% in the late surgery group showing at least a 2 grade improvement on the ASIA scale, and the benefit remained significant when adjusted for administration of steroid protocols and the degree of neurologic impairment.[20] Subsequent systematic reviews on the issue have noted marginal benefits in favor of early surgery, noting that the strength of the evidence remains relatively poor.[21,22,23] At this time, most centers continue to favor early (< 24 hours from injury) surgery for decompression and stabilization of acute spinal cord injuries, especially for incomplete injuries, in order to maximize their potential for neurologic recovery as well as to support early mobilization and rehabilitation and reduce complications associated with prolonged bedrest.

9.2 Traumatic Brain Injury

9.2.1 Introduction

Traumatic brain injury (TBI) is an unfortunately common event in the developed world, and often cited as one of the leading causes for mortality and long-term disability in young patients. Sources have quoted 2.5 million cases of TBI per year and 50,000 to 100,000 deaths annually in the United States alone, with associated costs approaching $100 billion. The leading cause of these injuries includes falls, motor vehicle accidents, and assault.[24,25,26] Not only are these injuries common, but the pathophysiology is extremely complex. With the emergence of neurocritical care as a distinct medical subspecialty over the past several decades, the progress in treating this challenging patient population has been slow but steady. An understanding of the mechanisms of injury and appropriate medical care are essential to maximize outcomes in this difficult patient population.[27] Classification of TBI is commonly based on the Glasgow Coma Scale (GCS) score, shown in ▶ Table 9.2. This classification is useful because outcomes in terms of morbidity and mortality correlate with this classification, and it provides a simple framework that allows quick communication between care providers across multiple disciplines and specialties. With that in mind, it should be understood that the GCS is a very simple classification scheme, and that injuries to the central nervous system can be quite different despite an identical GCS score. Thus, further understanding the mechanisms and pathophysiology behind TBI is critical.[27] Key to this is the difference between primary and secondary injury.

Table 9.2 Glasgow Coma Scale

Category	Behavior	Score
Eye opening	Spontaneously	4
	To command	3
	To painful stimulus	2
	None	1
Verbal	Oriented	5
	Confused speech	4
	Inappropriate speech	3
	Incomprehensible	2
	None	1
Motor	Follows commands	6
	Localizes pain	5
	Withdraws to pain	4
	Decorticate/flexor posturing	3
	Decerebrate/extensor posturing	2
	None	1

Mild TBI: 13–15, Moderate TBI: 9–12, Severe TBI: 3–8

Abbreviation: TBI, traumatic brain injury.

- **Primary injury:** Direct tissue injury related to the force of impact. The injury can be blunt or penetrating, with resulting injuries either focal (e.g., subdural hematoma or parenchymal contusion) or diffuse (e.g., diffuse axonal injury) and result in largely irreparable tissue damage.
- **Secondary injury:** Progressive injury to surrounding brain parenchyma as a result of functional and metabolic derangements in the traumatized brain. This represents tissue that can potentially be salvaged by appropriate neuro-critical care protocols. Examples include:[27,28,29]
  - Loss of cerebrovascular autoregulation
  - Abnormal neuronal circuitry with imbalance in excitatory/inhibitor throughput
  - Metabolic derangements
- Historically, the two most important parameters associated with expanding secondary injury have been hypotension and hypoxia.[30,31] Commonly quoted

thresholds to maintain are systolic blood pressure > 90, and Pa O2 > 60 mm Hg. Treatment aimed at avoiding falling below these values should be aggressive in all phases of care, including pre-hospital, as even transient episodes below these thresholds have been associated with worse functional outcome and higher mortality.

- Arrival at an appropriately equipped trauma center begins the intense hospital phase of TBI care. ATLS protocols should be strictly adhered to. Systemic injuries should be evaluated and the patient stabilized efficiently, with particular attention paid to blood pressure and oxygenation. Of note, aggressive hyperventilation should not be pursued prophylactically, as this may lead to severe vasoconstriction and worsening ischemic damage to at-risk penumbra.[24] Home medications and lab values should be reviewed, particularly for anticoagulant and antiplatelet medication. Once stable, a noncontrast computed tomography (CT) scan of the head should be performed and reviewed immediately for the presence of hematomas that warrant surgical evaluation. Guidelines have been published to help streamline decision-making. While each case is unique, in general acute subdural hematomas associated with clot thickness > 10 mm, midline shift > 5 mm, and/or abnormal pupillary function should be evacuated. An epidural hematoma with clot volume > 30 mm^3, midline shift > 5 mm, and/or abnormal pupillary function should be strongly considered for evacuation regardless of GCS. Parenchymal hematomas > 50 mm^3 should always be considered for decompression, and the threshold for surgery is lower for lesions in the temporal lobe or associated with significant midline shift of basal cistern effacement. Posterior fossa hemorrhages should prompt a very low threshold for suboccipital craniectomy for clot size > 3 cm, distortion of the fourth ventricle, obstructive hydrocephalus, and basal cistern or brainstem mass effect.
- In surgical patients, the threshold for leaving the bone flap off (i.e., craniectomy) should be low, especially for acute subdural hematomas, which are often associated with more severe parenchymal injury and swelling compared to an epidural hematoma.[24,26,32] This is being further evaluated by the RESCUE-ASDH trial, results of which are not yet published.[33] Additionally, in the setting of intracranial hemorrhage, antiplatelet and anticoagulant agents should be reversed. This may require consultation with a hematologist to discuss reversal options for some newer anticoagulant agents.
- Upon completion of an ATLS evaluation and with no emergent operative interventions planned, the patient should be quickly transferred to a neuro- or surgical intensive care unit (ICU). Invasive monitoring, usually with arterial and central venous lines, is often indicated. Aggressive avoidance of hypotension and hypoxia is the rule. With that in mind, all administered fluids should be isotonic or hypertonic, as hypotonic fluids may exacerbate cerebral edema due to blood–brain barrier disruption in the setting of TBI. Further, blood transfusion thresholds higher than 7 g/dL showed no benefit

at 6 months in a randomized trial.[34] Historically, an intracranial pressure (ICP) monitor is placed in those with GCS < 9 and an abnormal head CT. However, due to low quality evidence, the most recent guidelines make no statement on selecting patients for ICP monitoring, or on open versus continuous cerebrospinal fluid (CSF) drainage, and they stress that the clinical judgment of treating physicians should select which patients are at risk for elevated ICP.[25,35] Although the BEST TRIP study suggested severe TBI patients could be successfully managed without ICP monitor placement, the accepted practice in many severe TBI patients is to directly assess ICP.[31] Options for this include the following:

- Epidural and subdural monitors
- Direct parenchymal monitors
- Intraventricular monitor (aka external ventricular drain or EVD)
- EVD placement is often considered the gold standard due to the ability to both monitor ICP and therapeutically drain CSF as needed; however, all of the above options provide acceptable ICP measurements.[26] Additionally, ICP monitors allow for calculation of cerebral perfusion pressure (CPP), by the formula:

$$CPP = \text{Mean arterial pressure (MAP)} - ICP$$

CPP should be maintained between 50 and 70 mm Hg to ensure adequate metabolic supply to the brain. Ancillary invasive monitoring techniques, such as jugular bulb oximetry, direct brain tissue oxygen monitors, and microdialysis catheters, also exist, although discussion of these is beyond the scope of this chapter.[26,36,37,38 39]

9.2.2 Management of Elevated ICP

Prolonged elevated ICP is associated with worse outcomes.[25,40,41] Thus, timely management is critical. Any acute change in ICP should prompt an urgent head CT to evaluate for surgical lesions and the degree of parenchymal edema. If an external ventricular drain is placed, CSF should be drained to bring ICP < 20 if possible. Medical management of elevated intracranial pressures should proceed in stepwise fashion, and include:

- Patient positioning
  - Head of bed elevated by > 30 degrees
  - Head midline position
  - Ensure hard cervical collars are not too tight and avoid neck kinking to optimize venous outflow
- Adequate pain control
- Adequate sedation to decrease metabolic demand of brain parenchyma with optimization of blood pressure for cerebral blood flow

- Use of hyperosmolar therapy can be used to reduce intracranial pressure in severe TBI patients[42,43]
- Assess serial bladder pressures when appropriate for early identification of abdominal compartment syndrome[24]

Further details on the medical management of elevated ICP can be found in Chapter 6. For the surgical management in severe TBI, there have been two prospective, randomized clinical trials evaluating the role of decompressive craniectomy.[44,45] The consensus is that while ICP is likely reduced with craniectomy, this comes at a high risk of poor long-term functional recovery, and frank discussions with family members is required to make sure that expectations are reasonable prior to pursuing this treatment modality. Given the lack of clarity in the data, the most recent Brain Trauma Foundation Guidelines only recommend that if craniectomy is pursued, a large decompressive hemicraniectomy should be pursued compared to a smaller flap, with the anterior-posterior dimension often quoted as 12 to 15 cm.[35] Another consideration in the treatment of ICP is hypothermia, either on a prophylactic basis for neuroprotection after severe TBI or as a therapy for refractory ICP elevations. Two recent reviews on the topic suggested reduced mortality and poor neurologic outcome in patients with severe TBI treated with hypothermia, but there was significant heterogeneity in a variety of therapeutic parameters and much of the data was of relatively low quality leaving the authors to suggest its use only in carefully constructed research settings.[46,47]

9.2.3 Other Post-TBI Considerations

A variety of other miscellaneous considerations in the post-TBI patient often arise. Skull fractures are not uncommon, and may be classified as open or closed, linear or comminuted, and depressed or nondepressed. Conservative care is generally the rule, with the exception being surgical washout and elevation of open fractures depressed > 5 mm beyond the adjacent inner table or greater than the thickness of the calvarium.[26,48] The primary goal of surgery is to reduce the likelihood of infection and as such a course of broad-spectrum antibiotics is recommended, and a secondary goal is improved cosmesis.[26,48,49] Post-TBI hydrocephalus is an additional concern, with incidence reports varying widely. It should be considered in any post-TBI patient with neurologic decline or less-than-anticipated recovery, especially in the setting of ventriculomegaly.[26,50,51,52] CSF diversion procedures may offer benefit for such patients. Post-TBI CSF leaks are also worth mentioning, which are quoted to complicate up to 2% of TBI cases.[26,53] Those at particularly high risk are those harboring fractures of the frontal or ethmoidal sinuses as well as the temporal bone. Infections including meningitis/encephalitis are the primary concern, but thankfully most leaks resolve spontaneously. Persistent leaks may require a period of lumbar drainage to allow the torn dura to scar, or direct surgical repair. The role of prophylactic antibiotics in this setting is unclear, and no clear guidelines have been published.[26,53,54]

9.3 Paroxysmal Sympathetic Hyperactivity (PSH)

Many patients with TBI display signs of autonomic instability during their recovery period, which is quoted to be as high as 33% incidence in severe TBI.[55,56] This can last up to months after the injury, and is associated with worse outcomes. There are many names used to describe the syndrome; some of the more common ones are sympathetic storming and dysautonomia; however, in 2014 a consensus agreed upon the name Paroxysmal Sympathetic Hyperactivity, along with the definition and diagnostic criteria.[57]

The clinical syndrome consists of the following features:
- Tachycardia
- Tachypnea
- Diaphoresis
- Hyperthermia
- Hypertension
- Dystonic posturing

Given the features found with the clinical syndrome it is a diagnosis of exclusion.[58] ▶ Table 9.3 lists features shared with other conditions.

Various theories regarding pathophysiology have been postulated, with recent studies supporting the "excitatory:inhibitory ratio model" in which relative disconnection of cortical inhibitory circuits leads to overexcitation of more caudal excitatory pathways, which in turn drives recovery of inhibitory centers.[55] This leads to the classic manifestation of symptoms with often minimally or even non-nociceptive external stimuli such as tracheal suctioning or even simple patient movement by nursing staff. Symptoms are generally noted at the time sedation is lifted. Treatment of dysautonomia is geared toward avoiding triggers, and limiting both sympathetic tone and its effects on end organs. The overall evidence base is of low quality, with no randomized controlled trials. Typical regimens to control dysautonomia focus on preventing episodes for starting via opioids, often in the form of either as required or continuous infusions or morphine or fentanyl, propofol, and benzodiazepines. Beta-blockers such as propranolol, labetalol, and metoprolol as well as alpha-2 agonists such as clonidine are often used to treat the clinical manifestations of the storming episode. Other agents, such as baclofen and gabapentin, have also been used for treatment of spasticity, allodynia, and dystonia. Such treatment regimens are important to institute as early as possible because extended

Table 9.3 Other medical conditions that share features with PSH. (Adapted from Blackman et al.[58])

Medical condition	Mental status	Temperature	HR	RR	BP	Pupil size	Sweating	Agitation	Posturing	CPK
Paroxysmal sympathetic hyperactivity	↓	↑	↑	↑	↑	↑	+	+	↑	NA
Malignant hyperthermia	↓	↑	↑	↑	±↑	Normal	NA	+	++ (rigid)	↑
NMS	↓	↑	↑	↑	↑/↓	Normal	+	+	++ (rigid)	↑
Increased ICP	↓	Normal	↓	↓	↑	±↑	NA	-	±	NA
Central fever	±↓	↑	↑	↑	NA	NA	NA	NA	NA	NA
Infection	±↓	↑	↑	↑	↑/↓	Normal	±	NA	NA	NA
Narcotic withdrawal	±↓	NA	↑	↑	NA	↑	+	NA	NA	NA
Autonomic dysreflexia*	NA	↑	↑	↑	↑	NA	+	NA	NA	NA

*Seen in spinal cord injury

Abbreviations: BP, blood pressure; CPK, Creatine phosphokinase; ICP, intracranial pressure; HR, heart rate; NMS, neuroleptic malignant syndrome; PSH, paroxysmal sympathetic hyperactivity; RR, respiratory rate; TBI, traumatic brain injury.

courses of dysautonomia have been associated with worse outcomes and even mortality in patients with TBI.[55,56]

References

[1] Wyndaele M, Wyndaele JJ. Incidence, prevalence and epidemiology of spinal cord injury: what learns a worldwide literature survey? Spinal Cord. 2006; 44(9):523–529

[2] Rahimi-Movaghar V. Efficacy of surgical decompression in the setting of complete thoracic spinal cord injury. J Spinal Cord Med. 2005; 28(5):415–420

[3] DeVivo MJ. Causes and costs of spinal cord injury in the United States. Spinal Cord. 1997; 35 (12):809–813

[4] Oyinbo CA. Secondary injury mechanisms in traumatic spinal cord injury: a nugget of this multiply cascade. Acta Neurobiol Exp (Warsz). 2011; 71(2):281–299

[5] Tanhoffer RA, Yamazaki RK, Nunes EA, et al. Glutamine concentration and immune response of spinal cord-injured rats. J Spinal Cord Med. 2007; 30(2):140–146

[6] Liverman TC, Joy EJ, Johnson TR. Spinal Cord Injury: Progress, Promise, and Priorities. Washington D.C.: National Academy of Sciences; 2005

[7] Velmahos GC, Toutouzas K, Chan L, et al. Intubation after cervical spinal cord injury: to be done selectively or routinely? Am Surg. 2003; 69(10):891–894

[8] Saadeh YS, Smith BW, Joseph JR, et al. The impact of blood pressure management after spinal cord injury: a systematic review of the literature. Neurosurg Focus. 2017; 43(5):E20

[9] Bracken MB, Shepard MJ, Hellenbrand KG, et al. Methylprednisolone and neurological function 1 year after spinal cord injury. Results of the National Acute Spinal Cord Injury Study. J Neurosurg. 1985; 63(5):704–713

[10] Bracken MB, Shepard MJ, Collins WF, Jr, et al. Methylprednisolone or naloxone treatment after acute spinal cord injury: 1-year follow-up data. Results of the Second National Acute Spinal Cord Injury Study. J Neurosurg. 1992; 76(1):23–31

[11] Bracken MB, Shepard MJ, Holford TR, et al. Administration of methylprednisolone for 24 or 48 hours or tirilazad mesylate for 48 hours in the treatment of acute spinal cord injury. Results of the Third National Acute Spinal Cord Injury Randomized Controlled Trial. JAMA. 1997; 277 (20):1597–1604

[12] Hamamoto Y, Ogata T, Morino T, Hino M, Yamamoto H. Real-time direct measurement of spinal cord blood flow at the site of compression: relationship between blood flow recovery and motor deficiency in spinal cord injury. National Acute Spinal Cord Injury Study. Spine. 2007; 32 (18):1955–1962

[13] Xu K, Chen QX, Li FC, Chen WS, Lin M, Wu QH. Spinal cord decompression reduces rat neural cell apoptosis secondary to spinal cord injury. J Zhejiang Univ Sci B. 2009; 10(3):180–187

[14] Pollard ME, Apple DF. Factors associated with improved neurologic outcomes in patients with incomplete tetraplegia. Spine. 2003; 28(1):33–39

[15] McKinley W, Meade MA, Kirshblum S, Barnard B. Outcomes of early surgical management versus late or no surgical intervention after acute spinal cord injury. Arch Phys Med Rehabil. 2004; 85 (11):1818–1825

[16] Sapkas GS, Papadakis SA. Neurological outcome following early versus delayed lower cervical spine surgery. J Orthop Surg (Hong Kong). 2007; 15(2):183–186

[17] Pointillart V, Petitjean ME, Wiart L, et al. Pharmacological therapy of spinal cord injury during the acute phase. Spinal Cord. 2000; 38(2):71–76

[18] La Rosa G, Conti A, Cardali S, Cacciola F, Tomasello F. Does early decompression improve neurological outcome of spinal cord injured patients? Appraisal of the literature using a meta-analytical approach. Spinal Cord. 2004; 42(9):503–512

[19] Fehlings MG, Perrin RG. The timing of surgical intervention in the treatment of spinal cord injury: a systematic review of recent clinical evidence. Spine. 2006; 31(11) Suppl:S28–S35, discussion S36

[20] Fehlings MG, Vaccaro A, Wilson JR, et al. Early versus delayed decompression for traumatic cervical spinal cord injury: results of the Surgical Timing in Acute Spinal Cord Injury Study (STASCIS). PLoS One. 2012; 7(2):e32037

[21] Fehlings MG, Tetreault LA, Wilson JR, et al. A clinical practice guideline for the management of patients with acute spinal cord injury and central cord syndrome: recommendations on the timing (≤24 hours versus >24 hours) of decompressive surgery. Global Spine J. 2017; 7(3) Suppl:195S–202S

[22] Wilson JR, Tetreault LA, Kwon BK, et al. Timing of decompression in patients with acute spinal cord injury: a systematic review. Global Spine J. 2017; 7(3) Suppl:95S–115S

[23] Piazza M, Schuster J. Timing of surgery after spinal cord injury. Neurosurg Clin N Am. 2017; 28 (1):31–39

[24] Vella MA, Crandall ML, Patel MB. Acute management of traumatic brain injury. Surg Clin North Am. 2017; 97(5):1015–1030

[25] Abou El Fadl MH, O'Phelan KH. Management of traumatic brain injury: an update. Neurol Clin. 2017; 35(4):641–653

[26] Adams H, Kolias AG, Hutchinson PJ. The role of surgical intervention in traumatic brain injury. Neurosurg Clin N Am. 2016; 27(4):519–528

[27] McGinn MJ, Povlishock JT. Pathophysiology of traumatic brain injury. Neurosurg Clin N Am. 2016; 27(4):397–407

[28] Cohen AS, Pfister BJ, Schwarzbach E, Grady MS, Goforth PB, Satin LS. Injury-induced alterations in CNS electrophysiology. Prog Brain Res. 2007; 161:143–169

[29] Sharp DJ, Scott G, Leech R. Network dysfunction after traumatic brain injury. Nat Rev Neurol. 2014; 10(3):156–166

[30] Miller JD, Sweet RC, Narayan R, Becker DP. Early insults to the injured brain. JAMA. 1978; 240 (5):439–442

[31] Chesnut RM, Marshall LF, Klauber MR, et al. The role of secondary brain injury in determining outcome from severe head injury. J Trauma. 1993; 34(2):216–222

[32] Bullock MR, Chesnut R, Ghajar J, et al. Surgical Management of Traumatic Brain Injury Author Group. Surgical management of acute epidural hematomas. Neurosurgery. 2006; 58(3) Suppl:S7–S15, discussion Si–iv

[33] Kolias AG, Adams H, Timofeev I, et al. Decompressive craniectomy following traumatic brain injury: developing the evidence base. Br J Neurosurg. 2016; 30(2):246–250

[34] Robertson CS, Hannay HJ, Yamal JM, et al. Epo Severe TBI Trial Investigators. Effect of erythropoietin and transfusion threshold on neurological recovery after traumatic brain injury: a randomized clinical trial. JAMA. 2014; 312(1):36–47

[35] Carney N, Totten AM, O'Reilly C, et al. Management of Severe Traumatic Brain Injury. 4th ed. Brain Trauma Foundation, Coma Guidelines. 2016. Available at: https://braintrauma.org/uploads/03/12/guidelines_for_management_of_severe_TBI_4th_edition.pdf

[36] Lazaridis C, Robertson CS. The role of multimodal invasive monitoring in acute traumatic brain injury. Neurosurg Clin N Am. 2016; 27(4):509–517

[37] Bouzat P, Marques-Vidal P, Zerlauth JB, et al. Accuracy of brain multimodal monitoring to detect cerebral hypoperfusion after traumatic brain injury. Crit Care Med. 2015; 43(2):445–452

[38] Citerio G, Oddo M, Taccone FS. Recommendations for the use of multimodal monitoring in the neurointensive care unit. Curr Opin Crit Care. 2015; 21(2):113–119

[39] Le Roux P, Menon DK, Citerio G, et al. Neurocritical Care Society, European Society of Intensive Care Medicine. Consensus summary statement of the International Multidisciplinary Consensus Conference on Multimodality Monitoring in Neurocritical Care: a statement for healthcare professionals from the Neurocritical Care Society and the European Society of Intensive Care Medicine. Intensive Care Med. 2014; 40(9):1189–1209

[40] Alali AS, Fowler RA, Mainprize TG, et al. Intracranial pressure monitoring in severe traumatic brain injury: results from the American College of Surgeons Trauma Quality Improvement Program. J Neurotrauma. 2013; 30(20):1737–1746

[41] Badri S, Chen J, Barber J, et al. Mortality and long-term functional outcome associated with intracranial pressure after traumatic brain injury. Intensive Care Med. 2012; 38(11):1800–1809

[42] Mangat HS, Chiu YL, Gerber LM, Alimi M, Ghajar J, Härtl R. Hypertonic saline reduces cumulative and daily intracranial pressure burdens after severe traumatic brain injury. J Neurosurg. 2015; 122(1):202–210

[43] Cottenceau V, Masson F, Mahamid E, et al. Comparison of effects of equiosmolar doses of mannitol and hypertonic saline on cerebral blood flow and metabolism in traumatic brain injury. J Neurotrauma. 2011; 28(10):2003–2012

[44] Cooper DJ, Rosenfeld JV, Murray L, et al. DECRA Trial Investigators, Australian and New Zealand Intensive Care Society Clinical Trials Group. Decompressive craniectomy in diffuse traumatic brain injury. N Engl J Med. 2011; 364(16):1493–1502

[45] Hutchinson PJ, Kolias AG, Timofeev IS, et al. RESCUEicp Trial Collaborators. Trial of decompressive craniectomy for traumatic intracranial hypertension. N Engl J Med. 2016; 375(12):1119–1130

[46] McIntyre LA, Fergusson DA, Hébert PC, Moher D, Hutchison JS. Prolonged therapeutic hypothermia after traumatic brain injury in adults: a systematic review. JAMA. 2003; 289(22):2992–2999

[47] Sydenham E, Roberts I, Alderson P. Hypothermia for traumatic head injury. Cochrane Database Syst Rev. 2009(2):CD001048

[48] Bullock MR, Chesnut R, Ghajar J, et al. Surgical Management of Traumatic Brain Injury Author Group. Surgical management of depressed cranial fractures. Neurosurgery. 2006; 58(3) Suppl: S56–S60, discussion Si-iv

[49] Ali B, Ghosh A. Antibiotics in compound depressed skull fractures. Emerg Med J. 2002; 19 (6):552–553

[50] Guyot LL, Michael DB. Post-traumatic hydrocephalus. Neurol Res. 2000; 22(1):25–28

[51] Paoletti P, Pezzotta S, Spanu G. Diagnosis and treatment of post-traumatic hydrocephalus. J Neurosurg Sci. 1983; 27(3):171–175

[52] Tribl G, Oder W. Outcome after shunt implantation in severe head injury with post-traumatic hydrocephalus. Brain Inj. 2000; 14(4):345–354

[53] Friedman JA, Ebersold MJ, Quast LM. Post-traumatic cerebrospinal fluid leakage. World J Surg. 2001; 25(8):1062–1066

[54] Rimmer J, Belk C, Lund VJ, Swift A, White P. Immunisations and antibiotics in patients with anterior skull base cerebrospinal fluid leaks. J Laryngol Otol. 2014; 128(7):626–629

[55] Meyfroidt G, Baguley IJ, Menon DK. Paroxysmal sympathetic hyperactivity: the storm after acute brain injury. Lancet Neurol. 2017; 16(9):721–729

[56] Deepika A, Mathew MJ, Kumar SA, Devi BI, Shukla D. Paroxysmal sympathetic hyperactivity in pediatric traumatic brain injury: a case series of four patients. Auton Neurosci. 2015; 193:149–151

[57] Baguley IJ, Perkes IE, Fernandez-Ortega JF, Rabinstein AA, Dolce G, Hendricks HT, Consensus Working Group. Paroxysmal sympathetic hyperactivity after acquired brain injury: consensus on conceptual definition, nomenclature, and diagnostic criteria. J Neurotrauma. 2014; 31(17):1515–1520

[58] Blackman JA, Patrick PD, Buck ML, Rust RS, Jr. Paroxysmal autonomic instability with dystonia after brain injury. Arch Neurol. 2004; 61(3):321–328

10 Neuromuscular and Other Neurologic Emergencies

Danielle Wilhour and Alison L. Walsh

Abstract

Prompt recognition, diagnosis, and treatment of neuromuscular conditions in the critical care setting are crucial as specific therapies and supportive care can prevent mortality and mitigate morbidity. Neuromuscular disorders are diseases that affect the peripheral nervous system from the anterior horn cells, peripheral nerves, and neuromuscular junction to the muscles. Many of these patients present with rapidly advancing or severe weakness which can lead to respiratory failure. Possessing the acumen to quickly and accurately identify neuromuscular emergencies is therefore essential. This chapter will discuss high-yield information on identification and management of various neuromuscular disorders.

Keywords: Guillain-Barré syndrome, acute inflammatory demyelinating polyradiculoneuropathy, myasthenia gravis, botulism, organophosphate toxicity, neuromuscular junction, neuroleptic malignant syndrome, serotonin syndrome

10.1 Guillain-Barré Syndrome (GBS)/Acute Inflammatory Demyelinating Polyradiculoneuropathy (AIDP)

10.1.1 Definition

- Acute immune-mediated polyradiculoneuropathy characterized by flaccid ascending weakness with areflexia, and, when severe, neuromuscular respiratory failure.[1,2,3,4]
- Monophasic course with symptom onset to nadir of weakness < 4 weeks.[3]
- Most often caused by demyelination and occasionally caused by axonal type.[4]

10.1.2 Epidemiology

- Worldwide incidence of 1 to 2 per 100,000 per year.[3]
- Median age is 53 years old with a ratio of men to women of 1.78.[2,3]
- Mortality ranges between 3 and 13% with higher mortality in patients who require mechanical ventilation.[7]

• Respiratory failure, pneumonia, autonomic dysautonomia, and cardiac arrest are the most common causes of death in these patients.[7]

10.1.3 Differential Diagnosis

Bilateral strokes, posterior fossa structural lesion, transverse myelitis, compressive myelopathy, anterior spinal artery syndrome, poliomyelitis, acute infectious myelitis (West Nile virus, coxsackie, echovirus), Lyme disease, botulism, myasthenia gravis (MG), neuromuscular blocking agents, acute viral myositis, acute inflammatory or metabolic myopathies, periodic paralysis, and psychogenic symptoms

10.1.4 Common Clinical Presentation

• Two-thirds of cases are preceded by respiratory infection or gastroenteritis days to weeks before (most commonly *Campylobacter jejuni*, cytomegalovirus [CMV], Epstein-Barr virus [EBV], varicella-zoster virus [VZV], and *Mycoplasma pneumoniae*).[3,4]
• **Initial symptoms:** Numbness, paresthesias, weakness, dysautonomia, and pain in limbs.[1,3]
• **Cardinal features:** Progressive, bilateral, and symmetric ascending weakness of the limbs with hypo/areflexia which progresses over days to weeks.[3,4]
• Dysautonomia occurs in 70% of patients.[4] Dysautonomia is characterized by wide fluctuations in blood pressure and respiratory rate, tachyarrhythmias, bradyarrhythmias, urine retention, diaphoresis, and gastric slowing causing ileus.

10.1.5 Diagnosis

See ▶ Table 10.1.

10.1.6 GBS Variants

• **GBS/AIDP:** Areflexia, mild sensory changes, distal paresthesias, loss of deep tendon reflexes (DTR), ascending paralysis, respiratory failure, and autonomic dysautonomia
• **Acute motor axonal neuropathy (AMAN):** Acute, flaccid ascending paralysis associated with GM1 and GD1a ganglioside antibodies
• **Acute motor and sensory axonal neuropathy (AMSAN):** Loss of DTR, distal weakness, and sensory symptoms (GM1 and GD1a antibodies)
• **Miller-Fisher syndrome (MFS):** Ophthalmoplegia, ataxia, areflexia (GQ1b and GT1a antibodies)

Table 10.1 Diagnostic criteria for GBS/AIDP[2]

Required features	Supportive features	Unlikely GBS
• Progressive weakness of > 1 limb, the trunk, bulbar and facial muscles, or ophthalmoplegia • Hyporeflexia or areflexia	• Symptom progression over days to 4 weeks • Relative symmetry • Mild sensory symptoms or signs • Cranial nerve involvement • Recovery 2–4 weeks after plateau • Autonomic dysfunction • No fever at the onset • CSF has ↑ protein with WBC < 10/mm^3 • GBS electrodiagnostic abnormalities	• Sensory level • > 50 WBC in CSF • Asymmetry of weakness • Severe and persistent bowel and bladder dysfunction

Abbreviations: AIDP, acute inflammatory demyelinating polyradiculoneuropathy; CSF, cerebrospinal fluid; GBS, Guillain-Barré syndrome; WBC, white blood cell.

- **Bickerstaff encephalitis:** Encephalopathy, ophthalmoplegia, and ataxia with areflexia to hyperreflexia (GQ1b and GT1a antibodies)

10.1.7 Ancillary Testing

- Autoimmune and infectious workup (can be presenting sign of human immunodeficiency virus [HIV])
- Serum ganglioside antibodies (GM1, GD1a, GQ1b, and GT1a) when considering a GBS variant
- Lumbar puncture can rule out infectious diseases or malignancy.[3,4]
  - Albuminocytologic dissociation (elevated cerebrospinal fluid [CSF] protein with normal CSF white blood cell [WBC]) seen in 50% of patients' CSF in the first week and proportion increases with time.[3,4]
- Nerve-conduction studies (NCS) help confirm the presence, pattern, and severity of neuropathy.
  - Prolonged F-wave latencies, prolonged distal motor latencies, temporal dispersion, conduction block, and slow motor nerve conduction velocities (typically in demyelinating range).[1]
  - Note that NCS are usually not performed immediately and can be delayed by up to 2 weeks.

10.1.8 Complications of GBS

- **Cardiac:** Labile blood pressure (70%), hypertension, hypotension, arrhythmias, tachycardia, bradycardia (4%), atrioventricular (AV) blocks, and asystole

- **Pulmonary:** Respiratory failure, pneumonia, aspiration, atelectasis, and mucus plugging
  - Ventilator support is required by 20 to 30% of patients.[5]
- **Gastrointestinal:** Gastroparesis and adynamic ileus
- **Genitourinary:** Bladder dysfunction, retention, and incontinence
- **Endocrine:** Syndrome of inappropriate antidiuretic hormone secretion (SIADH) (monitor sodium and fluid status)
- **Hematologic:** Venous thromboembolism and pulmonary embolism
- **Neuropathic pain (40–50%):** Use gabapentin or carbamazepine in acute phase.

10.1.9 Management

- Monitor respiratory function closely. Intubation may be required if vital capacity (VC) is < 20 mL/kg and maximum negative inspiratory force (NIF) is < 30 cm H_2O (or a reduction of 50% from baseline VC or NIF).[1]
- Treatment with intravenous immunoglobulin (IVIG) or plasma exchange hastens recovery from GBS if initiated within 4 weeks of the onset of symptoms. Combining these two treatments is not beneficial.[1,6] See ▶ Table 10.2.
- Corticosteroid treatment is not effective and therefore not recommended.[1,6]

10.1.10 Prognosis

- At 1 year
  - 84% of patients will be able to walk.
  - 5 to 10% of patients have incomplete recovery.

Table 10.2 Medications used in treatment of GBS

	Dosing	Adverse effects	Contraindications
IVIG	2 g/kg over 2–5 days	Headache, chills, dizziness, rash, myalgias, CHF exacerbation, aseptic meningitis, acute renal failure, thrombotic events, and anaphylaxis	Hypersensitivity reactions, selective IgA deficiency, and coagulation disorders
Plasma exchange	Five exchanges (3–5 L of plasma each) every other day for 10 days	Coagulopathy, fever, hypocalcemia, hypotension, cardiac arrhythmias, myocardial infarction, hemolysis, and myalgias Catheter complications such as infection pneumothorax and local hematoma	Patients taking ACE inhibitors, hemodynamic instability

Abbreviations: ACE, angiotensin-converting enzyme; CHF, congestive heart failure; GBS, Guillain-Barré syndrome; IVIG; intravenous immunoglobulin.

○ 4 to 5% of patients with GBS die despite intensive care.[1,7]
• Relapses can occur in approximately 10% of patients.

10.2 Myasthenia Gravis

10.2.1 Definition

• Autoimmune disorder affecting postsynaptic neuromuscular transmission at the neuromuscular junction (NMJ), producing characteristic variable and fatigable weakness in skeletal muscles.[8,9,10,11]
• Myasthenic crisis is a complication of MG with worsening muscle weakness, resulting in respiratory failure that often requires intubation and mechanical ventilation.[11,12,13]

10.2.2 Epidemiology

• Prevalence is about 20 per 100,000.[10]
• **Bimodal distribution with age of onset:** Early peak in the 2nd and 3rd decades (female predominance) and late peak in the 6th to 8th decades (male predominance).[14]
• The median time from onset of MG to first myasthenic crisis is 8 to 12 months. However, myasthenic crisis may be the initial presentation of MG in 20% of patients.[11]

10.2.3 Differential Diagnosis

Lambert-Eaton myasthenic syndrome, GBS, organophosphate toxicity, botulism, congenital myasthenia syndromes, thyroid ophthalmopathy, mitochondrial disorders, myotonic dystrophy, skull-based tumors, and motor neuron disease.

10.2.4 Clinical Presentation of Generalized Myasthenia Gravis

• Presents with several days/weeks of worsening ptosis, diplopia, bulbar symptoms, extremity weakness, and/or shortness of breath.[9]
• **Physical examination findings:** Ptosis, inability to sustain upgaze, normal pupillary reflexes, bulbar weakness, flaccid dysarthria, neck flexor/extensor weakness, proximal > distal limb weakness, tachypnea, intact sensation, and decreased reflexes.[10]

10.2.5 Diagnosis

- Diagnosis is based on history and physical examination and supported by electrophysiologic and serologic studies.
- Electrophysiologic studies
  - **Repetitive nerve stimulation:** Low rates of repetitive stimulation (2–5 Hz) deplete acetylcholine and cause > 10% decrement in compound muscle action potential (CMAP) amplitude (80% sensitive for generalized MG).[9,10]
  - **Single fiber electromyography (EMG):** Increased jitter or variation in contraction time between pairs of muscle fibers (95% sensitive, nonspecific).[9,10]
- Serologic antibody tests are positive in > 90% of MG patients.
  - Acetylcholine receptor (AChR) antibodies
    - Present in 85% of patients with generalized MG[9,10]
    - Highly specific for MG (> 99%)
    - Correlate with thymic hyperplasia and thymoma
  - **Muscle-specific kinase (MuSK) antibodies:** Found in 40% of patients with generalized MG who are negative for AChR antibodies.[9]
  - **Low-density lipoprotein receptor-related protein 4 (LRP4) antibodies:** Found in 18% of patients with generalized MG who are negative for AChR and MuSK.[9]
- **Ancillary tests:** CT of chest with contrast to evaluate for thymoma

Myasthenic Crisis

- **Precipitating factors:** Infection (38%), medication changes (particularly initiation and withdrawal of corticosteroids), aspiration pneumonitis, upper airway obstruction, pregnancy, surgery, and disease progression.[11,12]
- For one-third of the patients, no precipitating factor can be found.

Cholinergic Crisis

Increase in anticholinergic medications that can lead to weakness associated with signs of increased cholinergic activity (miosis, salivation, lacrimation, bradycardia, diarrhea).[11]

10.2.6 Management of Myasthenic Crisis

- **Supportive care:** Aspiration precautions, temporary nil per os (NPO) with nasogastric tube feedings, frequent monitoring with NIF and VC, and ventilatory support. ABGs are insensitive.
- Treatment typically consists of high-dose steroids with either IVIG or plasma exchange. See ▶ Table 10.3.

Table 10.3 Treatment of myasthenia crises

	Dosing	Adverse effects	Contraindications
IVIG	2 g/kg over 2–5 days	Headache, chills, dizziness, CHF exacerbation, aseptic meningitis, acute renal failure, thrombotic events, and anaphylaxis	Hypersensitivity reactions, selective IgA deficiency, and coagulation disorders
Plasma exchange	Five exchanges (3–5 L of plasma each) every other day	Bleeding, fever, hypocalcemia, hypotension, cardiac arrhythmias, myocardial infarction, hemolysis, and myalgias. Catheter complications such as infection and thrombosis	Patients taking ACE inhibitors, hemodynamic instability
Pyridostigmine	Initial dose 15–30 mg four times per day; increase to goal 30–90 mg four times per day	Abdominal cramping, and diarrhea; others are increased salivation, bronchial secretions, nausea, diaphoresis, bradycardia, and myalgias	GI or GU obstruction; caution with bronchial asthma
Steroids	60–100 mg per day or 1–1.5 mg/kg daily	Hyperglycemia, insomnia, mania, hypertension, dyspepsia, and hypokalemia	Relative contraindications: Infection, poorly controlled diabetes, and severe osteoporosis

Abbreviations: ACE, angiotensin-converting enzyme; CHF, congestive heart failure; GI, gastrointestinal; GU, genitourinary; IVIG; intravenous immunoglobulin.

- ○ Plasma exchange is more efficacious than IVIG but has higher complication rate.[11]
- Thymic tumors are found in 32% of patients with myasthenic crises, which should be treated with thymectomy when myasthenic crisis is resolved.[11]

10.2.7 Prognosis

- Overall, the outcome for patients with myasthenic crisis is good if therapeutic measures are instituted quickly. Extubation failure rate is around 27%. Mortality rate is approximately 5%.[12,13]
- One-third of patients with myasthenic crisis will experience a recurrent episode.

10.3 Botulism

10.3.1 Definition

Rare but potentially life-threatening neuroparalytic syndrome caused by neurotoxin of the bacterium *Clostridium botulinum*.[15,16]

10.3.2 Epidemiology

Approximately 110 cases of botulism are reported each year in USA. Of these cases, around 72% are infant botulism, 25% are foodborne botulism (typically from improperly canned foods), and 3% are wound botulism.[15]

10.3.3 Pathophysiology

- *C. botulinum* is a gram-positive, rod-shaped, spore-forming, anaerobic bacterium.[15]
- Spores of *C. botulism* produce a very potent toxin which blocks neurotransmitter release at peripheral cholinergic nerve terminals. [17]
- Toxin binds irreversibly to receptors on presynaptic membrane of NMJ. It is internalized by endocytosis, and then cleaves SNARE proteins preventing transmitter exocytosis. This blocks the release of acetylcholine from the presynaptic motor nerve terminal resulting in skeletal muscle paralysis and autonomic dysfunction.[18]

10.3.4 Differential Diagnosis

Stroke, GBS, MG, Lambert-Eaton myasthenic syndrome, diphtheric polyneuropathy, poliomyelitis, tick paralysis, hypermagnesemia, and curare poisoning.

10.3.5 Clinical Presentation

- Neuromuscular symptoms begin 2 to 36 hours after exposure. Weakness progresses for several days then plateaus. Fatal respiratory paralysis may occur rapidly.[18,19,20]
- **Classic triad:** Afebrile, symmetrical descending flaccid paralysis, and intact mental status.
- **Physical examination findings:** Fixed dilated pupils with impaired pupillary reflex, ptosis, ophthalmoplegia, facial weakness, dysarthria, dysphagia, dry mouth, urinary retention, postural hypotension, and intact sensation.[15]

Table 10.4 Treatment of botulism

	Dosing	Adverse effects
Trivalent equine serum botulinum antitoxin	Adults: One vial IV Children (1–17 years): 20–100% of vial	Headache, fever, chills, rash, itching, nausea, anaphylaxis (3%), and serum sickness (20%)
Botulism Immune Globulin Intravenous (Human)	Infants (< 12 months): 1 mL/kg	Erythematous rash

Abbreviation: IV, intravenous.

10.3.6 Diagnosis

- Cultures and toxin assay of suspected food, wound, and stool for *C. botulinum*
- Lumbar puncture to rule out other causes; CSF analysis is benign in botulism
- Electrophysiologic testing shows abnormal single fiber EMG (routine motor and sensory studies normal)
  - In at least two muscles, > 20% facilitation of CMAP amplitude during tetanic stimulation; prolonged post-tetanic facilitation > 120 seconds; absence of post-activation exhaustion.[15,18]

10.3.7 Management (▶ Table 10.4)

- When botulism is suspected, contact the State Health Department or CDC immediately.[21]
- For infant botulism, administer human-derived botulism immune globulin (BIG-IV).[22]
- For wound botulism, administer antitoxin if able, as well as penicillin G 3 million units IV every 4 hours or metronidazole 500 mg IV every 8 hours, debride wound, and give tetanus booster if appropriate.
- For foodborne toxin, administer botulinum antitoxin if able.[23]
- Intubate patients with worsening upper airway competency and those with a VC < 30% of predicted.

10.3.8 Prognosis

With prompt attention and supportive care, mortality in botulism ranges from < 5 to 10%.

10.4 Organophosphate Toxicity

10.4.1 Definition

Organophosphates are potent cholinesterase inhibitors capable of causing severe cholinergic toxicity following cutaneous exposure, inhalation, or ingestion.[24,25,26]

10.4.2 Epidemiology

- Acute poisoning from organophosphates causes over 300,000 fatalities annually worldwide, which is more than any other class of drug or chemical.[24,27]
- In the USA, there were more than 8,000 reported exposures to these agents in 2008.[27]

10.4.3 Pathophysiology

Organophosphorus compounds bind to acetylcholinesterase (AchE) and render this enzyme nonfunctional. This inhibition leads to an overabundance of acetylcholine at the NMJ, which activates both nicotinic receptors in the central nervous system (CNS) and peripheral nervous system (PNS) as well as muscarinic receptors in the autonomic nervous system.[24,25]

10.4.4 Differential Diagnosis

Gastroenteritis; asthma; myxedema coma; hypoglycemia; diabetic ketoacidosis; sepsis; meningoencephalitis; GBS; spider, scorpion, or snake bite; consumption of muscarine-containing mushrooms; narcotic overdose; phencyclidine (PCP) overdose; and nicotine overdose.

10.4.5 Clinical Presentation

- Activation of muscarinic receptors: Salivation, lacrimation, urination, diarrhea, gastric emptying, bradycardia, bronchorrhea, and bronchospasm.[24,25]
- Activation of nicotinic receptors:
  - **PNS:** Fasciculations, muscle weakness, and paralysis.
  - **CNS:** Agitation, confusion, central respiratory depression, seizures, and coma.[24]

10.4.6 Diagnosis

- Made on clinical grounds when patient presents with symptoms of cholinergic excess.[24]

Table 10.5 Treatment of organophosphate overdose

	Dosing	Mechanism
Atropine	2–5 mg IV/IM bolus Double dose every 3–5 minutes until bronchial secretions and wheezing stopped	Competes with acetylcholine at muscarinic receptors, preventing cholinergic activation
Pralidoxime (2-PAM)	2 g IV or 600 mg IM May repeat in 30 minutes or give continuous infusion at 8 mg/kg/hour	Reactivates acetylcholinesterase by displacing organophosphate enzyme from receptor site
Diazepam	Diazepam 10 mg IV as needed	Decreases neurocognitive dysfunction Repeat if seizures occur

Abbreviations: IM, intramuscular; IV, intravenous.

- Serum measurement of red blood cell (RBC) acetylcholinesterase to confirm diagnosis.[25]

10.4.7 Management

- Deliver 100% oxygen via facemask; early intubation often required (avoid succinylcholine).[24,28]
- **Decontamination:** Aggressive dermal and ocular irrigation. Bag and discard clothing.[24]
- Administer atropine concurrently with pralidoxime. See ▶ Table 10.5.

10.4.8 Prognosis

Using a cut off for Glasgow coma score (GCS) ≤ 13, patients can be divided into a high-risk group with a 37% case fatality rate and a low-risk group with only 4% mortality.[29]

10.5 Neuroleptic Malignant Syndrome (NMS) and Serotonin Syndrome (SS)

10.5.1 Definition

- NMS is a rare but life-threatening idiosyncratic reaction to antipsychotic drugs characterized by fever, altered mental status, muscle rigidity, and autonomic instability.[30]

- SS is a potentially life-threatening condition associated with increased serotonergic activity in the CNS which causes mental status changes, autonomic instability, hyperreflexia, and clonus.[30]

10.5.2 Epidemiology

- The incidence of NMS has declined recently because of awareness to 0.1 to 0.2%.[30,31,32]
  - Both age and gender distributions correspond with the distribution of the exposure to neuroleptic agents.[32]
- The true incidence of SS is unknown because many cases go unrecognized, although increased incidence parallels the increasing use of serotonergic agents in medicine.[31]
  - Observed in all age groups, including newborns and the elderly.[34]

10.5.3 Pathogenesis

- NMS is due to decreased dopamine activity in CNS either from blockade of D_2 receptors of hypothalamic and nigrostriatal pathways or reduced dopamine signaling resulting from sudden withdrawal of dopaminergic agents.[30,35,36]
- SS is due to excess serotonergic activity causing an increase in the $5HT_{1A}$ and $5HT_{2A}$ receptors due to therapeutic medications, drug interactions, and intentional overdose.[31]

10.5.4 Differential Diagnosis

Malignant hyperthermia, anticholinergic toxicity, drugs of abuse (cocaine, amphetamine, 3,4-methylenedioxymethamphetamine [MDMA], PCP), drug withdrawal of alcohol, benzodiazepines, or baclofen, delirium tremens, thyrotoxicosis, acute renal failure, meningoencephalitis, and heat stroke.[33]

10.5.5 Clinical Presentation

See ▶ Table 10.6.

10.5.6 Diagnosis

Levenson's clinical criteria for diagnosis of NMS:
- A high probability of NMS is suggested if patient has all three major criteria or two major and four minor criteria if supported clinically
  - **Major:** Fever, rigidity, and elevated creatinine phosphokinase concentration

Table 10.6 Presentation of toxidromes

	Serotonin syndrome	Neuroleptic malig-nant syndrome	Anticholinergic toxidrome
Medication history	Pro-serotonergic drug	Dopamine agent	Anticholinergic agent
Time to development	<12 hours	1–3 days	<12 hours
Vital signs	↑ BP, ↑ HR, ↑ RR, ↑ temp (>41.1℃)	↑ BP, ↑ HR, ↑ RR, ↑ temp (>41.1℃)	↑ BP, ↑ HR, ↑ RR, ↑ temp (<38.8℃)
Muscle tone	Rigid	Rigid	Normal
Mucosa/skin	Wet	Wet	Dry
Pupil size	Increased	Normal	Increased
Bowel sounds	Increased	Normal/decreased	Decreased
Reflexes	Increased	Bradyreflexia	Normal
Mental status	Agitated, coma	Stupor, coma	Agitated, delirium

○ **Minor:** Tachycardia, abnormal blood pressure, altered consciousness, dia-phoresis, and leukocytosis[36]

Hunter criteria for serotonin syndrome—serotonergic agent plus one of the following:
• Spontaneous clonus
• Inducible clonus with agitation or diaphoresis
• Ocular clonus with agitation or diaphoresis
• Tremor and hyperreflexia
• Hypertonia and temperature > 38 °C (100 °F) and ocular clonus or inducible clonus[31]

10.5.7 Management (▶ Table 10.7)

• The single most important treatment is to stop the causative agent. However, in cases where the cause is due withdrawal of dopaminergic therapy, it is recommend that the medication be resumed.[36,37] See ▶ Table 10.8.
• For NMS, dantrolene and bromocriptine may be used alone or in combina-tion along with benzodiazepines. Electroconvulsive therapy has been reported to improve some of the symptoms of NMS.[36]
• For serotonin syndrome, cyproheptadine is used along with benzodiazapam.[38]

Table 10.7 Medications for neuroleptic malignant syndrome and serotonin syndrome

	Mechanism	Dose
Dantrolene (NMS)	Skeletal muscle relaxant Inhibits calcium release from the sarcoplasmic reticulum	1 to 2.5 mg/kg IV followed by 1 mg/kg every 6 hours up to a maximum dose of 10 mg/kg/d • Discontinue when symptoms stop
Bromocriptine (NMS)	D_2 receptor agonist	2.5 mg po every 8–12 hours, titrated up to a response or max dose of 40 mg/day. • Continue for 10 days followed by slow taper
Benzodiazepine (NMS/SS)	GABAa agonist	Lorazepam 2–4 mg IV or diazepam 5–10 mg IV
Cyproheptadine (SS)	Serotonin 2a antagonist	Initial dose: 12 mg, then 2 mg every 2 hours if symptoms continue Maintenance: 8 mg every 6 hours

Abbreviations: IV, intravenous; NMS, neuroleptic malignant syndrome; SS, serotonin syndrome.

10.5.8 Complications

- The need for aggressive and supportive care is essential. Complications are common and can be fatal.
- **Cardiac**: Cardiac arrhythmias (torsades de pointes and cardiac arrest), myocardial infarction, and cardiomyopathy
  - Maintain cardiorespiratory stability with antiarrhythmic agents or pacemaker.
  - Lower blood pressure with short-acting agents such as nitroprusside and esmolol.
- **Pulmonary**: Respiratory failure from chest wall rigidity, aspiration pneumonia, and pulmonary embolism
  - Mechanical ventilation may be required.
- **Renal**: Dehydration, electrolyte imbalance, acute renal failure, and rhabdomyolysis[36]
  - Maintain euvolemic state using IV fluids.
- **Hematologic**: Deep venous thrombophlebitis, thrombocytopenia, and disseminated intravascular coagulation (DIC)[36]
  - Prophylaxis with subcutaneous heparin
- **Infectious disease**: Fever and sepsis
  - Use cooling blankets
- **Psychiatric:** Agitation
  - Use benzodiazepines, avoid mechanical restraints[31]

Table 10.8 Drugs associated with NMS and SS

Drugs associated with NMS
- Typical neuroleptics:
  - Haloperidol, fluphenazine, chlorpromazine, prochlorperazine, trifluoperazine, thioridazine, perphenazine, and promazine
- Atypical neuroleptics:
  - Clozapine, risperidone, olanzapine, quetiapine, and aripiprazole
- Antidopaminergic agents:
  - Metoclopramide, droperidol, promethazine, prochlorperazine, tetrabenazine, reserpine, amoxapine, and diatrizoate
- Withdrawal of: Levodopa, dopamine agonists, amantadine, tolcapone, and lithium

Drugs associated with serotonin syndrome
- Monoamine oxidase inhibitors
  - Irreversible inhibitors: Phenelzine, tranylcypromine, iproniazid, and isocarboxazid
  - Reversible inhibitors of monoamine oxidase A: Moclobemide
  - Nonpsychotropic drugs: Linezolid, methylene blue (methylthioninium chloride)
- Serotonin releasing agents
  - Sympathomimetics: Amphetamine, methamphetamine, and methylphenidate
  - Synthetic stimulants: MDMA and LSD
  - SSRIs: Fluoxetine, fluvoxamine, paroxetine, citalopram, sertraline, and escitalopram
  - SNRIs: Venlafaxine, desvenlafaxine, and duloxetine
  - TCAs: Clomipramine and imipramine
  - Opioid analgesics: Tramadol, fentanyl, dextromethorphan, and pethidine
  - Anti-emetics: Ondansetron and metoclopramide
  - Herbal products: St John's wart (Hypericum perforatum), and panax ginseng
- Miscellaneous: Lithium, ritonavir, valproate, tryptophan, buspirone, and mirtazapine

Abbreviations: LSD, lysergic acid diethylamide; MDMA, 3,4-methylenedioxymethamphetamine; NMS, neuroleptic malignant syndrome; SS, serotonin syndrome; SNRIs, serotonin-norepinephrine reuptake inhibitors; SSRIs, selective serotonin reuptake inhibitors; TCAs, tricyclic antidepressants.

10.5.9 Prognosis

- For NMS, mean recovery times are 2 to 14 days and most patients recover fully.[30]
  - Reported mortality rates for NMS are 5 to 20%. Disease severity and the occurrence of medical complications such as renal failure are the strongest predictors of mortality.
- For SS, prognosis is favorable if condition is treated early. Symptoms typically resolve over 24 hours, but persist longer in 40% of patients.[39]

References

[1] Rabinstein AA. Acute neuromuscular respiratory failure. Continuum (Minneap Minn). 2015; 21 5 Neurocritical Care:1324–1345

[2] Fokke C, van den Berg B, Drenthen J, Walgaard C, van Doorn PA, Jacobs BC. Diagnosis of Guillain-Barré syndrome and validation of Brighton criteria. Brain. 2014; 137(Pt 1):33–43

[3] Yuki N, Hartung HP. Guillain-Barré syndrome. N Engl J Med. 2012; 366(24):2294–2304

[4] Dimachkie MM, Barohn RJ. Guillain-Barré syndrome and variants. Neurol Clin. 2013; 31 (2):491–510

[5] Walgaard C, Lingsma HF, Ruts L, et al. Prediction of respiratory insufficiency in Guillain-Barré syndrome. Ann Neurol. 2010; 67(6):781–787

[6] Cornblath DR, Hughes RA. Treatment for Guillain-Barré syndrome. Ann Neurol. 2009; 66 (5):569–570

[7] van den Berg B, Bunschoten C, van Doorn PA, Jacobs BC. Mortality in Guillain-Barre syndrome. Neurology. 2013; 80(18):1650–1654

[8] Gilhus NE. Myasthenia gravis. N Engl J Med. 2016; 375(26):2570–2581

[9] Nicolle MW. Myasthenia gravis and Lambert-Eaton myasthenic syndrome. Continuum (Minneap Minn). 2016; 22 6, Muscle and Neuromuscular Junction Disorders:1978–2005

[10] Jayam Trouth A, Dabi A, Solieman N, Kurukumbi M, Kalyanam J. Myasthenia gravis: a review. Autoimmune Dis. 2012; 2012:874680

[11] Wendell LC, Levine JM. Myasthenic crisis. Neurohospitalist. 2011; 1(1):16–22

[12] Lacomis D. Myasthenic crisis. Neurocrit Care. 2005; 3(3):189–194

[13] Chaudhuri A, Behan PO. Myasthenic crisis. QJM. 2009; 102(2):97–107

[14] Alshekhlee A, Miles JD, Katirji B, Preston DC, Kaminski HJ. Incidence and mortality rates of myasthenia gravis and myasthenic crisis in US hospitals. Neurology. 2009; 72(18):1548–1554

[15] Cherington M. Botulism: update and review. Semin Neurol. 2004; 24(2):155–163

[16] Sobel J. Botulism. Clin Infect Dis. 2005; 41(8):1167–1173

[17] Maselli RA. Pathogenesis of human botulism. Ann N Y Acad Sci. 1998; 841:122–139

[18] Cherington M. Clinical spectrum of botulism. Muscle Nerve. 1998; 21(6):701–710

[19] Cox N, Hinkle R. Infant botulism. Am Fam Physician. 2002; 65(7):1388–1392

[20] Schmidt RD, Schmidt TW. Infant botulism: a case series and review of the literature. J Emerg Med. 1992; 10(6):713–718

[21] Shapiro RL, Hatheway C, Swerdlow DL. Botulism in the United States: a clinical and epidemiologic review. Ann Intern Med. 1998; 129(3):221–228

[22] Arnon SS, Schechter R, Maslanka SE, Jewell NP, Hatheway CL. Human botulism immune globulin for the treatment of infant botulism. N Engl J Med. 2006; 354(5):462–471

[23] Robinson RF, Nahata MC. Management of botulism. Ann Pharmacother. 2003; 37(1):127–131

[24] King AM, Aaron CK. Organophosphate and carbamate poisoning. Emerg Med Clin North Am. 2015; 33(1):133–151

[25] Eddleston M, Buckley NA, Eyer P, Dawson AH. Management of acute organophosphorus pesticide poisoning. Lancet. 2008; 371(9612):597–607

[26] Peter JV, Sudarsan TI, Moran JL. Clinical features of organophosphate poisoning: a review of different classification systems and approaches. Indian J Crit Care Med. 2014; 18(11):735–745

[27] Bronstein AC, Spyker DA, Cantilena LR, Jr, Green JL, Rumack BH, Giffin SL. 2008 Annual Report of the American Association of Poison Control Centers' National Poison Data System (NPDS): 26th Annual Report. Clin Toxicol (Phila). 2009; 47(10):911–1084

[28] Sungur M, Güven M. Intensive care management of organophosphate insecticide poisoning. Crit Care. 2001; 5(4):211–215

[29] Davies JO, Eddleston M, Buckley NA. Predicting outcome in acute organophosphorus poisoning with a poison severity score or the Glasgow coma scale. QJM. 2008; 101(5):371–379

[30] Berman BD. Neuroleptic malignant syndrome: a review for neurohospitalists. Neurohospitalist. 2011; 1(1):41–47

[31] Boyer EW, Shannon M. The serotonin syndrome. N Engl J Med. 2005; 352(11):1112–1120

[32] Pelonero AL, Levenson JL, Pandurangi AK. Neuroleptic malignant syndrome: a review. Psychiatr Serv. 1998; 49(9):1163–1172

[33] Strawn JR, Keck PE, Jr, Caroff SN. Neuroleptic malignant syndrome. Am J Psychiatry. 2007; 164 (6):870–876

[34] Mills KC. Serotonin syndrome: a clinical update. Crit Care Clin. 1997; 13(4):763–783

[35] Carbone JR. The neuroleptic malignant and serotonin syndromes. Emerg Med Clin North Am. 2000; 18(2):317–325, x

[36] Bhanushali MJ, Tuite PJ. The evaluation and management of patients with neuroleptic malignant syndrome. Neurol Clin. 2004; 22(2):389–411

[37] Mason PJ, Morris VA, Balcezak TJ. Serotonin syndrome: presentation of 2 cases and review of the literature. Medicine (Baltimore). 2000; 79(4):201–209

[38] Gillman PK. The serotonin syndrome and its treatment. J Psychopharmacol. 1999; 13(1):100–109

[39] Birmes P, Coppin D, Schmitt L, Lauque D. Serotonin syndrome: a brief review. CMAJ. 2003; 168 (11):1439–1442

11 Brain Tumor Postoperative Management

Richard F. Schmidt, Nikolaos Mouchtouris, Muaz Qayyum, James J. Evans, and Christopher Farrell

Abstract

In this chapter, we discuss the critical care management of patients with brain tumors. Given that many patients with brain tumors present to the intensive care unit (ICU) in the perioperative period, significant attention is given to the perioperative management of these patients, addressing commonly encountered conditions that can complicate their stay in the ICU. Furthermore, we will discuss other factors that may require critical care management, including cerebral edema, cerebrospinal fluid (CSF) leakage, hormonal dysregulation, and pituitary apoplexy. We outline the pathophysiology, clinical presentation, diagnostic evaluation, and management for each of these conditions to prepare the intensivist to safely manage this complex patient population.

Keywords: cerebral edema, cerebrospinal fluid leak, pneumocephalus, pituitary apoplexy, postoperative complications, brain tumor

11.1 Introduction

Brain tumors encompass a wide variety of pathologies that can present in a highly variable fashion depending on the location of the tumor, type of tumor, amount of surrounding edema, and involvement of vascular structures. The management of brain tumors is highly complex, involving extensive inpatient and outpatient treatment strategies. This chapter will focus exclusively on the critical care management of patients with brain tumors, specifically on important clinical factors in the perioperative management of these patients. The topics covered include perioperative complication avoidance, treatment of tumor-associated cerebral edema, diagnosis and management of cerebrospinal fluid (CSF) leakage, and specific concerns for sellar region tumors, including acute endocrinopathies and pituitary apoplexy. Armed with the information in this chapter, the neuro-intensivist should be able to manage routine postoperative intensive care unit (ICU) admissions in addition to diagnosing and treating potentially devastating complications.

11.1.1 Clinical Presentation

The clinical presentation of the patient varies and depends on the size and location of the tumor. Slow growing tumors can grow for years before a patient becomes symptomatic while a smaller metastatic tumor can be fast growing and have early signs and symptoms. ▶ Table 11.1 details some of the presenting symptoms. An understanding of involved cortical and subcortical structures, cranial nerves, vascular structures, and bony anatomy is important in identifying nuances in examination changes and allows for the neurointensivist to anticipate, mitigate, and manage potential complications in the perioperative period.

Table 11.1 Clinical presentation considerations and concerns

Symptoms	Considerations	Concerns
Headache	• New onset • Atypical • Progressive over period of time • Associated with additional finding • Worse with coughing, laying down or bending over, and Valsalva maneuvers	• Mass effect • Increased intracranial pressure • Hydrocephalus • Venous thrombosis
Nausea and vomiting	• Intractable • No associated systemic findings (fever, diarrhea, abdominal pain) • Association with headache • Relief of headache after vomiting	• Mass effect on the fourth ventricle • Hydrocephalus
Seizure	• New onset • Refractory to medical therapy	• Surgical resection may be delayed with status epilepticus • May require multiple medications to manage
Focal neurologic deficit	• New motor weakness • New speech/language deficit • Ataxia • Sensory deficits • Hyperreflexia/spasticity	• Symptoms depend on location • May be related to surrounding cerebral edema • Often occur in association with other symptoms
Encephalopathy	• Psychomotor slowing • Confusion with common daily events	• Cerebral edema • Mass effect • Increased intracranial pressure • Hydrocephalus

11.1.2 Tumor Classification

There are two main classifications of brain tumors: metastatic and primary brain. Metastatic brain tumors are the most common tumor in adults. These tumors arise from outside the brain. According to the American Brain Tumor Foundation, the incidence of metastatic brain tumors is estimated between 200,000 and 300,000 people per year. Although any cancer has the potential to metastasize to the brain, it is most common with the following:

• Lung
• Breast
• Melanoma
• Colorectal
• Renal cell
• Lymphoma

Primary brain tumors can be further classified into benign or malignant, with benign occurring almost twice as frequently as malignant. They can be classified as intra-axial, extra-axial, and intraventricular (see ▶ Table 11.2).

• Infra-axial tumors arise from cells within the brain parenchyma itself, i.e., glial cells.
• Extra-axial tumors arise from structures outside the brain, i.e., dura, cranial nerves, and bone.
• Intraventricular tumors arise from cells within the ventricles.

They can be further categorized into supratentorial and infratentorial. Distinctions between the two are important when considering associated anatomic structures and potential perioperative complications.

Table 11.2 Tumors by location

Intra-axial	Extra-axial	Intraventricular
Astrocytoma	Chordoma	Ependymoma
Oligodendroglioma	Craniopharyngioma	Subependymoma
Ganglioglioma	Meningioma	Choroid plexus papilloma
Medulloblastoma	Pituitary adenoma	Central neurocytoma
Hemangioblastoma	Schwannoma	
Metastases	Epidermoid	
	Metastases	

Supratentorial Tumors

- Higher incidence of pre- or postoperative seizures[15]
- May grow to larger sizes before exhibiting clinically significant mass effect
- Risk of venous injury causing venous infarction or possible catastrophic hemorrhage
- Potential for injury to anterior circulation arteries or branches causing hemorrhage or ischemia

Infratentorial Tumors

- Composed of the contents of the posterior fossa (cerebellum, brainstem, fourth ventricle, cerebral aqueduct, and origin of cranial nerves III–XII)
- Limited space available to accommodate postoperative swelling
- At risk for rapid clinical decompensation and cranial nerve involvement
- Potential for injury to posterior circulation arteries or branches causing hemorrhage or ischemia
- Tumors may invade or exhibit mass effect on the brainstem reticular activating system or the fourth ventricle potentially compromising a patient's level of consciousness or causing hydrocephalus

11.2 Postoperative Care and Complications (▶ Table 11.3)

Most patients who undergo surgical intervention for brain tumors experience a relatively uneventful postoperative stay. The rate of postoperative complications is estimated to be around 3 to 4% based on National Inpatient Database sampling. Furthermore, certain at-risk populations may experience significantly higher rates of postoperative morbidity:[1,2]

- Patients > 70 years of age
- Preoperative Karnofsky Performance score < 80
- High intraoperative blood loss (≥ 350 mL)
- Drop in hemoglobin of ≥ 2 g/dL preoperative to postoperative

11.2.1 Airway Management

Patients are typically extubated in the operating room once they are awake and following commands or exhibiting purposeful movement.[3] However, prolonged operative times and brain retraction during surgery may result in an extended postanesthetic recovery period during which the patient might be at increased risk for respiratory compromise.[3] Extended intubation times are not uncommon. In patients with delayed emergence from anesthesia, a screening

Table 11.3 Postoperative management following brain tumor resection

	Considerations	Management
Airway management	Prolonged intubation Risk factors for prolonged intubation (COPD, asthma) Lower cranial nerve/bulbar dysfunction/vocal cord injury Prolonged anesthetic effect (patients with renal or liver dysfunction baseline)	• Serial neurologic checks • Sedation vacation • Pulmonary toilet • CT of head, if delayed extubation with poor neurologic exam • Consider ENT evaluation prior to extubation
Antibiotic prophylaxis and postoperative infection	Endoscopic transphenoidal surgery, especially if nasal packing Comorbidities • Diabetes, obesity, poor nutritional status	• Standard prophylaxis as per institutional guidelines • Aggressive workup if concern for wound infection/meningitis, including CSF sampling and broad-spectrum antibiotics
Blood pressure control and postoperative hemorrhage	Patient age > 40 years Incompletely resected or biopsied tumors Tumor pathology plays important role (frozen tissue diagnosis) Astrocytic, vascularized, cystic, and/or malignant tumors carry increased post-op bleeding risk	• Systolic BP > 90 and < 140 • Mean arterial BP > 65 and < 100 • Continuous infusion of antihypertensive to avoid fluctuations in blood pressure
Cerebral edema	Can be both vasogenic (tumor related) and cytotoxic (secondary to ischemia) Can be symptomatic or asymptomatic Concerning when mass effect and potential ICP crisis Corticosteroids (decadron) preferred Steroids may be held until post operatively if tumor is concerning for lymphoma Tumor debulking may worsen edema	• Continue intravenous steroids 4–8 mg every 6 hours • Maintain normal serum Na (135–145 mEq/Dl) • Malignant edema can be managed with mannitol or hypertonic saline • Head of bed > 30 degrees

(Continued)

Table 11.3 (*Continued*) Postoperative management following brain tumor resection

	Considerations	Management
CSF leak	High flow (ventricular/cisternal entry) vs. low flow Signs of intracranial hypotension • Rhinorrhea • Positional headache (worse when sitting or standing) • Nausea • Neck stiffness Development of infection/meningitis Development of tension pneumocephalus Send β2-transferrin but don't delay treatment while waiting for results Delay in management can increase the risk of meningitis	• Sinus precautions (for transphenoidal) • CTH to evaluate for pneumocephalus (Mt. Fuji sign) • Antibiotics if suspected of infection • Notify neurosurgeon, may need CSF diversion (lumbar drain, external ventricular drain, ventriculoperitoneal shunt) • Primary operative repair
Diabetes insipidus	• Hourly urine output, urine specific gravity • Cognitive status—ability to respond to thirst • Serum sodium levels • Involvement of pituitary stalk (likely permanent if transected) • Triphasic response	• Supportive measures—readily available water • Hormone supplementation—DDAVP
Fluid resuscitation	Need to know intraoperative ins/outs Prolonged surgery has higher insensible losses	• Crystalloid replacement • Blood products when indicated • Blood pressure may not be initially affected due to intraoperative pressor use • Hemoglobin may not be reflective of hypovolemia initially
Hypocortisolemia	• Secreting vs. nonsecreting pituitary tumors • Tracking AM cortisol levels—best evaluation hypothalamic pituitary axis • Possible cardiovascular collapse if untreated	• Hormone supplementation • Dexamethasone does not affect endogenous cortisol level measurements

(*Continued*)

Table 11.3 (*Continued*) Postoperative management following brain tumor resection

	Considerations	Management
Hyponatremia	Often due to SIADH in the setting of tumor Can be chronic with euvole-mic state Preoperative management with crystalloid fluids preferred	• In SIADH, manage with free water restriction • Avoid rapid correction over 24 hours, no more than 8–10 mEq/dL
Pain management	Poorly controlled pain can contribute to elevated blood pressure Pain can be associated with nausea and vomiting	• Minimize use of narcotics in order to maintain neurologic exam • Consider 1000 mg IV acet-aminophen every 6 hours during the first 24 hours when available • Avoid NSAIDs and aspirin to minimize risk of bleeding
Seizure prophylaxis	History of prior seizures Not required for posterior fossa (infratentorial) tumors Supratentorial tumors predis-posed to seizures	• Continue any preoperative AEDs • No standard guidelines • Consider short course when possible • Consider side effect profile and drug–drug interactions when selecting agent • For prolonged encephalopathy post-op continuous EEG mon-itoring is recommended • Enteral access may be needed if no IV formulation is available
VTE prophylaxis	Malignant tumors (GBM) • Higher risk if age > 60 years, large tumor burden, and/or on chemotherapy or bevacizumab Limb paresis Admission screening when possible	• SCDs in all patients, minimum 20 hours/day • Low-dose heparin/LMW heparin generally tolerated at 24 hours

Abbreviations: AEDs, antiepileptic drugs; BP, blood pressure; COPD, chronic obstructive pulmonary disease; CSF, cerebrospinal fluid; CT, computed tomography; DDAVP, D-amino D-arginine vasopressin; EEG, electroencephalography; ENT, ear, nose, and throat; GBM, glioblastomas; IV, intravenous; LMW, low molecular weight; NSAIDs, nonsteroidal anti-inflammatory drugs; SCDs, sequential compression devices; SIADH, syndrome of inappropriate antidiuretic hormone secretion.

computed tomography (CT) scan of the head is typically performed to rule out acute perioperative complications, such as a hematoma, followed by further monitoring if needed. Minimizing post-operative sedation and regular pulmonary toilet are important in preparing for extubation. Occasionally, patients develop airway edema which can delay extubation. Consider ear, nose, and throat (ENT) evaluation if concern. Patients with infratentorial lesions and suspected lower cranial nerve deficits require particular attention to limit the potential risk for aspiration due to insufficient airway protection.[3] This also applies to patients with tumors of the pons, medulla, or fourth ventricle, as involvement of brainstem parenchyma or edema in this region may exacerbate vocal cord and pharyngeal muscle dysfunction. These patients require close monitoring to limit the risk for aspiration and further respiratory compromise.

11.2.2 Blood Pressure Control and Postoperative Hemorrhage

Postoperative hemorrhage is associated with a 3.3 times increased risk of inpatient hospital mortality and can be seen in 1.1 to 4.4% of cases, 88% of which occur within 6 hours of surgery.[1,4] While postoperative hemorrhage is often considered a result of insufficient intraoperative hemostasis, perioperative hypertension has been suggested to play a role as well by increasing dynamic stress on fragile bod vessels in the operative bed.[4,5] Patients aged > 40 years, with astrocytic tumors, giant tumors, and partially resected or biopsied tumors, especially highly vascularized, cystic, and/or malignant tumors, are at an increased risk of postoperative hemorrhage.[6,7,8] Minimally invasive procedures, such as stereotactic biopsies, may have hemorrhage rates as high as 5%, especially within high-risk locations, such as the pineal region.[7] Furthermore, patients with a recurrent malignant gliomas and who have taken bevacizumab are also at an increased risk of perioperative hemorrhage.[9]

While there are no standardized parameters for blood pressure management, maintaining systolic blood pressure less than 140 mm Hg and mean arterial pressure less than 100 mm Hg have been reported to prevent spontaneous hematoma expansion, and are often used as guidelines for protection against postoperative bleeding following resection.[5,10] Furthermore, adequate control of postoperative pain and nausea, as well as an appropriate bowel regimen are recommended to limit blood pressure spikes from discomfort, retching, and Valsalva.[3]

11.2.3 Seizure Prophylaxis

Evidence based on a meta-analysis of high-quality randomized controlled trials suggests that seizure prophylaxis in the postoperative setting does not provide any significant benefit.[11] However, there are numerous criticisms to this assertion. Postoperative seizures have the greatest risk of occurring within 48 hours of surgery and can be present in 1 to 12% of cases. Furthermore, the potential consequences of postoperative seizure can be devastating, including malignant cerebral edema and hemorrhage.[4] The vast majority of studies looking at perioperative seizure prophylaxis investigated older antiepileptic drugs (AEDs), such as phenytoin, which are known to have a more deleterious side effect profile, particularly in regards to their action on the cytochrome P450 enzyme complex.[11] Currently, there has been only one meta-analysis that has incorporated a study of more modern AEDs, specifically levetiracetam, which is known to have a far more limited side effect profile.[12] Levetiracetam is associated with rare behavioral disturbances, with dose limiting side effects seen in as few as 2.4% of patients.[13] Additionally, newer agents, such as lacosamide, have yet to be studied regarding effectiveness for perioperative seizure prophylaxis in this population. Therefore, while there is limited data to suggests routine use of seizure prophylaxis following brain tumor resection, a thorough assessment of individual risks and benefits must be considered. Populations that are at an increased risk of seizures should be given additional consideration for starting seizure prophylaxis, namely patients with oligodendrogliomas, gangliogliomas, dysembryoplastic neuroepithelial tumors (DNET),[8] glioblastomas (GBM) of the frontal lobe, non-skull base meningiomas, and meningiomas with significant peritumoral edema.[8,14,15] Generally, a short course of a recent generation AED, such as levetiracetam, is well-tolerated in patients for whom prophylaxis is deemed appropriate, and patients with history of seizure should have their AED maintained postoperatively.[4,11,12] Patients with posterior fossa lesions are unlikely to require any seizure protection due to the inherent lack of cortical involvement.

11.2.4 Venous Thromboembolism Prophylaxis

Venous thromboembolism (VTE) remains the most common adverse event affecting brain tumor patients in the postoperative setting, occurring in 3 to 26% of patients in the perioperative period.[4,16] Unfortunately, there is a dearth of literature to provide meaningful guidance on balancing this risk with the risk of postoperative hemorrhage. The use of sequential compression devices (SCDs) in neurosurgical patients has been well described and is currently recommended for all postoperative patients.[17] The optimal timing and dose of chemical thromboprophylaxis with either heparin or low-molecular-weight heparins (i.e., enoxaparin) remain unclear; however, most practitioners agree that starting low-dose prophylactic anticoagulation in the acute postoperative period is generally acceptable. Patients with significantly increased risk of thromboembolic complications, such as those with a mechanical heart valve, hypercoagulability, or history of deep vein thrombosis, initiation of mechanical and chemical thromboprophylaxis should be started as soon as possible.[4,18] Patients with a paretic limb, patients on bevacizumab for recurrent GBM, and patients with malignant gliomas who are > 60 years old, are on active chemotherapy, and/or have a larger tumor burden, have also been showed to be at an increased risk for VTE.[19,20] Ultimately, the timing for restarting thromboprophylactic medication must be based on the individual patient's risk profile for both hemorrhage and thromboembolism.[4,19,20]

11.2.5 Antibiotic Prophylaxis and Postoperative Infection

Routine use of postoperative antibiotics has been shown to reduce the risk of surgical site infections, including a reduction in postoperative meningitis in neurosurgical patients.[21,22] Therefore, perioperative antibiotic use for approximately 24 hours postoperatively is universally recommended, with specific agents determined by institutional guidelines to account for local antibiotic resistances. Patients who undergo transsphenoidal surgery warrant special consideration, with studies suggesting up to 7 days of antibiotics, while nonabsorbable packing is in place, to prevent bacterial overgrowth and development of toxic shock syndrome.[10] Other patients who may be at an increased risk for postoperative infection include those with advanced age, extended length of surgery, and factors that may affect wound healing such as obesity, diabetes/hyperglycemia, and poor nutritional status.[23]

An important consideration regarding the workup for postoperative infection is the potential for aseptic (chemical) meningitis. The underlying etiology of this phenomenon is not clearly understood but is suspected to be an inflammatory response to the presence of external substances in the CSF such as blood, bone dust, tumor, and/or cystic contents. The clinical presentation of aseptic meningitis is highly variable, but largely mimics the symptoms of bacterial meningitis such as headache, neck stiffness, photophobia, and possibly fever. There are no clear risk factors for aseptic meningitis; however, resection of certain cystic tumors, such as epidermoid cysts and craniopharyngiomas, have been suggested to play a role in postoperative meningeal inflammation, especially if there is spillage of cystic contents intraoperatively or incomplete resection of the cyst wall.[24,25,26,27] Due to the largely ambiguous presentation of aseptic meningitis, patients exhibiting meningeal symptoms in the postoperative setting, particularly those with fever, CSF leak, or wound breakdown, should be expeditiously evaluated for bacterial meningitis with CSF sampling and started on broad-spectrum antibiotics while cultures are pending. There is no agreed upon standard for the diagnosis of aseptic meningitis based on CSF specimens. However, negative CSF cultures in low-risk patients may favor an aseptic etiology.[26] These patients may be treated conservatively for aseptic meningitis at the practitioners' discretion with corticosteroids to reduce meningeal inflammation and possibly serial lumbar puncture or CSF diversion in cases of persistent symptoms or elevated intracranial pressure (ICP).[26]

11.2.6 Cerebral Edema

Cerebral edema is commonly seen in patients harboring brain tumors and warrants careful management to avoid devastating complications. A more detailed discussion on the management of cerebral edema can be found in Chapter 6. therefore, only information as it pertains to brain tumor patients will be discussed. Vasogenic edema, which results from the disruption of the blood–brain barrier (BBB) and affects mostly the white matter, is the most common form of edema seen in brain tumors. Pathophysiologically, this is the result of the accumulation of inflammatory cytokines, leukotrienes, prostaglandins, vascular endothelial growth factor (VEGF), and matrix metalloproteinases (MMPs), which ultimately result in BBB breakdown and extravasation of plasma into the surrounding brain parenchyma.[28,29,30,31,32,33] Surgical debulking relieves tumor mass effect and may improve surrounding edema. However, the timing of edema resolution is highly variable and may temporarily worsen following operative manipulation. Brain retraction and intraoperative venous compromise may also lead to venous congestion, worsening cerebral edema. Furthermore, cytotoxic edema from cerebral infarction my also occur in cases of injury to crucial draining veins, such as the veins of Trolard, Labbe, basal vein of Rosenthal, the dural sinuses, or in cases with intraoperative arterial compromise.

Symptomatic cerebral edema in the postoperative period is present in approximately 7.7 to 9.5% of patients.[4,34,35] Patients with cerebral edema require careful monitoring to mitigate the development of transient neurologic deficits and prevent potentially life-threatening elevations in ICP.[36] Early manifestations of elevated ICP secondary to cerebral edema include headaches, nausea, vomiting, diplopia (from cranial nerve VI palsy), and papilledema.[36] Focal neurologic deficits, impaired consciousness, aphasia, and seizures can also be seen as edema progresses. With the onset of any new neurologic deficit, emergent noncontrast CT of the head should be obtained to assess for alternative potential etiologies such as cerebral infarction or hemorrhage that may require emergent intervention.[28] Radiographic evidence of midline shift, sulcal effacement, and basal cistern obliteration can help assess the severity of the edema and potential for elevated ICPs. Magnetic resonance imaging (MRI) may also be used to better characterize the nature and extent of the edema, particularly T2 and fluid-attenuated inversion recovery (FLAIR) sequences.

Postoperatively, patients should have their head of bed elevated at a minimum of 30 degrees angle to increase venous outflow and decrease the hydrostatic pressure in the cranial vault to limit the potential for worsening edema.[37,38] Pharmacologically, steroids have been extensively used in the

159

treatment of vasogenic edema, with dexamethasone being the most common agent. Corticosteroids can be administered 1 to 2 days before resection to reduce the edema preoperatively in symptomatic patients and are routinely administered intraoperatively. Steroids have been shown to result in neurologic improvement within the first 24 to 72 hours after initiation.[39,40] Postoperatively and/or upon improvement of symptoms, steroids should tapered to a low maintenance dose or weaned entirely as tolerated.[4] Acute exacerbations in cerebral edema and ICP elevation should prompt interventions to improve cerebral perfusion and oxygenation, reduce the metabolic demands of the brain, and decrease ICP. Algorithms for the management of ICP crisis are beyond the scope of this chapter, but treatment should be initiated as soon as possible to limit the potential for permanent neurologic injury or death.

11.2.7 CSF Leak

CSF leakage is a potential complication of brain tumor resection that can significantly prolong the postoperative ICU course. A variety of etiologies can lead to CSF leakage, including the presence of hydrocephalus, inadequate dural closure, and disruption of bony and soft tissue structures secondary to tumor invasion or extensive skull base surgical approaches.[4,41] Rates of CSF leak have been reported to range from 2 to 16% following transsphenoidal surgery[10,42,43] and up to 32% for posterior fossa surgeries.[44,45,46] High-flow CSF leaks occur when CSF cisterns and/or ventricles are entered during surgery and are much more likely to result in postoperative CSF leakage compared to low-flow leaks.[10] Communication of operative factors between the surgeon and the ICU team is crucial in establishing the risk for postoperative CSF leak and the necessary treatment measures. For example, high-flow leaks may require more aggressive early intervention in order to resolve completely.[10,47]

Depending on the site of surgical intervention, CSF leakage may manifest as clear fluid drainage from the wound or as rhinorrhea, with patients often complaining of a metallic or salty taste. Sampling of draining fluid for β2-transferrin can be helpful for establishing the presence of a CSF leak when the diagnosis is uncertain. β2-transferrin testing, however, typically does not yield rapid results and waiting for laboratory confirmation may lead to unnecessary delays in initiating treatment.[41] In patients who have undergone transsphenoidal surgery, endoscopic exploration can sometimes be useful in isolating the source of the leak. Also, CT or MRI may be useful in identifying the site of an anatomical defect and potential CSF egress site, although small defects along the skull base may be missed on even thin-cut imaging. Other diagnostic tools available include radioactive cisternography, CT cisternogram, and intrathecal fluorescein administration, but these diagnostic interventions are used less frequently due to their invasive nature. Occasionally, a CSF leak may present solely as symptomatic intracranial hypotension, manifesting as positional headaches, nausea, and/or neck stiffness. Lastly, patients with prolonged CSF leaks may present with meningitis due to communication between the environment and the intracranial space. Therefore, patients with a CSF leak and clinical suspicion for meningitis should be evaluated emergently with CSF sampling and treated with antibiotics until the presence or absence of infection is confirmed.

Initial prevention of CSF leak involves patient positioning and basic postoperative care. Patients should be positioned with their head elevated and patients who have undergone a transsphenoidal resection should be placed on strict precautions to try and limit pressure gradients across the cranial defect into the sinonasal cavity. These precautions include sneezing with their mouth open and avoiding blowing their nose.[10] Furthermore, all patients should be started on stool softeners and antiemetic medication to help avoid straining, which may result in transient ICP elevation and failure of intraoperative CSF leak repair.

Many patients with an established leak can be successfully managed with temporary CSF diversion, typically via a lumbar drain or external ventriculostomy, to allow the communicating defect to heal.[10,47] In patients with CSF leaks following posterior fossa surgery, several studies support the use of lumbar drainage for at least 5 days with good results.[10,48,49] On the contrary, in patients with CSF leaks following endoscopic transsphenoidal surgery, less than 24% are able to be treated conservatively with lumbar drainage alone, and many of these patients require operative intervention for definitive leak repair.[10,42,43] Patients with persistent CSF leaks should also be evaluated for the presence of hydrocephalus. Increased ICPs from hydrocephalus will not only prevent healing of dural defects but may also lead to long-term consequences if not managed appropriately. Diagnosis revolves around a constellation of clinical and radiographic findings, such as altered mental status, neurologic deficit, and ventriculomegaly; however, some patients may be asymptomatic. If hydrocephalus is suspected, alternative methods of CSF diversion, such as external ventricular drainage or ventriculoperitoneal shunt insertion, may be required.[41]

Tension pneumocephalus is a rare but potentially life-threatening condition in which air enters the cranial cavity via a one-way valve mechanism, resulting in progressively increased ICP as air enters and cannot escape. Tension pneumocephalus is frequently associated with a CSF leak, most commonly following transnasal surgery, and can exhibit a rapidly progressive course, resulting in severe clinical and neurologic sequelae.[50,51] Increased ICPs from tension pneumocephalus can result in brain herniation, air embolism, and/or cardiac arrest in cases where it is not recognized or treated rapidly.[51,52] On imaging, tension pneumocephalus may present as the "Mount Fuji sign" (▶ Fig. 11.1), seen when intracranial air compresses the bilateral frontal lobe convexities, exhibiting a "peak" at the frontal poles, or as the "air bubble sign" in which numerous air bubbles are found throughout the basal cisterns.[50,51,53] Management of tension pneumocephalus relies primarily on operative intervention. Burr hole decompression may allow release of the built-up air; however, ultimate treatment

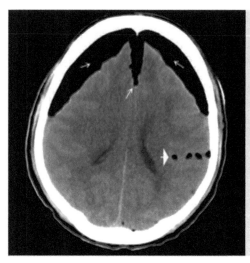

Fig. 11.1 Mount Fuji sign and air bubble sign. (Reproduced with permission from Sebastian B and Moideen J. Mount Fuji is Not as "Active" as We Think. Indian Journal of Neurosurgery 2018; 07(03):278–279.)

typically involves focal repair of the bony defect or site of CSF leak to prevent further air entry.[50,53,54]

11.3 Specific Concerns for Sellar and Parasellar Tumors

11.3.1 Hormonal Dysregulation

Pituitary surgery is often performed without complication. However, even without direct injury to the hypothalamic-pituitary axis (HPA), removal of sellar and parasellar tumors can result in postoperative endocrinopathy related to traction on normal tissues. In general, patients with preoperative pituitary dysfunction should be continued on hormonal replacement postoperatively.[47] Patients with suppressed preoperative adrenal function may require stress-dose corticosteroids in the perioperative period.[55,56] Dexamethasone is frequently preferred for supplementation, as it will not directly affect serum cortisol measurements, exhibiting only a suppressive effect on the adrenal axis.[47] To assess for endogenous corticosteroid function, morning cortisol testing is typically performed on postoperative day 1 or 2. Patients with values < 10 μg/L often require long-term glucocorticoid replacement; however, there is no standardized protocol and the exact management varies between practitioners. Patients treated for Cushing's disease require unique consideration as they may experience a rapid decrease in cortisol levels following tumor resection, resulting in adrenal crisis without adequate replacement.[47,56] On the other hand, adrenocorticotropic hormone (ACTH)-secreting tumors that are sub-totally resected may continue to experience elevated levels of cortisol production and supplemental steroid administration may be contraindicated. Therefore, communication between the treating surgeon, endocrinologist, and intensivist is critical to anticipate and avoid hormone related complications. Clinical signs of hypocortisolemia include hypotension, nausea, and lethargy, and given the potential for rapid decline, hormonal replacement should be initiated in suspected patients while laboratory test results are pending.[47]

Postoperative diabetes insipidus (DI) is a relatively frequent complication of pituitary surgery, occurring in up to 12 to 24% of postoperative patients.[47,57] However, this is often a transient occurrence, with only 1 to 2% of patients needing permanent hormone supplementation.[57] Monitoring for postoperative DI involves strict monitoring of fluid balance in all patients. Polyuria is a hallmark sign of DI. Monitoring the patient's ins and outs becomes critical. There is no consensus as to what amount of urine output becomes concerning, thresholds of > 30 mL/kg/day, > 2 mL/kg/hour to > 250–500 mL/hour have been reported.[75] The practice at our institution is a patient with urine outputs of greater than 250 cc for 2 to 3 consecutive hours should obtain a urine specific gravity, urine osmolality, serum osmolality, and serum sodium concentration. Urine specific gravity values < 1.005 and urine osmolality of < 300 mOsm/kg with serum osmolality of > 300 mOsm/kg in the setting of high fluid output typically are indicative of DI.[47,75] Management of DI varies greatly depending on the extent of fluid balance and the patient's clinical examination. Patients with moderate losses who are alert and able to drink free water can typically maintain a normal sodium level and overall fluid balance due to appropriate activation of their thirst mechanism. However, patients with depressed mental status, those with elevated sodium levels, or those who are otherwise unable to keep up with extensive fluid losses may require pharmacologic support in the form of D-amino D-arginine vasopressin (DDAVP), an analog of antidiuretic hormone (ADH) that acts on V2 receptors in the kidneys.[47] DDAVP can be delivered either intravenously or intranasally; however, careful consideration for the side of any packing or mucosal grafts is needed in patients who have recently undergone transsphenoidal surgery.[57] Furthermore, practitioners must be aware of a possible bi- or tri-phasic response in DI (▶ Fig. 11.2), which may occur over 1 to 2 weeks postoperatively in up to 5 and 1.1% of patients, respectively.[58,59] This triphasic response is believed to be due to (1) initial DI from decreased secretion of ADH from injured cells, followed by (2) a period of syndrome of inappropriate antidiuretic hormone secretion (SIADH), resulting in hyponatremia as injured cells degenerate or necrose, releasing ADH in the blood stream, and (3) persistent DI in patients with permanently injured posterior pituitary or pituitary stalk who cannot return to physiologic ADH secretion.[47,58,59] Careful monitoring of fluid balance, urine specific gravity, and electrolytes is critical throughout this period to maintain adequate treatment of DI while ensuring overcorrection does not occur in periods of SIADH.

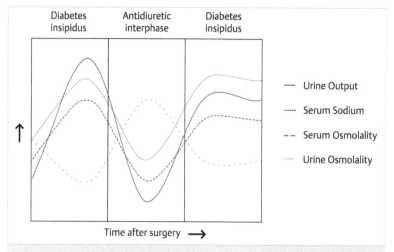

Fig. 11.2 Triphasic response of diabetes insipidus. (Reproduced with permission from Schreckinger M, Szerlip N, Mittal S. Diabetes insipidus following resection of pituitary tumors. Clin Neurol Neurosurg. 2013; 115(2):121–126.)

11.3.2 Pituitary Apoplexy

Although pituitary apoplexy is generally considered a preoperative condition, it is a potentially fatal condition and should be mentioned. Pituitary apoplexy is caused by rapid expansion of a mass within the sella turcica due to hemorrhage or infarction. The incidence of apoplexy ranges from 0.6 to 27.2% of pituitary adenomas, resulting from the formation of abnormal venous sinuses that are prone to rupture.[60],[61],[62],[63],[64],[65],[66],[67],[68] Factors that can predispose to apoplexy include pregnancy, fluctuating hypertension, anticoagulant therapy, surgery, recent head injury, or sudden increases in ICP. Additionally, rapid growth of the tumor may compress its blood supply or extend beyond it, resulting in tissue ischemia and subsequent infarct.

Patients with acute pituitary apoplexy may present with:

- New onset of visual field defects: Decreased visual acuity, diplopia, and ophthalmoplegia
- Altered mental status secondary to increased ICP
- Dizziness
- Headaches
- Hypotension
- Cardiac dysrhythmias
- Meningismus (neck pain, photophobia, nausea, and/or vomiting)[69]

Suspicion of pituitary apoplexy warrants prompt endocrine serologic evaluation and imaging of the brain, including MRI or thin-cut CT imaging and neurosurgical consultation.

Initial management involves establishing hemodynamic stability through administration of IV fluids and administration of glucocorticoids. Hormone replacement therapy with DDAVP and levothyroxine should be initiated depending on the hormonal deficiencies present, but these are often less acute in nature than hypocortisolemia. Surgical decompression is required in patients with new-onset neurologic deficits, including decreased visual acuity and/or visual fields, diplopia, and reduced level of consciousness.[70] Improved recovery of vision has been seen in patients who underwent surgery within 6 to 8 days from the onset of apoplexy, with complete resolution of visual deficits achieved in 43 to 64% of patients. Normal pituitary hormonal function was seen in 19% of patients at a median of 49 months.[71,72,73,74]

11.4 Conclusion

The management of brain tumor patients in the ICU requires a tailored approach to each individual patient, focusing on the specific pathology and nature of their treatment. Frequently, these patients are managed in the ICU during the perioperative period. As such, a detailed understanding of postoperative management and potential complications that can occur in these patients is imperative. Armed with a robust understanding of the variability and complexity of the perioperative management of patients with brain tumors, an astute neurointensivist can help prevent disaster and lay the foundation for a safe recovery.

References

[1] De la Garza-Ramos R, Kerezoudis P, Tamargo RJ, Brem H, Huang J, Bydon M. Surgical complications following malignant brain tumor surgery: an analysis of 2002–2011 data. Clin Neurol Neurosurg. 2016; 140:6–10

[2] Asano K, Nakano T, Takeda T, Ohkuma H. Risk factors for postoperative systemic complications in elderly patients with brain tumors. Clinical article. J Neurosurg. 2009; 111(2):258–264

[3] Jellish WS, Murdoch J, Leonetti JP. Perioperative management of complex skull base surgery: the anesthesiologist's point of view. Neurosurg Focus. 2002; 12(5):e5

[4] Wong JM, Ziewacz JE, Ho AL, et al. Patterns in neurosurgical adverse events: open cerebrovascular neurosurgery. Neurosurg Focus. 2012; 33(5):E15

[5] Steiner T, Bösel J. Options to restrict hematoma expansion after spontaneous intracerebral hemorrhage. Stroke. 2010; 41(2):402–409

[6] Edzhelat Fl. [Hemorrhage in cerebral gliomas]. Vestn Khir Im I I Grek. 1998; 157(6):66–67

[7] Nishihara M, Sasayama T, Kudo H, Kohmura E. Morbidity of stereotactic biopsy for intracranial lesions. Kobe J Med Sci. 2011; 56(4):E148–E153

[8] Vecht CJ, Kerkhof M, Duran-Pena A. Seizure prognosis in brain tumors: new insights and evidence-based management. Oncologist. 2014; 19(7):751–759

[9] Abrams DA, Hanson JA, Brown JM, Hsu FP, Delashaw JB, Jr, Bota DA. Timing of surgery and bevaci-zumab therapy in neurosurgical patients with recurrent high grade glioma. J Clin Neurosci. 2015; 22(1):35–39

[10] Tien DA, Stokken JK, Recinos PF, Woodard TD, Sindwani R. Comprehensive postoperative manage-ment after endoscopic skull base surgery. Otolaryngol Clin North Am. 2016; 49(1):253–263

[11] Sayegh ET, Fakurnejad S, Oh T, Bloch O, Parsa AT. Anticonvulsant prophylaxis for brain tumor sur-gery: determining the current best available evidence. J Neurosurg. 2014; 121(5):1139–1147

[12] Komotar RJ, Raper DM, Starke RM, Iorgulescu JB, Gutin PH. Prophylactic antiepileptic drug ther-apy in patients undergoing supratentorial meningioma resection: a systematic analysis of efficacy. J Neurosurg. 2011; 115(3):483–490

[13] Rosati A, Buttolo L, Stefini R, Todeschini A, Cenzato M, Padovani A. Efficacy and safety of levetira-cetam in patients with glioma: a clinical prospective study. Arch Neurol. 2010; 67(3):343–346

[14] Xue H, Sveinsson O, Tomson T, Mathiesen T. Intracranial meningiomas and seizures: a review of the literature. Acta Neurochir (Wien). 2015; 157(9):1541–1548

[15] Su X, Chen HL, Wang ZY, Lan Q. Relationship between tumour location and preoperative seizure incidence in patients with gliomas: a systematic review and meta-analysis. Epileptic Disord. 2015; 17(4):397–408

[16] Brandes AA, Scelzi E, Salmistraro G, et al. Incidence of risk of thromboembolism during treatment high-grade gliomas: a prospective study. Eur J Cancer. 1997; 33(10):1592–1596

[17] Skillman JJ, Collins RE, Coe NP, et al. Prevention of deep vein thrombosis in neurosurgical patients: a controlled, randomized trial of external pneumatic compression boots. Surgery. 1978; 83 (3):354–358

[18] Niemi T, Armstrong E. Thromboprophylactic management in the neurosurgical patient with high risk for both thrombosis and intracranial bleeding. Curr Opin Anaesthesiol. 2010; 23(5):558–563

[19] Marras LC, Geerts WH, Perry JR. The risk of venous thromboembolism is increased throughout the course of malignant glioma: an evidence-based review. Cancer. 2000; 89(3):640–646

[20] Li X, Huang R, Xu Z. Risk of adverse vascular events in newly diagnosed glioblastoma multiforme patients treated with bevacizumab: a systematic review and meta-analysis. Sci Rep. 2015; 5:14698

[21] Barker FG, II. Efficacy of prophylactic antibiotics against meningitis after craniotomy: a meta-anal-ysis. Neurosurgery. 2007; 60(5):887–894, discussion 887–894

[22] Stulberg JJ, Delaney CP, Neuhauser DV, Aron DC, Fu P, Koroukian SM. Adherence to surgical care improvement project measures and the association with postoperative infections. JAMA. 2010; 303(24):2479–2485

[23] Walcott BP, Redjal N, Coumans JV. Infection following operations on the central nervous system: deconstructing the myth of the sterile field. Neurosurg Focus. 2012; 33(5):E8

[24] Koutourousiou M, Seretis A. Aseptic meningitis after transsphenoidal management of Rathke's cleft cyst: case report and review of the literature. Neurol Sci. 2011; 32(2):323–326

[25] Lopes M, Capelle L, Duffau H, et al. [Surgery of intracranial epidermoid cysts. Report of 44 patients and review of the literature]. Neurochirurgie. 2002; 48(1):5–13

[26] O'Malley MR, Haynes DS. Assessment and management of meningitis following cerebellopontine angle surgery. Curr Opin Otolaryngol Head Neck Surg. 2008; 16(5):427–433

[27] Rajput D, Srivastva A, Kumar R, Mahapatra A. Recurrent chemical meningitis in craniopharyng-ioma without reduction in size of cyst: case report of two cases and review of the literature. Turk Neurosurg. 2012; 22(2):233–236

[28] Esquenazi Y, Lo VP, Lee K. Critical care management of cerebral edema in brain tumors. J Intensive Care Med. 2017; 32(1):15–24

[29] Rosenberg GA, Yang Y. Vasogenic edema due to tight junction disruption by matrix metalloprotei-nases in cerebral ischemia. Neurosurg Focus. 2007; 22(5):E4

[30] Gerstner ER, Duda DG, di Tomaso E, et al. VEGF inhibitors in the treatment of cerebral edema in patients with brain cancer. Nat Rev Clin Oncol. 2009; 6(4):229–236

[31] Heiss JD, Papavassiliou E, Merrill MJ, et al. Mechanism of dexamethasone suppression of brain tumor-associated vascular permeability in rats: involvement of the glucocorticoid receptor and vascular permeability factor. J Clin Invest. 1996; 98(6):1400–1408

[32] Chio CC, Baba T, Black KL. Selective blood-tumor barrier disruption by leukotrienes. J Neurosurg. 1992; 77(3):407–410

[33] Taketo MM. Cyclooxygenase-2 inhibitors in tumorigenesis (Part II). J Natl Cancer Inst. 1998; 90 (21):1609–1620

[34] Cabantog AM, Bernstein M. Complications of first craniotomy for intra-axial brain tumour. Can J Neurol Sci. 1994; 21(3):213–218

[35] Ciric I, Ammirati M, Vick N, Mikhael M. Supratentorial gliomas: surgical considerations and immediate postoperative results. Gross total resection versus partial resection. Neurosurgery. 1987; 21(1):21–26

[36] Lin AL, Avila EK. Neurologic emergencies in the patients with cancer. J Intensive Care Med. 2017; 32(2):99–115

[37] Raslan A, Bhardwaj A. Medical management of cerebral edema. Neurosurg Focus. 2007; 22(5):E1–2

[38] Feldman Z, Kanter MJ, Robertson CS, et al. Effect of head elevation on intracranial pressure, cerebral perfusion pressure, and cerebral blood flow in head-injured patients. J Neurosurg. 1992; 76 (2):207–211

[39] Ryken TC, McDermott M, Robinson PD, et al. The role of steroids in the management of brain metastases: a systematic review and evidence-based clinical practice guideline. J Neurooncol. 2010; 96(1):103–114

[40] Soffietti R, Cornu P, Delattre JY, et al. EFNS guidelines on diagnosis and treatment of brain metastases: report of an EFNS Task Force. Eur J Neurol. 2006; 13(7):674–681

[41] Illing EA, Woodworth BA. Management of frontal sinus cerebrospinal fluid leaks and encephaloceles. Otolaryngol Clin North Am. 2016; 49(4):1035–1050

[42] D'Anza B, Tien D, Stokken JK, Recinos PF, Woodard TR, Sindwani R. Role of lumbar drains in contemporary endonasal skull base surgery: meta-analysis and systematic review. Am J Rhinol Allergy. 2016; 30(6):430–435

[43] Kassam AB, Prevedello DM, Carrau RL, et al. Endoscopic endonasal skull base surgery: analysis of complications in the authors' initial 800 patients. J Neurosurg. 2011; 114(6):1544–1568

[44] Locatelli D, Vitali M, Custodi VM, Scagnelli P, Castelnuovo P, Canevari FR. Endonasal approaches to the sellar and parasellar regions: closure techniques using biomaterials. Acta Neurochir (Wien). 2009; 151(11):1431–1437

[45] Kassam A, Horowitz M, Carrau R, et al. Use of Tisseel fibrin sealant in neurosurgical procedures: incidence of cerebrospinal fluid leaks and cost-benefit analysis in a retrospective study. Neurosurgery. 2003; 52(5):1102–1105, discussion 1105

[46] Kumar A, Maartens NF, Kaye AH. Evaluation of the use of BioGlue in neurosurgical procedures. J Clin Neurosci. 2003; 10(6):661–664

[47] Ausiello JC, Bruce JN, Freda PU. Postoperative assessment of the patient after transsphenoidal pituitary surgery. Pituitary. 2008; 11(4):391–401

[48] Altaf I, Vohra AH, Shams S. Management of cerebrospinal fluid leak following posterior cranial fossa surgery. Pak J Med Sci. 2016; 32(6):1439–1443

[49] Fishman AJ, Hoffman RA, Roland JT, Jr, Lebowitz RA, Cohen NL. Cerebrospinal fluid drainage in the management of CSF leak following acoustic neuroma surgery. Laryngoscope. 1996; 106 (8):1002–1004

[50] Kankane VK, Jaiswal G, Gupta TK. Posttraumatic delayed tension pneumocephalus: Rare case with review of literature. Asian J Neurosurg. 2016; 11(4):343–347

[51] Thiagarajah S, Frost EA, Singh T, Shulman K. Cardiac arrest associated with tension pneumocephalus. Anesthesiology. 1982; 56(1):73–75

[52] Cipriani NA, Hong C, Rosenblum J, Pytel P. Air embolism with pneumocephalus. Arch Neurol. 2009; 66(9):1172–1173

[53] Çelikoğlu E, Hazneci J, Ramazanoğlu AF. Tension pneumocephalus causing brain herniation after endoscopic sinus surgery. Asian J Neurosurg. 2016; 11(3):309–310

[54] DelGaudio JM, Ingley AP. Treatment of pneumocephalus after endoscopic sinus and microscopic skull base surgery. Am J Otolaryngol. 2010; 31(4):226–230

[55] Dumont AS, Nemergut EC, II, Jane JA, Jr, Laws ER, Jr. Postoperative care following pituitary surgery. J Intensive Care Med. 2005; 20(3):127–140

[56] AbdelMannan D, Selman WR, Arafah BM. Peri-operative management of Cushing's disease. Rev Endocr Metab Disord. 2010; 11(2):127–134

[57] Nemergut EC, Zuo Z, Jane JA, Jr, Laws ER, Jr. Predictors of diabetes insipidus after transsphenoidal surgery: a review of 881 patients. J Neurosurg. 2005; 103(3):448–454

[58] Hensen J, Henig A, Fahlbusch R, Meyer M, Boehnert M, Buchfelder M. Prevalence, predictors and patterns of postoperative polyuria and hyponatraemia in the immediate course after transsphenoidal surgery for pituitary adenomas. Clin Endocrinol (Oxf). 1999; 50(4):431–439

[59] Loh JA, Verbalis JG. Diabetes insipidus as a complication after pituitary surgery. Nat Clin Pract Endocrinol Metab. 2007; 3(6):489–494

[60] Bills DC, Meyer FB, Laws ER, Jr, et al. A retrospective analysis of pituitary apoplexy. Neurosurgery. 1993; 33(4):602–608, discussion 608–609

[61] Randeva HS, Schoebel J, Byrne J, Esiri M, Adams CB, Wass JA. Classical pituitary apoplexy: clinical features, management and outcome. Clin Endocrinol (Oxf). 1999; 51(2):181–188

[62] Wakai S, Fukushima T, Teramoto A, Sano K. Pituitary apoplexy: its incidence and clinical significance. J Neurosurg. 1981; 55(2):187–193

[63] Nielsen EH, Lindholm J, Bjerre P, et al. Frequent occurrence of pituitary apoplexy in patients with non-functioning pituitary adenoma. Clin Endocrinol (Oxf). 2006; 64(3):319–322

[64] Mou C, Han T, Zhao H, Wang S, Qu Y. Clinical features and immunohistochemical changes of pituitary apoplexy. J Clin Neurosci. 2009; 16(1):64–68

[65] Fraioli B, Esposito V, Palma L, Cantore G. Hemorrhagic pituitary adenomas: clinicopathological features and surgical treatment. Neurosurgery. 1990; 27(5):741–747, discussion 747–748

[66] Riedl M, Clodi M, Kotzmann H, et al. Apoplexy of a pituitary macroadenoma with reversible third, fourth and sixth cranial nerve palsies following administration of hypothalamic releasing hormones: MR features. Eur J Radiol. 2000; 36(1):1–4

[67] Carral San Laureano F, Gavilán Villarejo I, Olveira Fuster G, Ortego Rojo J, Aguilar Diosdado M. [Pituitary apoplexy: retrospective study of 9 patients with hypophyseal adenoma]. Med Interna. 2001; 18(11):582–586

[68] Deb S. Clinical significance of pituitary apoplexy. J Indian Med Assoc. 1998; 96(10):302–303, 307

[69] Liu ZH, Chang CN, Pai PC, et al. Clinical features and surgical outcome of clinical and subclinical pituitary apoplexy. J Clin Neurosci. 2010; 17(6):694–699

[70] Baldeweg SE, Vanderpump M, Drake W, et al. Society for Endocrinology Clinical Committee. Society for Endocrinology Endocrine Emergency Guidance: emergency management of pituitary apoplexy in adult patients. Endocr Connect. 2016; 5(5):G12–G15

[71] Agrawal D, Mahapatra AK. Visual outcome of blind eyes in pituitary apoplexy after transsphenoidal surgery: a series of 14 eyes. Surg Neurol. 2005; 63(1):42–46, discussion 46

[72] Chuang CC, Chang CN, Wei KC, et al. Surgical treatment for severe visual compromised patients after pituitary apoplexy. J Neurooncol. 2006; 80(1):39–47

[73] Semple PL, Webb MK, de Villiers JC, Laws ER, Jr. Pituitary apoplexy. Neurosurgery. 2005; 56 (1):65–72, discussion 72–73

[74] Sibal L, Ball SG, Connolly V, et al. Pituitary apoplexy: a review of clinical presentation, management and outcome in 45 cases. Pituitary. 2004; 7(3):157–163

[75] Schreckinger M, Szerlip N, Mittal S. Diabetes insipidus following resection of pituitary tumors. Clin Neurol Neurosurg. 2013; 115(2):121–126

12 Brain Death in Adults

Rodney D. Bell, Norman Ajiboye, and Yu Kan Au

Abstract

Since the passage of the Uniform Determination of Death Act of 1981, the concept of brain death has become widely accepted. Actual policies for determination of brain death have been developed by local institutions and vary with personnel and equipment availability. Unfortunately, there is great variability.[1] Legal requirements for the declaration of brain death differ by states and hospital policy, while protocols for determining brain death vary by institutions. Brain death is defined as the irreversible cessation of cerebral function due to an identified proximate cause. Reversible causes of coma must be excluded. A properly performed brain death examination establishes the diagnosis in the absence of ancillary tests. The presence of confounders in the brain death examination necessitates ancillary testing. The preferred ancillary tests are cerebral angiography, cerebral scintigraphy, transcranial Doppler, and electro-encephalogram (EEG). This chapter describes the clinical evaluation of brain death as per Thomas Jefferson University protocol. Reversible causes of coma are discussed. The brain death examination is described. The indications and proper selection of ancillary testing in brain death evaluation are presented.

Keywords: brain death, apnea test, irreversible coma, brainstem reflexes, cerebral edema

12.1 Definition of Brain Death[2,3,4,5]

Irreversible cessation of cerebral function due to an identified proximate cause. According to the American Academy of Neurology, brain death is defined as "irreversible loss of function of the brain including the brainstem."

12.2 Clinical Evaluation[2,3,4,5]

Clinical evaluation of brain death involves establishing a proximate cause and irreversibility. A proximate cause of brain death can be established through history, examination, and neuroimaging. Irreversibility is established through exclusion of reversible causes and proper performance of the brain death examination.

12.2.1 Establishing the Proximate Cause of Coma

- History, examination, laboratory testing, and neuroimaging should help inform the cause of coma.
- Neuroimaging usually demonstrates structural lesions such as a mass or stroke causing significant midline shift, or profound diffuse cerebral edema.
- Normal neuroimaging may be seen early after certain conditions such as cardiopulmonary arrest. In these cases, repeat neuroimaging may reveal structural lesions.
- Exclude reversible causes prior to clinical examinations (▶ Table 12.1).

12.2.2 Clinical Examination to Establish Irreversibility

General Examination

- No awakening; coma (no responsiveness)
- No cerebral motor response to noxious stimuli in all four limbs:
  - No decerebrate or decorticate posturing
  - Spinal reflexes such as tendon reflex or triple-flexion may be present[2,3,4,6]

Table 12.1 Reversible causes of coma

Reversible causes	Clinical evaluations
Profound hypothermia	Core body temperature should be $\geq 36\,°C$ (96.8 °F).
Drug intoxication/ CNS depressants effect	Ensure there is no history of CNS depressants use. Check drug screen. If prior CNS depressants were used: • Calculate clearance using five times the drug's half-life (assuming normal hepatic and renal function). • Confirm drug plasma levels below the therapeutic. • Hypothermia and shock liver (i.e., after cardiopulmonary resuscitation for cardiac arrest) may delay drug metabolism; therefore, there should be adequate time prior to initiating the formal examination. • The legal alcohol limit for driving (blood alcohol content 0.08%) is a practical threshold below which an examination to determine brain death could reasonably proceed.
Neuromuscular blockade	Often patients are paralyzed for procedures or intubation. The presence of a train of four twitches with maximal ulnar nerve stimulation confirms the absence of neuromuscular blockade.
Severe metabolic disturbance	Rule out profound acid–base, endocrine, or electrolyte disturbances. Note there is no standard for metabolic disturbances. It is physician's preference.

Abbreviation: CNS, central nervous system.

- No facial movements to noxious stimuli, including blinking
- No spontaneous respiration (patient is not overbreathing on ventilator)
- Confounder: High cervical cord lesion may abolish motor response[5]

Absence of Cranial Nerve Reflexes

Confounder: Pre-existing cranial neuropathies or neuromuscular disease may render cranial nerve examination unreliable (▶ Table 12.2).

Absence of Respiratory Drive[2,3,4,5,7]

The apnea test relies on rapidly increasing $PaCO_2$ to > 60 or 20 mm Hg above baseline to trigger the respiratory drive center in the medulla (▶ Table 12.3 and ▶ Table 12.4).

12.3 Ancillary Tests[2,3,4,9]

In the United States, ancillary tests are not required for the diagnosis of brain death in adults. Ancillary tests are indicated when clinical examination is unreliable or when apnea test cannot be completed (▶ Table 12.5). Existing ancillary tests either measure cerebral blood flow or cerebral electrical activity.

- Preferred tests include cerebral angiography, cerebral scintigraphy, transcranial ultrasound (TCDs), and electroencephalogram (EEG).
- Ancillary tests that are being investigated but are still awaiting validation include cerebral CT angiography and MR angiography, as well as evoked potentials (▶ Table 12.6).[2,10]

12.4 Legal

In the United States, the Uniform Determination of Death Act mandates the determination of death in accordance with accepted medical standards at the national, regional, or local level, which leads to institutional variations in brain death protocols.[1]

Check with local laws and hospital policies regarding required number of clinical examinations and requirements regarding medical specialist allowed to perform examination (any physician vs. intensive care physician vs. neurologist vs. neurosurgeon, etc.). The indication of ancillary testing will vary based on hospital policy and availability.

Any patient who had been pronounced brain dead by neurologic criteria should be evaluated for suitability for organ donation (see ▶ Fig. 12.1). Involvement of the organ procurement organization will vary by hospital.

Table 12.2 Evaluation of cranial nerves

Cranial nerve	Examination	Confounders
CN II, III	Pupil unreactive and midposition or dilated	Pre-existing pupillary abnormalities renders the examination unreliable. Medication may influence pupil size.
CN III, VI, VIII	Absence of spontaneous ocular movements Absence of oculocephalic reflex (doll's eyes) • Rapid lateral head turn from midline to 90 degrees on both sides • Ocular movements should be absent Absence of vestibulo-ocular reflex (caloric testing) • Elevate head to 30 degrees • Inspect ear canal prior to testing, ensure that ear canal is patent • Inject 50 mL of ice water into each ear canal • Observe for 1 minute after each irrigation • Allow for 5-minute interval between the irrigation of each ear • Ocular movements should be absent	Chemosis, eyelid edema, and other structural abnormalities may impair ocular movements. Placing the patient in a cervical collar due to traumatic injury will not allow for the oculocephalic reflex to be performed. The lack of vestibulo-ocular reflex would be considered adequate; however, both should be performed when able. Obstructed ear canal may render the caloric testing inaccurate. Inspect ear canal prior to testing. Pre-existing lesions from trauma (e.g., skull base fractures) or medication intoxication may abolish the vestibulo-ocular reflex.
CN V, VII	Absence of corneal reflex Absence of facial movement to noxious stimulation	No grimace or response to noxious stimulation
CN IX, X	Absence of gag reflex (both sides) to stimulation of posterior pharynx Absence of cough reflex to stimulation of the trachea through in-line suctioning	

12.5 Management of the Brain-Dead Patient for Organ Donation

Maintain physiologic goals to prepare organs for transplantation.[17,18,19]
• Continuous hemodynamic monitoring
• Placement of arterial and/or central venous catheter may be needed if not already in place

Table 12.3 Evaluation of respiratory drive prerequisites

	Prerequisites for apnea test	Comments
1	Core body temperature ≥ 36 °C (96.8 °F)	Carbon dioxide production rate is slowed in hypothermia secondary to decreased metabolic rate.[5]
2	Pre-oxygenate for a minimum of 10 minutes prior to initiation of the apnea test to target PaO2 > 200 mm Hg	Pre-oxygenation minimizes the risk of early desaturation during the apnea test.[5,7,8]
3	Euvolemia (or exclusion of hypovolemia)	Minimize the risk of hypotension during the apnea test.
4	Systolic pressures > 100 mm Hg	Minimize the risk of hypotension during the apnea test. Vasopressors should be at the bedside during the test if needed.
5	PaCO2 within normal range (35–45 mm Hg)	Adjustments to the ventilator may be necessary in order to obtain proper PaCO2.
6	No prior evidence of CO_2 retention such as history of COPD or severe obesity	Chronic CO_2 retention may blunt the respiratory drive stimulated by rapid increase in PaCO2.[5,7] If present requires confirmatory test.

Abbreviation: COPD, chronic obstructive pulmonary disease.

- Central venous pressure (CVP) monitoring with CVP goal of 5 to 10 mm Hg
- Maintain euvolemia
  - Diabetes insipidus is common after brain herniation and careful attention should be paid to urine output hourly and sodium changes
    - Goal is to maintain urine output less than or equal to 300 mL/hour
    - Desmopressin (DDVAP) 2 to 4 mcg/day IV or vasopressin 50 units/100 mL (0.5 units/mL). Start between 1 and 5 units/hour and titrate to desired urine output (UOP).
- Maintain temperature between 36 and 38 °C
- Maintain systolic blood pressure (SBP) above 100 mm Hg
- Frequent labs to assess electrolytes and replete as needed
- Thyroid protocol may be applied in certain circumstances:
  - Levothyroxine 20 mcg IV bolus; followed by infusion 200 mcg/500 mL NSS (0.4 mcg/mL); start at 20 mcg/hour and titrate to SBP > 100 mm Hg (max dose 40 mcg/hour)
  - Solumedrol 2 grams IV bolus
  - Dextrose 50% 1 amp (50 mL) IV bolus

Table 12.4 Performance of apnea test

	Apnea test	Comments
1	Disconnect ventilator and provide O_2 via cannula into the trachea at approximately the level of the carina at a flow rate of 6 LPM.	Baseline blood gas should have CO_2 in normal range as described in Table 12.3.
2	Observe for respiratory movements. If respiratory movements are present, replace ventilator and abort test.	Bring patient's gown to the pelvic area exposing the chest and upper abdomen. Note that carotid pulsations in the neck and chest can often be seen and should not be misconstrued for respiratory movement.
3	Continue the test for 8 minutes. During that time the SaO2 should be maintained by > 90% and the SBP > 100 mm Hg. Vasopressors should be used to maintain SBP and O_2 flow can be increased to continue proper saturation.	If unable to maintain these measures, a blood gas should be drawn and the patient should be placed back on the ventilator. If PaCO2 > 60 or 20 mm Hg above baseline, then the apnea test is considered positive (confirmation of lack of respiratory drive).
4	After 8 minutes, draw arterial blood gas. The test can be continued while waiting for the results if the patient remains stable. If the initial blood gas does not meet criteria another gas can be sent.	If the patient is unable to tolerate the full test and/or the blood gas does not show a PaCO2 > 60 or 20 mm Hg above baseline, the test is considered inconclusive. The test can be repeated later if labs and vitals remain stable.
5	If the test is unable to be performed or remains inconclusive then an ancillary test should be performed.	

Abbreviation: SBP, systolic blood pressure.

Table 12.5 Indications for ancillary testing

	Indications for ancillary tests[2,4,5,9]
1	Reversible causes cannot be excluded, e.g., severe metabolic disturbance cannot be corrected.
2	Clinical examination may be unreliable due to presence of confounders as listed Table 12.4.
3	Inability to achieve prerequisite conditions for apnea testing as listed Table 12.4.
4	Inability to complete an apnea test.
5	Use of extracorporeal membrane oxygenation (ECMO).

Table 12.6 Ancillary tests

List of ancillary tests	Confirmatory findings	Comments
Cerebral angiography	Positive study is marked by absence of cerebral perfusion after contrast injection into the common carotid and vertebral artery origins bilaterally from the aorta.[2,4,11]	Considered "gold standard" in assessing intracranial blood flow Disadvantages: Invasive procedure, requires two injections at least 20 minutes apart, requires transport, difficult to coordinate in hemodynamically unstable patients, potential for allergic reaction to contrast
Cerebral scintigraphy Nuclear Medicine Technetium Scan	Confirmatory finding is characterized by the "hollow skull" appearance with visualized flow only in the external carotid circulation.[12,13]	Advantages: Includes its long history of use Disadvantages: Lack of availability, time consuming, requires transport, lack of uptake with hypothermia and barbiturates, difficult to coordinate in hemodynamically unstable patients
EEG	Confirmatory finding is characterized by electrocerebral silence demonstrated by an isoelectric pattern, as well as a lack of reactivity to visual, auditory, and sensory stimuli.	Testing requirements include[2,14]: • Sensitivity settings of at least 2 μV for a testing duration of at least 30 minutes. • Interelectrode impedances should be under 10,000 Ohms and over 100 Ohms. • Interelectrode distances should be at least 10 cm. Advantages: Performed on bedside, noninvasive, quick Disadvantages: Affected by electrical artifact, susceptible to false positives
Transcranial Dopplers	Positive findings include oscillating flow which represents reversal of diastolic flow and small systolic peaks in early systole which represent lack of net forward flow.[15,16]	Advantages: Safe, noninvasive, inexpensive, performed on bedside Disadvantages: Operator dependence, lack of acoustic window in some patients, bilateral anterior and posterior vessels must be insonated[4] Absence of flow is not reliable as it may indicate absence of suitable acoustic window

Abbreviation: EEG, electroencephalogram.

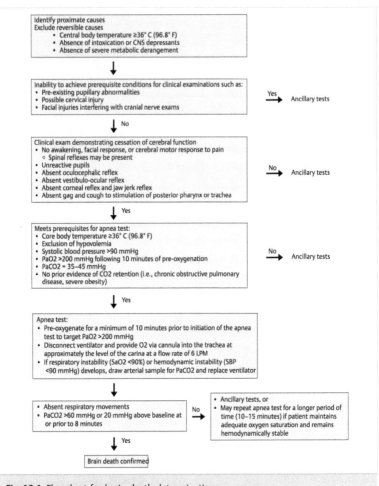

Fig. 12.1 Flowchart for brain death determination.

- Regular insulin 20 units IV bolus
- Vasopressin 1 unit IV bolus
- Obtain serum quantitative beta human chorionic gonadotropin (HCG) (for all female donors over the age of 10)
- For potential lung donors, perform O_2 challenge, to be completed every 4 hours, or more often if indicated

○ **O$_2$ challenge:** Draw baseline arterial blood gas (ABG), place patient on FiO$_2$ 100% and positive end-expiratory pressure (PEEP) 5 cm H$_2$O for 20 minutes, then repeat ABG.

References

[1] Powell T, Zisfein J, Halperin J. Variability of brain death determination guidelines in leading US neurologic institutions. Neurology. 2008; 71(22):1839–1840, author reply 1839–1840

[2] Thomas Jefferson University policy for determination of death by neurologic criteria in adults

[3] The Quality Standards Subcommittee of the American Academy of Neurology. Practice parameters for determining brain death in adults (summary statement). Neurology. 1995; 45(5):1012–1014

[4] Wijdicks EFM, Varelas PN, Gronseth GS, Greer DM, American Academy of Neurology. Evidence-based guideline update: determining brain death in adults: report of the Quality Standards Subcommittee of the American Academy of Neurology. Neurology. 2010; 74(23):1911–1918

[5] Wijdicks EF. Brain death guidelines explained. Semin Neurol. 2015; 35(2):105–115

[6] Saposnik G, Basile VS, Young GB. Movements in brain death: a systematic review. Can J Neurol Sci/Journal Canadien des Sciences Neurologiques. 2009; 36(2):154–160

[7] Scott JB, Gentile MA, Bennett SN, Couture M, MacIntyre NR. Apnea testing during brain death assessment: a review of clinical practice and published literature. Respir Care. 2013; 58(3):532–538

[8] Yee AH, Mandrekar J, Rabinstein AA, Wijdicks EF. Predictors of apnea test failure during brain death determination. Neurocrit Care. 2010; 12(3):352–355

[9] Kramer AH. Ancillary testing in brain death. Semin Neurol. 2015; 35(2):125–138

[10] Welschehold S, Boor S, Reuland K, et al. Technical aids in the diagnosis of brain death: a comparison of SEP, AEP, EEG, TCD and CT angiography. Dtsch Arztebl Int. 2012; 109(39):624–630

[11] Savard M, Turgeon AF, Gariépy J-L, Trottier F, Langevin S. Selective 4 vessels angiography in brain death: a retrospective study. Can J Neurol Sci. 2010; 37(4):492–497

[12] Sinha P, Conrad GR. Scintigraphic confirmation of brain death. Semin Nucl Med. 2012; 42(1):27–32

[13] Munari M, Zucchetta P, Carollo C, et al. Confirmatory tests in the diagnosis of brain death: comparison between SPECT and contrast angiography. Crit Care Med. 2005; 33(9):2068–2073

[14] American Clinical Neurophysiology Society. Guideline 3: minimum technical standards for EEG recording in suspected cerebral death. J Clin Neurophysiol. 2006; 23(2):97–104

[15] Sharma D, Souter MJ, Moore AE, Lam AM. Clinical experience with transcranial Doppler ultrasonography as a confirmatory test for brain death: a retrospective analysis. Neurocrit Care. 2011; 14 (3):370–376

[16] Chang JJ, Tsivgoulis G, Katsanos AH, Malkoff MD, Alexandrov AV. Diagnostic accuracy of transcranial Doppler for brain death confirmation: systematic review and meta-analysis. AJNR Am J Neuroradiol. 2016; 37(3):408–414

[17] Gift of Life Donor Program. Organ donor evaluation and standard orders for the adult

[18] Rech TH, Moraes RB, Crispim D, Czepielewski MA, Leitão CB. Management of the brain-dead organ donor: a systematic review and meta-analysis. Transplantation. 2013; 95(7):966–974

[19] McKeown DW, Bonser RS, Kellum JA. Management of the heartbeating brain-dead organ donor. Br J Anaesth. 2012; 108 Suppl 1:i96–i107

13 Sodium Dysregulation

M. Kamran Athar and Christian Bacheler

Abstract

Disorders of sodium regulation leading to either hyponatremia or hypernatremia are seen frequently in the critical care setting, and have particular importance in the setting of neurologic injury, surgery, and disease. This chapter is split into two major sections: hyponatremia and hypernatremia. For each, a basic overview with important features are provided, followed by a list of possible causes, an approach to the diagnosis (with specific focus on neurologically relevant etiologies such as syndrome of inappropriate antidiuretic hormone secretion (SIADH), cerebral salt wasting (CSW), and diabetes insipidus), and finally our recommendations on the general approach to treatment. Useful terminology and equations are also provided throughout the chapter that may assist in the bedside management while rounding in the critical care unit.

Keywords: hyponatremia, hypernatremia, SIADH, cerebral salt wasting, diabetes insipidus, hypertonic saline, free water deficit

13.1 Terminology

- **Tonicity:** total concentration of nonpenetrating solutes (effective plasma osmolality)
- **Osmolarity:** total concentration of penetrating and nonpenetrating solutes (mOsm/L of solution = mmol/L)
- **Osmolality:** per kg of solvent (normal range: 275–290 mOsm/kg)
- **Calculation:** Serum Osmolality = 2 × Serum [Na] + Serum Glucose/18 + Blood urea nitrogen (BUN)/2.8

13.2 Hyponatremia Classification

Multiple factors are taken into consideration when classifying hyponatremia. In addition to serum sodium concentration, the patient's volume status and serum and urine osmolality should be taken into consideration. Hyponatremia is defined as serum $[Na^+] < 135$ mEq/L[1] with severity based on the concentration. Hyponatremia can be found in a wide range of hospitalized patients (1–15%) but is far more common in patients with neurologic injury ranging from 15 to 30% depending on the etiology.[23] Depending on the concentration, hyponatremia can be categorized by severity: Mild: 130–135 mEq/L, Moderate:

125–129 mEq/L; Severe: < 125 mEq/L. It can be broken into additional categories based on serum osmolality and urine Na + concentration (▶ Fig. 13.1).

13.2.1 Causes of Hyponatremia

There are multiple medical conditions associated with hyponatremia including surgery, critical illness, medications, and advanced age. Hyponatremia has also been associated in patients with traumatic brain injury, subarachnoid hemorrhage, meningitis, and brain tumors. ▶ Table 13.1 details various causes of hyponatremia.

13.2.2 Symptomatic Hyponatremia

Symptomatic hyponatremia typically occurs with a serum sodium concentration < 125 mEq/L. However, symptoms are more likely to occur when there is a rapid sodium change.[2] In chronic conditions where the sodium concentration decreases over months, the brain is able to adapt by decreasing tonicity and subsequently the patient may remain relatively asymptomatic despite moderate to severe degree of hyponatremia.[3]

- **Mild hyponatremia** ([Na] 130–135 mEq/L): Asymptomatic

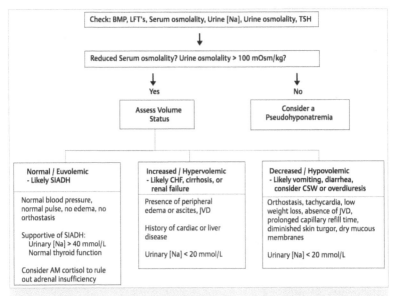

Fig. 13.1 Diagnostic approach to hyponatremia.

Table 13.1 Causes of hyponatremia based on classification

Causes of hyponatremia based on osmolality and volume status

Hypo-osmolar euvolemia	Hypo-osmolar hypervolemia	Hypo-osmolar hypovolemia		Normo-osmolar "pseudohyponatremia"	Hyper-osmolar
		Renal Na + losses	Extrarenal losses		
SIADH	Congestive heart failure			Severe hypertriglyceridemia	Hyperglycemia
Hypothyroid	Acute or chronic renal failure	Diuretic use	Vomiting	Hyperproteinemia	Hypertonic infusions
PAIN	Nephrotic syndrome	Cerebral salt wasting	Diarrhea	Mannitol infusion	Hypertonic saline
Thiazide diuretics	Cirrhosis	Adrenal insufficiency	Excessive sweating	Ethanol ingestion	
Water intoxication	Pregnancy	Renal tubular acidosis	"Third space" losses	Isotonic fluids • Glucose • Glycerol • Sorbitol • Glycine	

Abbreviation: SIADH, syndrome of inappropriate antidiuretic hormone secretion.

- **Moderate hyponatremia ([Na] 124–129 mEq/L):** Nausea, malaise, confusion, headache, vomiting, lethargy, and increasing disorientation as the sodium concentration drops[3,22]
- **Severe hyponatremia (typically [Na] < 125 mEq/L):** In addition to the above-mentioned, seizures, coma, permanent brain damage, respiratory failure, brainstem herniation, and death[3,22]

Seizures typically occur with serum sodium concentrations < 120 mEq/L. Although the absolute risk of seizure ranges from 2.5 to 10% depending on the serum concentration with the higher risk related to concentrations < 110 mEq/L.[4]

13.3 SIADH versus CSW

13.3.1 Syndrome of Inappropriate Antidiuretic Hormone Secretion (SIADH)

- Characterized by excessive antidiuretic hormone (ADH) release leading to increased renal water reabsorption, extracellular fluid (ECF) expansion, and hyponatremia. Due to a variety of causes (▶ Table 13.2), ADH is unable to be fully suppressed despite the condition of hypo-osmolality.[5]
- SIADH should be suspected in any patient with hyponatremia, hypo-osmolality, and a urine osmolality > 100 mOsm/kg, after the exclusion of thyroid, adrenal, and renal causes. In SIADH, the urine sodium concentration is usually above 40 mEq/L, the serum potassium concentration is normal, there is no acid-base disturbance, and the serum uric acid concentration is frequently low.[6]

13.3.2 Cerebral Salt Wasting (CSW)

- Hypovolemic hyponatremia observed in subarachnoid hemorrhage, head injury, neurosurgical procedures, stroke, meningitis, and neoplasms (primitive neuroectodermal tumors with intraventricular dissemination, carcinomatous meningitis, glioma, and primary CNS lymphoma).[5,8]
- Hyponatremia is commonly seen in stroke, and may be from either SIADH or CSW. In ischemic stroke, hyponatremia has been reported in up to 11.5% of ischemic strokes, and 15.6% of intracerebral hemorrhage (ICH).[9,10] One study revealed hyponatremia to be present in 36.4% of ischemic strokes and 51.9% of ICH (over the entire hospital stay), and was attributed to CSW in 44.2% of cases.[11]

Table 13.2 Causes of SIADH[2,3,6,7]

Malignancy	Neurologic/Neuropsychiatric	Drugs/Medications	Other medical causes
Pulmonary tumors	Encephalitis/Meningitis	AVP analogues • DDAVP • Oxytocin • Vasopressin	Infection
Renal Cell Ca	Subarachnoid hemorrhage	Antiseizure meds • Carbamazepine • Valproate	Acute respiratory failure
Mediastinal tumors	Traumatic brain injury	Chemotherapeutics • Vincristine • Vinblastine • Cisplatin	Cystic fibrosis
Lymphoma/Leukemia	Intracerebral hemorrhage	SSRI, TCAs, MAOIs	HIV
Pituitary tumors	Stroke	Antipsychotics • Haldol • Thiothixene • Thioridazine	Nausea
Prostate	Demyelinating/Neuroinflammatory disorders	Amiodarone	Acute psychosis
Prolactinoma	Hydrocephalus	Amitriptyline	Stress
Osteosarcoma	Acute intermittent porphyria	MDMA "ecstasy"	Hereditary

Abbreviations: AVP, arginine vasopressin; DDAVP, D-amino D-arginine vasopressin; HIV, human immunodeficiency virus; MAOIs, monoamine oxidase inhibitors; MDMA, 3,4-methylenedioxymethamphetamine; SIADH, syndrome of inappropriate antidiuretic hormone secretion; SSRI, selective serotonin reuptake inhibitor; TCAs, tricyclic antidepressants.

It is characterized by volume contraction from renal salt wasting (differentiated from the volume expanded state of SIADH). It is important to distinguish CSW from SIADH.

13.3.3 SIADH and CSW Diagnosis

Accurate determination of the patient's volume status is crucial to differentiate these syndromes (see ▶ Table 13.3 and ▶ Fig. 13.1). Physical examination and other clinical measures can be useful to assess volume status, with evidence of a hypovolemic state increasing the likelihood of a CSW diagnosis.

Table 13.3 Differentiating SIADH from CSW

Feature	SIADH	Cerebral salt wasting
Volume status	Euvolemia to mild hypervolemia	Hypovolemia
Serum [Na+]	Low	Low
Urine [Na+]	Increased (>40 mEq/L)	Increased (>40 mEq/L)
Serum osmolality	Low	Low
Urine osmolality	High (>100 mOsm/kg)	High (>100 mOsm/kg)
Urine output	Normal	Increased
Serum uric acid	Low	Normal or low
Serum bicarbonate	Normal or low	Increased
Central venous pressure	Normal or slightly elevated (6–10 cm H_2O)	Low (<6 cm H_2O)
BUN	Normal or low	Increased
Mechanism	Water retention due to increased ADH secretion	Excess secretion of water and sodium

Abbreviations: ADH, antidiuretic hormone; BUN, blood urea nitrogen; CSW, cerebral salt wasting; SIADH, syndrome of inappropriate antidiuretic hormone secretion.

13.4 Diagnostic Approach to Hyponatremia

- Initial testing considerations: Basic metabolic panel, hepatic function panel, serum osmolality, urine sodium, urine osmolality, and thyroid stimulating hormone (TSH)
- May also consider obtaining AM cortisol if adrenal insufficiency is suspected

Additional notes on serum osmolality:
- Correction for hyperglycemia: To calculate the "corrected" serum sodium, we recommend the use of the following ratio: The sodium concentration will fall by 1.7 mEq/L for each 100 mg/100 mL (5.5 mmol/L) increase in glucose concentration.[12]
- Correct for azotemia: Tonicity = Measured serum osmolality – (BUN ÷ 2.8)

Dividing the BUN by 2.8 converts mg/dL of urea nitrogen into mmol/L of urea, which is required when calculating osmolality. If blood urea is measured in units of mmol/L, simply subtract without dividing by 2.8.[13]

13.4.1 Hyponatremia Treatment: General Principles

- Risk of osmotic demyelination (formerly known as central pontine myelinolysis)
    - **High risk:** [Na] < 105 mEq/L, hypokalemia, alcoholism, malnutrition, and liver disease[14]
    - **Low risk:** Hyperacute hyponatremia (over a few hours) as they have not had time to develop brain adaptations that increase risk of osmotic demyelination
- **Goal:** Increase [Na +] by 6–8 mEq/L in 24 hours; 12–14 mEq/L in 48 hours.
- *Do not correct serum Na at a rate greater than 10 mEq/L in 24 hours* (and no more than 18 in first 48 hours)
- Recheck serum sodium every 4 hours for the first 24 hours, and at regular intervals thereafter until stabilized.

13.4.2 Acute Symptomatic Moderate to Severe Hyponatremia

Serum [Na] usually < 129 mEq/L with symptoms that can include confusion, nausea (without vomiting), headache, somnolence, and hallucinations. More severe symptoms include: vomiting, seizures, cardiorespiratory arrest, abnormal and deep somnolence, and coma (Glasgow coma score [GCS] < 8).

Treatment

Use 3% hypertonic saline infusion to raise the serum [Na]

- **Initial emergent therapy:** Over the first 4 to 6 hours, determine the rate to increase the serum [Na] by roughly 1 mEq/hour. It has been shown that a 4 to 6 mEq/L increase in Na concentration is adequate in the most seriously ill patients.[15]

Note: With more severe symptoms, a 100 mL bolus of 3% hypertonic saline can be considered.

- Check serum [Na] after 4 hours, and adjust rate of 3% hypertonic saline solution so that total rise in serum [Na] will not be greater than 10 to 12 mEq over the first 24-hour period.

Determining the Rate of 3% Hypertonic Saline Infusion

- Determine the desired change in serum [Na] (and thus, the desired [Na])
- Determine the desired timeframe to achieve this change
- Determine rate of 3% hypertonic saline infusion using the following approach:

Solve for the amount of fluid needed to reach the desired [Na] by using this formula:

(Current amount of sodium in patient*) $+ \dfrac{\text{(Sodium added with 3\% saline)}}{\text{(Total body water [TBW]+Amount of fluid added)}}$

$=$ Desired [Na]

Next, solve for the rate by dividing the amount of fluid added by the desired timeframe

Note: To determine current amount of sodium in patient, multiply the TBW by the current [Na]. TBW in L = Weight (kg) × 0.6 (or 0.5 in females)

Example of a Rate Calculation

Patient = 70 kg male, Current Serum [Na] = 115 mEq/L, Desired Serum [Na] = 120 mEq/L, Desired time = 5 hours

First determine how many liters (X) of 3% hypertonic saline is needed to be added to the patient to achieve 120 mEq/L.

[Current amount of sodium in patient] $+ \dfrac{\text{[Sodium added with 3\% saline]}}{\text{[TBW + Amount of fluid added]}}$ 1 L = 120 mEq

[TBW × 115 mEq/L + [(513 mEq/L) × X]
= 120 mEq *Solve for X...* X/TBW + X 1 L = 0.53 L

Divide the amount of 3% hypertonic saline (0.53 L in this example) by desired timeframe (5 hours)

Rate = 107 cc/hour[a]

13.4.3 Acute Asymptomatic Moderate Hyponatremia

We recommend using 3% hypertonic saline to raise the serum [Na] at a rate of 0.5 mEq/hour. Remember to check serum [Na] every 4 hours and to adjust rate as needed so as not to exceed a rise of 10 mEq over the first 24 hours.

13.4.4 Severe Chronic Mild-Moderate Hyponatremia

A slow intravenous infusion of 3% hypertonic saline at 15 to 30 mL/hour can be considered. Only replete the sodium back to around the patient's baseline level. The infusion rate should be titrated, aiming for a correction rate of 6 mEq/L per day.

---

[a]There are many easy-to-use calculators available online.

13.4.5 SIADH Treatment

- Fluid restriction is a mainstay of therapy in most patients with SIADH, with a suggested goal intake of less than 800 mL/day.[2] Beware of fluid restriction in the diagnosis of SIADH in aneurysmal SAH (as it may increase risk of delayed ischemic deficits and mortality).[16]
- ADH receptor antagonists (tolvaptan or conivaptan): If fluid restriction alone does not correct the hyponatremia, ADH receptor antagonists can be considered. We recommend tolvaptan, 15 or 30 mg given orally twice a day. Often may only need to give first two doses. If there is no oral access, we recommend parenteral conivaptan: An initial loading dose of 20 mg over 30 minutes is recommended. This is followed by a continuous infusion at a rate of 20 mg/day for up to 4 days.[17]
- Sodium should be monitored closely (every 6 hours) when starting treatment with one of these medications.
- Loop diuretic (furosemide 20 mg twice a day)—caution for hypokalemia and potential for kidney injury
- **Salt tablets:** they can be difficult for patients to swallow or tolerate.
- Correct underlying disease process.

13.4.6 CSW Treatment

- **Volume repletion with isotonic saline:** Can be given in small boluses (500 cc) if not contraindicated.
- If refractory, consider fludrocortisone (starting oral dose of 0.1–0.2 mg twice a day) and/or salt tabs.

13.4.7 Treatment of Hyponatremia in Patients with Subarachnoid Hemorrhage

- Avoid fluid restriction for the first 10 to 14 days due to potential risk for delayed cerebral ischemia.
- If hyponatremia is significant ([Na] < 130) and persistent (greater than 24 hours), we recommend to treat with hypertonic (3%) saline to both preserve cerebral perfusion and prevent complications from hyponatremia-induced brain swelling. We recommend administering with a calculated rate to raise the serum [Na] at roughly 0.5 mEq/hour.
- ADH receptor antagonists may be also be considered (as described above for SIADH treatment).

13.4.8 Treatment of Hyponatremia in Patients with Heart Failure

- Treat when serum [Na] < 120
- Fluid restriction
- Can consider ADH receptor antagonists and/or loop diuretics (furosemide 20 mg twice a day, or if already on a loop diuretic, increasing the dose)

13.5 Hypernatremia

- Typically defined as a serum [Na] > 145 mEq/L.
- Frequently seen in the neonatal intensive care unit (NICU) setting, and most commonly from excess free water loss (or iatrogenic with hypertonic saline administration); however, the clinician should always consider other etiologies when it is not immediately evident. ▶ Table 13.4 details some of the causes of hypernatremia.
- Orthostatic hypotension and oliguria are typical findings, with other early signs being lethargy, irritability, and weakness. Severe symptoms include delirium, seizures, and coma (which are typically seen with serum [Na] > 158 mEq/L). Osmotic demyelination is uncommon, but can also be seen in severe hypernatremia.[3]

13.5.1 Central (Neurogenic) Diabetes Insipidus

- Characterized by an insufficient release of ADH. Symptoms include polyuria, nocturia, and polydipsia.
- **Causes:** Most often idiopathic (possibly due to autoimmune injury to the ADH-producing cells). Other causes include central herniation, brain death, tumors (pituitary adenoma and apoplexy, suprasellar germ cell tumors, hypothalamic tumors such as an eosinophilic granuloma, and rarely with a colloid cyst), mass lesions pressing on hypothalamus (ACom aneurysm), trauma (basal skull fractures), encephalitis or meningitis, drug induced (ethanol and phenytoin), granulomatous diseases (Wegener's, neurosarcoidosis involving hypothalamus), and inflammatory (autoimmune hypophysitis or lymphocytic infundibuloneurohypophysitis).[19]
- Another important cause of central diabetes insipidus (DI) is damage to the pituitary gland or the pituitary stalk following transsphenoidal pituitary surgery or removal of a craniopharyngioma. Postoperative DI generally follows three patterns[19]:
  1. Transient DI—duration 12 to 36 hours post-op
  2. "Prolonged" DI—duration of months, may be permanent
  3. "Triphasic response" (least common)

Table 13.4 Causes of hypernatremia (adapted from Adrogué and Madias[18])

Inadequate water intake	Excessive sodium	Renal loss	Drugs/Medications	GI loss	Skin loss
Impaired thirst	Excessive ingestion • Accidental • Intentional	Diabetes insipidus • Central neurogenic • Nephrogenic	Alcohol	Diarrhea	Burns
Inability to swallow water • Mechanical • Lack of access	Primary hyperaldosteronism	Loop diuretics	Phenytoin	Vomiting	Excessive sweating
	Cushing's syndrome	Impaired renal concentration	Lithium	Enterocutaneous fistula	Hyperthermia
	Sea water intake	Osmotic diuretics • Urea • Mannitol • Glucose	Amphotericin B	Nasogastric drainage	
	Hypertonic saline infusion	Post-obstructive diuresis	Conivaptan, tolvaptan		
		Polyuric phase of ATN	Aminoglycosides		

Abbreviation: ATN, acute tubular necrosis.

○ **Phase 1 (DI):** Injury to pituitary—reduced ADH levels for 4 to 5 days, polyuria/polydipsia

○ **Phase 2 (SIADH):** Cell death liberates ADH for next 4 to 5 days, normalization/water retention

○ **Phase 3 (DI):** Reduced or absent ADH secretion, can be transient or prolonged

13.5.2 Nephrogenic Diabetes Insipidus

• Characterized by normal ADH secretion but varying degrees of renal resistance to its water-retaining effect. This problem, in its mild form, is relatively common since most patients who are elderly or who have underlying renal disease have a reduction in maximum concentrating ability.

• Nephrogenic DI presenting in adults is almost always acquired with chronic lithium use and hypercalcemia being one of the most common causes of a defect severe enough to produce polyuria. Additional causes include urinary obstruction, renal disease (medullary cystic disease and interstitial nephritis), hypercalcemia, hypokalemia, drugs other than lithium (demeclocycline, foscarnet, methoxyflurane, amphotericin B, vasopressin V2-receptor antagonists), and those listed in ▸ Table 13.5.[3,7]

13.6 Diagnostic Approach to Hypernatremia

• Check urine and serum osmolality, urine output, basic metabolic panel, and serum calcium. Can consider AM cortisol, Sjögren antibodies, and angiotensin-converting enzyme (ACE) level.

• DI: Dilute urine (urine osmolality < 200 mOsm/L or specific gravity < 1.003), urine output > 250 cc/hour, normal or above-normal serum [Na], and normal adrenal function[19]

○ With high serum osmolality – > DI

– To differentiate central from nephrogenic DI, give 5 units of vasopressin (subcutaneous). In central DI, urine osmolality should double within 1 to 2 hours[19]

○ Low serum osmolality – > polydipsia

○ A water deprivation test can be performed if the diagnosis of DI is not clear. This will help determine if the patient can concentrate urine with dehydration.[19]

• Urine osmolality > 400 mmol/L indicates that the renal-conserving system is intact. Hypernatremia is caused when hypotonic fluid loss (sweating, diarrhea, respiratory, bowel) exceeds free water intake.[3]

Table 13.5 Causes of nephrogenic diabetes insipidus (adapted from Rose and Post[7])

Congenital disorders	Medications • Lithium • Colchicine • Fluoride • Demeclocycline • Amphotericin B • Methoxyflurane • Aminoglycosides
Polycystic kidney disease	Infiltration • Amyloidosis • Sjögren's syndrome
Hydronephrosis	Sarcoidosis
Distal renal tubular necrosis	Osmotic diuretics • Mannitol • Urea • Glucose
Sickle cell disease	Metabolic • Hypokalemia • Hypercalcemia
Fanconi syndrome	

13.6.1 Treatment

- Do not reduce serum [Na] by more than 10 mEq/L per 24-hour period.
- Recheck serum [Na] every 4 hours after the initiation of fluid repletion.
- Replace free water by oral means and with IV fluids (options include D5 W, ¼ NS, ½ NS).
- Limit the use of hypotonic fluids in the setting of brain injury and cerebral edema.
- Estimate Free Water deficit: $= (\text{Current TBW}) \times ((\text{Serum[Na]} / 140) - 1)/140$

Watson	Male TBW =	$2.447 - (0.09156 \times \text{age}) + (0.1074 \times \text{height}) + (0.3362 \times \text{weight})$
	Female TBW =	$-2.097 + (0.1069 \times \text{height}) + (0.2466 \times \text{weight})$
Hume-Weyers	Male TBW =	$(0.194786 \times \text{height}) + (0.296785 \times \text{weight}) - 14.012934$
	Female TBW =	$(0.34454 \times \text{height}) + (0.183809 \times \text{weight}) - 35.270121$

In a patient with acute hypernatremia, we recommend replacing the entire deficit in less than 24 hours. The hourly infusion rate should exceed the free water deficit divided by 24.

In a patient with chronic hypernatremia, a slower reduction in serum [Na] is recommended, with only a fraction of the water deficit replaced in 24 hours (i.e., enough water to lower the serum sodium by 10 mEq/L).

The same formula from the hyponatremia treatment, "General Principles" section earlier in this chapter, can be used to predict how much IV fluid is required to decrease the serum [Na] to a desired level (simply replace "513 mEq/L" with the [Na] of the chosen IV fluid). Formulas provided in ▶ Table 13.6a and characteristics of infusates listed in ▶ Table 13.6b may also be applied to calculate for hypernatremia.

Table 13.6 (a) Formulas for estimating changes in serum sodium concentration with infusate

Clinical situation	Formula (use table 13.6 (b) below for infusate values)
To estimate the change in serum sodium concentration with 1 liter of any sodium solution	$\text{Change in } [Na^+] = \dfrac{\text{infusate } [Na^+] - \text{serum } [Na^+]}{(TBW + 1)}$
To estimate the change in serum sodium concentration with 1 liter of any sodium solution also containing potassium	$\text{Change in } [Na^+] = \dfrac{(\text{infusate } [Na^+] + \text{infusate } [K^+]) - \text{serum } [Na^+]}{(TBW + 1)}$

Adapted from Adrogué HJ, Madias NE. Hyponatremia. N Engl J Med. 2000; 342(21):1581–1589

Table 13.6 (b) Infusate sodium concentrations (in mmol per liter)

5% Sodium chloride in water	885
3% Sodium chloride in water	513
0.9% Sodium chloride in water	154
Ringer's lactate	130
0.45% Sodium chloride in water	77
0.2% Sodium chloride in 5% dextrose in water	34
5% Dextrose in water	0

Adapted from Adrogué HJ, Madias NE. Hyponatremia. N Engl J Med. 2000; 342(21):1581–1589

13.6.2 Central DI Treatment

- **First line:** Desmopressin 0.1 mg given orally twice a day or nasal spray 2.5 mcg twice a day
- **Can also consider ADH-enhancing medications:** Clofibrate 500 mg given orally four times a day, chlorpropramide (increases renal sensitivity to ADH), and thiazide diuretics

13.6.3 Nephrogenic DI Treatment

- Thiazide diuretic (hydrochlorothiazide, 25 mg daily or twice a day)
- Low-salt and low-protein diet
- Other less common recommendations include:
  - Addition of a nonsteroidal anti-inflammatory drug (NSAID) (e.g., ibuprofen, indomethacin, or naproxen[20])
  - Addition of amiloride to a thiazide diuretic.[21] However, most studies have been done in the pediatric population[7] and are considered for refractory cases.

References

[1] Spasovski G, Vanholder R, Allolio B, et al. Clinical practice guideline on diagnosis and treatment of hyponatraemia. Intensive Care Med. 2014; 40(3):320–331

[2] Adrogué HJ, Madias NE. Hyponatremia. N Engl J Med. 2000; 342(21):1581–1589

[3] Cho KC. Electrolyte & acid-base disorders. In: Papadakis MA, McPhee SJ, Rabow MW, eds. Current Medical Diagnosis & Treatment 2017. New York, NY: McGraw-Hill; 2016

[4] Halawa I, Andersson T, Tomson T. Hyponatremia and risk of seizures: a retrospective cross-sectional study. Epilepsia. 2011; 52(2):410–413

[5] Verbalis JG, Goldsmith SR, Greenberg A, et al. Diagnosis, evaluation, and treatment of hyponatremia: expert panel recommendations. Am J Med. 2013; 126(10) Suppl 1:S1–S42

[6] Sterns RH. Pathophysiology and etiology of the syndrome of inappropriate antidiuretic hormone secretion (SIADH). In: UpToDate, Post TW, ed. UpToDate, Waltham, MA. (Accessed on February 1, 2017.)

[7] Rose B, Post T. Clinical Physiology of Acid-Base and Electrolyte Disorders. New York: McGraw-Hill Education; 2001:704,754, 782

[8] Yee AH, Burns JD, Wijdicks EF. Cerebral salt wasting: pathophysiology, diagnosis, and treatment. Neurosurg Clin N Am. 2010; 21(2):339–352

[9] Huang WY, Weng WC, Peng TI, et al. Association of hyponatremia in acute stroke stage with three-year mortality in patients with first-ever ischemic stroke. Cerebrovasc Dis. 2012; 34(1):55–62

[10] Kuramatsu JB, Bobinger T, Volbers B, et al. Hyponatremia is an independent predictor of in-hospital mortality in spontaneous intracerebral hemorrhage. Stroke. 2014; 45(5):1285–1291

[11] Kalita J, Singh RK, Misra UK. Cerebral salt wasting is the most common cause of hyponatremia in stroke. J Stroke Cerebrovasc Dis. 2017; 26(5):1026–1032

[12] Gennari FJ. Hypo-hypernatraemia: disorders of water balance. In: Davison AM, Cameron JS, Grünfeld J-P, Kerr DNS, Ritz E, Winearls CG, eds. Oxford Textbook of Clinical Nephrology. 2nd ed. Vol. 1. Oxford, England: Oxford University Press; 1998:175–200

[13] Sterns RH. Diagnostic evaluation of adults with hyponatremia. In: UpToDate, Post TW, ed. UpTo-Date, Waltham, MA. (Accessed on February 1, 2017.)

[14] Sterns RH, Hix JK, Silver SM. Management of hyponatremia in the ICU. Chest. 2013; 144 (2):672–679

[15] Sterns RH, Nigwekar SU, Hix JK. The treatment of hyponatremia. Semin Nephrol. 2009; 29 (3):282–299

[16] Wijdicks EF, Vermeulen M, Hijdra A, van Gijn J. Hyponatremia and cerebral infarction in patients with ruptured intracranial aneurysms: is fluid restriction harmful? Ann Neurol. 1985; 17 (2):137–140

[17] Gross P. Clinical management of SIADH. Ther Adv Endocrinol Metab. 2012; 3(2):61–73

[18] Adrogué HJ, Madias NE. Hypernatremia. N Engl J Med. 2000; 342(20):1493–1499

[19] Greenberg MS. Handbook of Neurosurgery. New York, NY: Thieme; 2010:15–17, 661

[20] Allen HM, Jackson RL, Winchester MD, Deck LV, Allon M. Indomethacin in the treatment of lith-ium-induced nephrogenic diabetes insipidus. Arch Intern Med. 1989; 149(5):1123–1126

[21] Knoers N, Monnens LAH. Amiloride-hydrochlorothiazide versus indomethacin-hydrochlorothia-zide in the treatment of nephrogenic diabetes insipidus. J Pediatr. 1990; 117(3):499–502

[22] Sprigings D, Chambers J. Acute Medicine: A Practical Guide to the Management of Medical Emer-gencies. 4th ed. Oxford; Malden, MA: Blackwell Science; 2008

[23] Diringer MN, Zazulia AR. Hyponatremia in neurologic patients: consequences and approaches to treatment. Neurologist. 2006; 12(3):117–126

14 Nutrition

Stephanie Dobak and Jacqueline S. Urtecho

Abstract
Brain injuries alter metabolism making glucose management and nutrient provision challenging. The main nutrition goal is to manage glycemic control and provide adequate nutrients to prevent or treat malnutrition. In this chapter, we will discuss the nutritional challenges of and recommendations for patients with brain injury.

Keywords: glucose, nutrition, enteral nutrition, parenteral nutrition, brain injury

14.1 Glucose Utilization

Hyperglycemia is common after brain injury, resulting from stress, inflammation, corticosteroids, diabetes mellitus, decreased insulin sensitivity, and increased gluconeogenesis from lactate clearance.[1] Early profound hyperglycemia is independently associated with poor prognosis after traumatic brain injury (TBI), stroke, and subarachnoid hemorrhage. Hyperglycemia has been associated with increased infection risk and critical illness polyneuropathy. In acute ischemic stroke there is evidence that persistent hyperglycemia is associated with worse outcome.[2] Yet hypoglycemia, which has been defined as blood glucose of < 60 or < 80 (mg/dL) depending on the study, also has deleterious effects. There are limited intensive insulin therapy (IIT) studies (blood glucose 80–120 (mg/dL)) specific to the neurologically injured patient population, and many of the most cited studies excluded patients with a neurologic injury. ▶ Table 14.1 summarizes key IIT studies. Of note, though the NICE-SUGAR trial observed more hypoglycemia events with IIT, this was not associated with Glasgow outcome score at 24 months post TBI.[3]

In summary, IIT may impair cerebral glucose metabolism after brain injury, and more liberal serum glucose goals may be needed. Although the ideal serum glucose target is still under debate, maintaining *a range of 140 to 180 mg/dL* and *avoiding hypoglycemia* are recommended.[2,4,5,6]

14.2 Nutrition in Critical Care

Brain injuries alter the body's metabolism of nutrients causing a hypermetabolic and hypercatabolic state. Inadequate nutrition leads to malnutrition, which is associated with:

Table 14.1 Intensive insulin therapy (IIT) RCTs

Trial (year)	N	Setting	Primary outcome	IIT group glucose range (mg/dL)	P-value
Van den Berghe (2006)	1,200	MICU	Hospital mortality	80–110	NS
HI-5 (2006)	240	CCU (AMI)	6 m mortality	<180	NS
Glucontrol[a] (2009)	1,101	MICU/SICU	ICU mortality	80–110	NS
Gandhi (2007)	400	OR (cardiac)	30 d mortality/ morbidity	80–100	NS
VISEP[b] (2008)	537	ICU (severe sepsis)	28 d mortality/ organ failure	80–110	NS
De La Rosa (2008)	504	MICU/SICU	28 d mortality	80–110	NS
Oddo (2008)	20	Neuro-ICU	Cerebral glucose metabolism	80–120	<0.01 (increased cerebral metabolic crisis with IIT)
NICE-SUGAR (2009)	6104	ICU	3 m mortality	81–108	<0.05 (increased mortality with IIT)
Vespa (2012)	13	ICU (TBI)	Brain metabolism	80–110	0.05 (increased cerebral metabolic crisis with IIT)

[a]Trial stopped early due to high rate of protocol violations.
[b]Trial ended early due to safety concerns (severe hypoglycemia and SAEs)
Abbreviations: CCU (AMI), coronary care unit (acute myocardial infarction); ICU, intensive care unit; MICU, medical intensive care unit; OR, operating room; RCT, randomized control trial; SAEs, serious adverse events; SICU, surgical intensive care unit; TBI, traumatic brain injury.

- Increased risk for infectious complications
- Prolonged need for mechanical ventilation
- Longer hospital and intensive care unit (ICU) length of stays

- Delayed wound healing
- Overall increased risk for morbidity and mortality[7,8]

Multiple factors play a role in determining calorie and protein needs and must be considered prior to devising a nutrition regimen:
- Acuity and degree of brain injury
- Medical history (e.g., diabetes, renal disease, heart disease)
- Surgical history (e.g., extensive bowel resection, bariatric surgery)
- Current medications (e.g., phenytoin, fluoroquinolones)
- Nutritional history (recent weight changes, intake, vitamin/mineral/herbal supplements)

14.3 Nutrition Status

14.3.1 Malnutrition

Patients should be evaluated on admission for the presence of malnutrition. *Malnutrition should not be based on body mass index (BMI) alone* as obese patients can be malnourished. The American Society for Parenteral and Enteral Nutrition (ASPEN)/Academy of Nutrition and Dietetics Malnutrition Consensus suggests using the following criteria to diagnose malnutrition:
- Insufficient energy intake (estimated percentage of usual intake)
- Weight loss ([usual body weight – current weight]/usual body weight × 100)
- Loss of muscle mass (in temples, clavicles, shoulders, scapulae, quadriceps, calves)
- Loss of subcutaneous fat (in orbital fat pads, triceps, over rib cage)
- Localized or generalized fluid accumulation (rule out other causes of edema/ascites)
- Diminished functional status (hand dynamometer strength and overall activity level)

▶ Table 14.2 identifies the criteria for moderate and severe malnutrition.[9] Note that there is no definition for mild malnutrition according to the guidelines.

It is important to recognize that patients with certain neurologic injuries remain at high risk for developing malnutrition. Some of these conditions include:
- Stroke
- Aneurysmal subarachnoid hemorrhage
- Brain tumors
- Spinal cord injury
- TBI
- Dementia
- Multiple sclerosis

Table 14.2 Criteria for diagnosing malnutrition in acute illness/injury [9] [a]

Malnutrition severity	Energy intake	% Weight loss	Muscle wasting	Subcutaneous fat wasting	Fluid accumulation	Grip strength
Severe	≤ 50% kcal of estimated energy requirement for ≥ 5 days	> 2% in 1 week > 5% in 1 month > 7.5% in 3 months	Moderate	Moderate	Moderate to Severe	Measurably reduced
Moderate	<75% of estimated energy requirement for >7 days	1–2% in 1 week 5% in 1 month 7.5% in 3 months	Mild	Mild	Mild	N/A

[a]two criteria must be met to diagnose

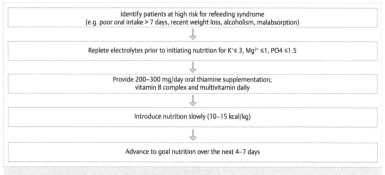

Fig. 14.1 Measures to prevent refeeding syndrome.

14.3.2 Refeeding Syndrome

It is important to screen for malnutrition prior to starting nutrition support. Initiating aggressive nutrition in the malnourished patient may result in refeeding syndrome. Refeeding syndrome is the potentially fatal intracellular shifts of fluids and electrolytes caused by the introduction of carbohydrates and subsequent insulin secretion. Measures must be taken to identify patients at refeeding syndrome risk, slowly advance nutrition, closely monitor electrolytes, and provide thiamine supplementation. ▶ Fig. 14.1 provides an algorithm for the prevention of refeeding syndrome.[11]

14.3.3 Nutrition-Related Laboratory Tests

Due to inflammation, serum protein markers (pre-albumin, albumin, transferrin) do not accurately reflect nutrition status during critical illness and may remain low despite adequate nutrition.[12] A 24-hour urine urea nitrogen measurement may help determine daily protein needs.

14.4 Nutrition Assessment

14.4.1 Calorie Needs

Calorie and protein assessments are needed to develop a nutrition plan, especially in the ICU. Indirect calorimetry (IC) is considered the gold standard in measuring resting energy expenditure (REE). IC calculates REE by measuring oxygen consumption and carbon dioxide production. Although considered to

Table 14.3 Variables affecting indirect calorimetry measurement[10]

Variable	Suggested limits	Reasoning
RQ	0.67–1.2	Values outside of range suggest technical errors
FiO_2	≤ 60%	Elevated FiO_2 can increase errors in measured VO_2
PEEP	< 12 cm H_2O; Not on APRV	High PEEP can increase FiO_2 variability
Activity (PT/OT, transport)	Conduct IC 1 to 2 hours after activity	Hyperventilation can lead to increased VCO_2, REE, RQ
Dialysis	Conduct IC ≥ 4 hours after HD N/A while on CRRT, ECMO	Filtration process removes CO_2, resulting in inaccurate RQ and underestimation of REE
Potential air leaks	No bronchopleural fistula or leaks in chest tube, trach, or ETT cuff	Gas losses result in erroneous data via reduced VO_2, VCO_2, REE measurements

Abbreviations: APRV, airway pressure release ventilation; CRRT, continuous renal replacement therapy; ECMO, extracorporeal membrane oxygenation; ETT, endotracheal tube; HD, hemodialysis; IC, indirect calorimetry; OT, occupational therapy; PEEP, positive end-expiratory pressure; PT, physical therapy; REE, resting energy expenditure; RQ, respiratory quotient.

be the gold standard, IC is expensive, requires trained personnel, and is contingent on many variables. ▶ Table 14.3 outlines the variables which affect IC.[10] Predictive equations (Penn State, Mifflin-St. Jeor, weight-based equations) using dry or usual weight to determine energy requirements are less reliable but often more feasible than IC. Caloric needs by weight category can be found in ▶ Table 14.4. It is important to know that caloric needs may increase from TBI, fever, or wounds and decrease from therapeutic hypothermia, barbiturate coma, paralytics, quadriplegia, or paraplegia, and this should be taken into consideration when determining nutritional goals.

14.4.2 Protein Needs

Protein requirements often increase following neurologic injury due to hypercatabolism. At this time, it is no longer recommended to restrict protein in the critically ill patient with acute kidney injury or liver failure.[5] Protein needs are typically calculated based on ideal body weight (as determined by the Hamwi method). ▶ Table 14.5 lists protein needs by clinical condition or therapy.

Table 14.4 Calorie needs determined by adult weight categories/BMI

Weight category	BMI	Calorie needs (kcal/kg)
Underweight	BMI < 18.5	30–40
Normal	18.5–24.9	25–30
Overweight	25–29.9	20–25
Obesity Class I	30–34.9	15–20
Obesity Class II	35–39.9	10–15
Obesity Class III (Morbid Obesity)	≥ 40	10–15

Abbreviation: BMI, body mass index.

Table 14.5 Protein needs by clinical condition or therapy[8]

Clinical condition	Protein needs by ideal weight (gm/kg)
Stroke; AKI; hepatic failure	1.2–2
HD	1.2–1.5
TBI	1.5–2.5
CRRT	2–2.5

Abbreviations: AKI, acute kidney injury; CRRT, continuous renal replacement therapy; HD, hemodialysis; TBI, traumatic brain injury.

14.4.3 Nutrition Support

Adequate oral intake is always the primary nutritional goal. When not feasible, enteral nutrition (EN) or parenteral nutrition (PN) should be initiated after achieving fluid resuscitation and hemodynamic stability. ▶ Fig. 14.2 lists an algorithm for determining the appropriate nutrition route.

14.4.4 Enteral Nutrition[8]

For patients with functional guts, the use of EN is currently recommended over PN.
• Early EN initiation (within 24–48 hours of admission) is associated with decreased
  ○ Gut permeability (supports intraepithelial cell tight junctions and villi height; stimulates blood flow and release of cholecystokinin, gastrin, and bile salts)

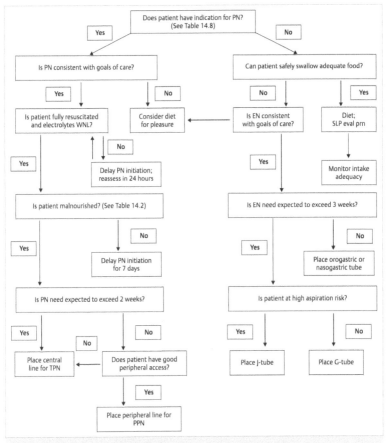

Fig. 14.2 Algorithm for determining appropriate route of nutrition.

- ○ Inflammatory cytokine release
- ○ **Clinical outcomes:** Infectious morbidity, mortality, hospital length of stay
- EN rate should be increased to provide > 80% calorie/protein goals within 48 to 72 hours.
- EN may need to be adjusted for certain medications (▶ Table 14.6). Consider modifying drug dosing to avoid frequent EN interruptions.
- ▶ Table 14.7 lists ways to troubleshoot EN complications.

Table 14.6 Common drug–nutrient interactions with continuous enteral nutrition

Drug	Interaction	Results	Prevention
Phenytoin	Drug adherence to tube wall Drug binds to protein and calcium salts	Decreased drug absorption	Monitor drug levels Hold EN 1 to 2 hours before and after administration if drug levels are low Dilute drug suspension Flush tube after administration
Carbamazepine	Drug may adhere to tube wall EN may alter drug solubility	Decreased drug absorption and bioavailability	Flush tube after administration Dilute drug suspension
Warfarin	Drug may bind to protein Drug may adhere to tube wall	Decreased drug absorption	Monitor INR; increase dose as needed Consider holding EN 1 hour before and after administration
Fluoroquinolones	Drug may compete with cations in EN	Decreased drug bioavailability	Hold EN 1 hour before and 2 hours after administration

Abbreviations: EN, enteral nutrition; INR, international normalized ratio.

There are few trials studying the most optimal way to feed brain injured patients. Initiating early EN at goal rates has been associated with decreased major complications, decreased post-injury inflammatory responses, and a trend toward accelerated neurologic recovery. Volume-based feeding protocols[5] (in which nurses are empowered to increase EN rates throughout the day to compensate for EN interruptions) are shown to increase EN delivery within all ICU settings. It is recommended that gastric residual volumes (GRVs) no longer be routinely monitored in the critically ill patient.[8] GRV monitoring requires additional nursing time and resources, and GRVs are not associated with pneumonia, regurgitation, or aspiration risk. At Thomas Jefferson University we have found the following to be efficacious:

- Starting early EN (within 24 hours of admission)
- Starting EN at goal rates (when refeeding risk is not present)
- Using standard EN
- Using a daily volume-based feeding regimen
- Not monitoring GRVs
- Addressing EN intolerance and resuming EN in a timely manner as per the ability

Table 14.7 Troubleshooting common gastrointestinal complications of EN

Complication	First steps to take	Cause	Treatment
Diarrhea (>4 liquid BMs/day)	Review medications Rule out infection Keep feeding	Hyperosmolar EN (>300 mOsm/L)	Change to isotonic EN
		Malabsorption	Change to peptide-based, MCT oil EN Consider soluble fiber supplement
		Medications	Decrease bowel regimen Eliminate sorbitol-containing solutions Review if on antibiotic therapy If infection ruled out, use antidiarrheal
		Infection (*C. diff*)	Antibiotics
Constipation (No BM >3 days when EN at goal rate)	Review enteral fluid intake Review fiber intake Order abdominal radiology to rule out obstruction	Inadequate fluid intake	Increase free water flush
		Inadequate fiber intake	Change to fiber-containing EN
		Fecal impaction	Enema; aggressive bowel regimen
		Ileus	If mild, trophic EN; if severe, hold EN
High gastric residuals (>500 mL) OR Nausea/ vomiting	Perform physical exam Order abdominal radiology Review medications Review blood sugars Evaluate aspiration risk	Delayed gastric emptying Gastroparesis	Consider prokinetic agent Consider post-pyloric feeds Decrease aspiration risk factors
		Narcotics	Decrease narcotics; increase bowel meds
		Consistently high blood sugars	Tighten glycemic control
Aspiration	Check HOB elevation Review medications Review aspiration history	Prone positioning	Elevate head of bed 30 to 45 degrees if able
		Decreased consciousness	Reduce sedatives if able
		History of aspiration	Consider post-pyloric feeds

Abbreviations: BM, bowel movement; C. diff, *Clostridioides difficile*; EN, enteral nutrition; HOB, head of bed; MCT, medium chaintriglyceride.

• Limiting fasting time to immediately prior to surgery for patients with protected airways

14.5 Specific EN Considerations[5]

The most appropriate EN therapy for brain injured patients continues to be debated. Below are recommendations from the SCCM/ASPEN guidelines for this population:

• **EN formula**: Standard (intact protein) EN formulation is typically tolerated and the use of immune-modulating EN formulations (containing arginine, eicosapentaenoic acid [EPA], docosahexaenoic acid [DHA], glutamine, and nucleic acid) should be considered.

• **Glutamine**: At this time, glutamine supplementation is not recommended.

• **Arginine:** There is not enough data to support routine supplementation of arginine.

• **Omega-3 fatty acids**: Use of EN formulas with EPA/DHA may be beneficial after TBI.

• **Fiber**: Avoid if there is high risk for bowel ischemia or severe dysmotility; if hemodynamically stable, 10 to 20 gm/day fermentable soluble fiber should be considered to decrease diarrhea.

• **Probiotics**: Routine use cannot be recommended due to lack of consistent outcome effect and heterogeneity of bacterial strains studied.

14.5.1 Parenteral Nutrition[5]

PN is available to meet nutrition needs when EN is not appropriate/tolerated. ▶ Table 14.8 lists PN indications. ▶ Table 14.9 lists the differences, pros and cons of peripheral PN (PPN) and total PN (TPN). SCCM/ASPEN recommend to:

• Provide PN immediately for severe malnutrition or high nutrition risk when diet/EN is not feasible.

• Withhold PN for 7 days in well-nourished patients.
  ○ Early PN initiation in well-nourished patients has been associated with increased risk for infectious morbidity and mortality.

• Use supplemental PN if unable to meet > 60% EN goals after 7 to 10 days.

14.6 Therapy-Specific Considerations

Certain therapies, such as barbiturate coma, therapeutic paralysis, and targeted temperature management (TTM) to hypothermia, may impact EN tolerance. ▶ Fig. 14.3, ▶ Fig. 14.4, ▶ Fig. 14.5 provide guides to feeding patients receiving these therapies. During barbiturate coma, Stevens et al noted that EN at goal rate can be tolerated, and feeding intolerance was not associated with

Table 14.8 Disease indications for parenteral nutrition use

Disease	Criteria for PN
Gastrointestinal fistula	Output > 500 mL/day Distal enteral access not accessible
Short bowel syndrome	< 200 cm remaining small bowel length > 50% losses of oral/EN intake < 1 L/day urine output
Inflammatory diseases (severe pancreatitis, severe infectious enteritis, Crohn's disease)	Failed oral/EN trial Need for bowel rest
Mechanical causes (small bowel obstruction, mesenteric ischemia)	Surgery not an option
Severe fat malabsorption	Fecal fat > 50% of 50 gm fat/day oral/EN intake
Severe gastric or intestinal motility disturbance (gastroparesis, scleroderma, prolonged ileus)	Unresponsive to prokinetic medications

Abbreviations: EN, enteral nutrition; PN, parenteral nutrition.

Table 14.9 Differences, and pros and cons of PPN and TPN

Route	Pros	Cons
PPN	• No risk for central line infection • Provides nutrition when time to return to GI function is unpredictable • Appropriate for mild-moderate malnutrition	• Requires good peripheral venous access • Duration limited by peripheral vein tolerance (10 days max) • Requires ability to tolerate higher fluid loads (2.5–3 L/day) • Osmolarity restriction (900 mOsm/L) limits nutrient delivery • May cause phlebitis
TPN	• Meets total nutrition needs through higher osmolarity loads (1,300–1,800 mOsm/L) • Appropriate for severe malnutrition • Can be provided for long term	• Requires central venous access • Risk for catheter-related venous thrombosis • Risk for central line associated blood stream infection • Long-term risk for bone and hepatobiliary disease

Abbreviations: GI, gastrointestinal; PPN, peripheral parenteral nutrition; TPN, total parenteral nutrition.

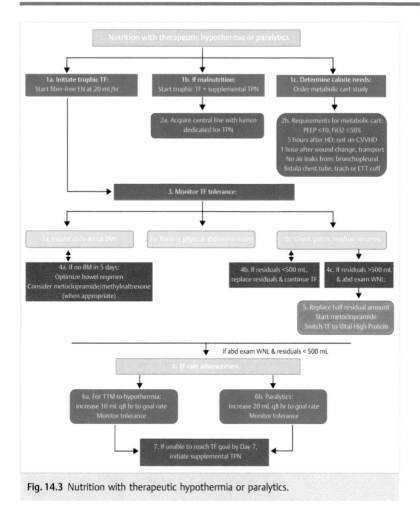

Fig. 14.3 Nutrition with therapeutic hypothermia or paralytics.

pentobarbital dosage, duration, or initiation time.[12] Conversely, Bochiccio et al noted EN intolerance in this population.[13] However, in this latter study intolerance was defined by a low GRV threshold (150 mL) and TF was initiated after coma was fully achieved (mean time to initiate coma was 3.8 ± 3 days). Ileus is propagated by delayed enteral feeding and prolonged fasting times.

There are few studies on EN tolerance with paralytics. Paralytics target skeletal muscle whereas the gastrointestinal (GI) tract is smooth muscle. Tamion et al noted that GI absorptive capacity is maintained and gastric emptying

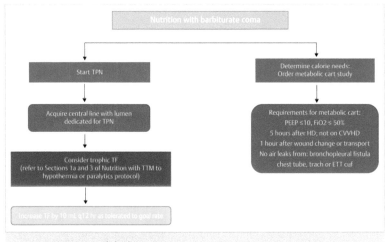

Fig. 14.4 Nutrition with barbiturate coma.

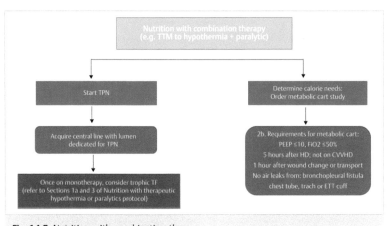

Fig. 14.5 Nutrition with combination therapy.

unaffected with the use of cisatracurium besilate.[14] If paralysis is being used in combination with other therapies, it may be prudent to implement a more conservative EN regimen.

There is also a paucity of trials studying EN during TTM to hypothermia. Ileus is common when body temperature is < 34 °F. We studied EN tolerance during

TTM to moderate hypothermia after intracranial hemorrhage. We noted that early EN is safe and EN intolerance is common but responsive to prokinetics.

If ileus refractory to prokinetics develops during these therapies, PN should be considered.

14.7 Conclusion

Head injuries typically alter glucose metabolism and increase calorie and protein needs. Maintaining a serum glucose range of 140 to 180 mg/dL and avoiding < 100 mg/dL is recommended. When feasible, EN is preferred over PN. EN should be initiated immediately once hemodynamic stability is attained. Standard EN formulas should be attempted first but if intolerance occurs, semi-elemental (peptide-based) EN formulas may improve tolerance. If EN is not appropriate, PN should be delayed for 7 days in the previously well-nourished patient. Omega-3 fatty acid supplementation may be beneficial in this population. Measures must be taken to prevent refeeding syndrome and iatrogenic malnutrition. Providing adequate nutrition support attenuates the acute phase response and improves clinical outcomes.

References

[1] Glenn TC, Martin NA, McArthur DL, et al. Endogenous nutritive support after traumatic brain injury: peripheral lactate production for glucose supply via gluconeogenesis. J Neurotrauma. 2015; 32(11):811–819

[2] Powers WJ, Rabinstein AA, Ackerson T, et al. American Heart Association Stroke Council. 2018 guidelines for the early management of patients with acute ischemic stroke: a guideline for healthcare professionals from the American Heart Association/American Stroke Association. Stroke. 2018; 49(3):e46–e110

[3] Finfer S, Chittock DR, Su SY, et al. NICE-SUGAR Study Investigators. Intensive versus conventional glucose control in critically ill patients. N Engl J Med. 2009; 360(13):1283–1297

[4] Torbey MT, Bösel J, Rhoney DH, et al. Evidence-based guidelines for the management of large hemispheric infarction: a statement for health care professionals from the Neurocritical Care Society and the German Society for Neuro-intensive Care and Emergency Medicine. Neurocrit Care. 2015; 22(1):146–164

[5] McClave SA, Taylor BE, Martindale RG, et al. Society of Critical Care Medicine, American Society for Parenteral and Enteral Nutrition. Guidelines for the provision and assessment of nutrition support therapy in the adult critically ill patient: Society of Critical Care Medicine (SCCM) and American Society for Parenteral and Enteral Nutrition (A.S.P.E.N.). JPEN J Parenter Enteral Nutr. 2016; 40(2):159–211

[6] Jacobi J, Bircher N, Krinsley J, et al. Guidelines for the use of an insulin infusion for the management of hyperglycemia in critically ill patients. Crit Care Med. 2012; 40(12):3251–3276

[7] Alberda C, Gramlich L, Jones N, et al. The relationship between nutritional intake and clinical outcomes in critically ill patients: results of an international multicenter observational study. Intensive Care Med. 2009; 35(10):1728–1737

[8] Corkins MR, Guenter P, DiMaria-Ghalili RA, et al. American Society for Parenteral and Enteral Nutrition. Malnutrition diagnoses in hospitalized patients: United States, 2010. JPEN J Parenter Enteral Nutr. 2014; 38(2):186–195

[9] White JV, Guenter P, Jensen G, Malone A, Schofield M, Academy Malnutrition Work Group, A.S.P.E. N. Malnutrition Task Force, A.S.P.E.N. Board of Directors. Consensus statement: Academy of Nutrition and Dietetics and American Society for Parenteral and Enteral Nutrition: characteristics recommended for the identification and documentation of adult malnutrition (undernutrition). JPEN J Parenter Enteral Nutr. 2012; 36(3):275–283

[10] Branson RD. Technical Aspects of Indirect Calorimetry. Critical Decisions. Burlington, VT: Saxe Healthcare Communications; 2001:2–5

[11] National Institute for Health and Clinical Excellence. Nutrition support for adults: oral nutrition support, enteral tube feeding and parenteral nutrition. https://www.nice.org.uk/guidance/cg32/chapter/1-Guidance. Published 2006. Accessed November 11, 2016

[12] Davis CJ, Sowa D, Keim KS, Kinnare K, Peterson S. The use of prealbumin and C-reactive protein for monitoring nutrition support in adult patients receiving enteral nutrition in an urban medical center. JPEN J Parenter Enteral Nutr. 2012; 36(2):197–204

[13] Stevens AM, Then JE, Frock KM, et al. Evaluation of feeding intolerance in patients with pentobarbital-induced coma. Ann Pharmacother. 2008;42(4):516–522.

[14] Bochicchio GV, Bochicchio K, Nehman S, Casey C, Andrews P, Scalea TM. Tolerance and efficacy of enteral nutrition in traumatic brain-injured patients induced into barbiturate coma. JPEN J Parenter Enteral Nutr. 2006;30(6):503–506.

[15] Tamion F, Hamelin K, Duflo A, Girault C, Richard JC, Bonmarchand G. Gastric emptying in mechanically ventilated critically ill patients: effect of neuromuscular blocking agent. Intensive Care Med. 2003;29(10):1717–1722.

15 Sedation

Akta Patel and Michelle Ghobrial

Abstract

Patients admitted to the neuroscience intensive care unit (neuro-ICU) may be one of the more complicated ICU populations to manage in regards to sedation, with respect to preservation and frequent assessment of the neurological examination. Providing adequate sedation to the patients in the neuro-ICU depends on determination of proper objective driven goals for sedation and the appropriate choice of agent based on the patient's physiology. Propofol and benzodiazepines are the most commonly used drugs to treat sedation in this population; however, dexmedetomidine has proven to be a noninferior agent of choice. Fentanyl is primarily an analgesic but has some sedative properties and is also often used as an option in the neuro-ICU. This chapter focuses on sedation in the neuro-ICU population and discusses advantages and disadvantages of the previously mentioned medications.

Keywords: neuro-ICU, intensive care unit, sedation, propofol, midazolam, dexmedetomidine, fentanyl

15.1 Introduction

Proper attention to sedation is an essential component of the care of critically ill patients in the intensive care unit (ICU). Patients admitted to the neuroscience ICU (neuro-ICU) may be one of the more complicated ICU populations to manage in regards to sedation, with respect to preservation and frequent assessment of the neurological examination.
- Sedation reduces the stress response, provides anxiolysis, improves tolerance of ventilatory support, decreases the cerebral metabolic rate of oxygen, and facilitates nursing care.
- Prolonged use of sedatives may result in drug accumulation, oversedation, delayed extubation, and lengthened ICU stay.
- Identifying underlying causes of agitation, such as pain, delirium, hypoxemia, hypoglycemia, hypotension, or withdrawal from alcohol and drugs, are important and treatment should be initiated prior to introducing sedatives.[1,2]

15.2 Indications for Sedation

- Neurologic injury: Traumatic brain injury (TBI), severe intracranial hypertension, status epilepticus, paroxysmal sympathetic hyperactivity, and withdrawal/intoxication from alcohol or drugs are a few common disease states which often require sedation.

- Patient safety: Cognitive dysfunction (dementia) and brain injury can cause agitation, restlessness, or combativeness prompting the use of sedation for the safety of the patient and staff.
- Patient comfort: Procedures such as intracranial pressure monitors, intravascular catheters, or targeted temperature management require the use of a short-acting sedative. Note that analgesia should be addressed before initiating sedation.

15.3 Complications of Sedation

- All sedation has risks. It is important to weight the risks and benefits before initiating sedatives in patients with a neurologic injury.
- Sedation can compromise a patient's neurologic examination which may be critical in patient populations like subarachnoid hemorrhage, stroke, or TBI.
- Sedation can also compromise normal physiology
  - **Cardiac**: Bradycardia, hypotension
  - **Pulmonary**: Respiratory depression, CO_2 retention
  - **Cerebral**: Low cerebral perfusion, decreased seizure threshold
- Duration of sedation may be prolonged in patients who have chronic disease states like kidney failure, heart failure, or hepatic failure. Sedation may also be prolonged in morbid obesity or when therapeutic temperature management is implemented.

15.4 Assessment of Sedation

- Sedation regimens must be individualized to account for differences in drug pharmacokinetic and pharmacodynamic properties.
  - Objective, goal-directed sedation is the recommended standard to avoid oversedation and when applicable promote earlier extubation.
  - In patients with neurologic injury, short-acting agents are preferred.
- Reliable assessment tools for sedation such as the Richmond Agitation Sedation Scale (RASS) have made titration of drugs more precise and cost effective. Details regarding the RASS Scale can be found in Chapter 1.
  - The RASS is a 10-point scale, validated and reliable in adult neuro-ICU patients, with four levels of anxiety or agitation (+ 1 to + 4), one level to denote a calm and alert state (0), and five levels of sedation (−1 to −5) culminating in unarousable (−5).[3,4,5](▶ Table 15.1)

Table 15.1 Richmond Agitation Sedation Scale (RASS)

Score		Description
+4	Combative	Violent, danger to staff
+3	Very agitated	Pulls or removes tube(s) or catheters; aggressive
+2	Agitated	Frequent nonpurposeful movement, fights ventilator
+1	Restless	Anxious, apprehensive, but not aggressive
0	Alert & calm	
−1	Drowsy	Awakens to *voice* (eye opening/contact) **>10 sec**
−2	Light sedation	Briefly awakens to *voice* (eye opening/contact) **<10 sec**
−3	Moderate sedation	Movement or eye opening to *voice*. **No eye contact**
−4	Deep sedation	No response to voice, but movement or eye opening to *physical* stimulation
−5	Unarousable	No response to *voice or physical* stimulation

Note: From Sessler et al.[3]

15.5 Choice of Sedative

- Propofol and benzodiazepines are among the most commonly used agents.
  - These drugs have both sedative and anterograde amnestic properties but often lack analgesic properties.[2]
- Dexmedetomidine has sedative, analgesic, anesthetic, and anxiolytic properties.
- Fentanyl is primarily an analgesic but has some sedative properties and is often used due to its short-acting duration in the neuro-ICU.
- A continuous infusion of these agents provides a more constant level of sedation and improved patients' comfort. It has been associated with prolonged mechanical ventilation and a longer ICU stay.
  - Thus, intermittent dosing along with daily interruption of sedatives allowing patients to "wake up" may improve outcomes.[6]
- ▶ Table 15.2 summarizes some of the pharmacological properties of some of the more commonly use sedative agents in the neuro-ICU.
- ▶ Table 15.3 provides studies of the agents being used for sedation in critically ill patients.

Table 15.2 Pharmacological properties of sedative agents

Drug	Onset	Duration	Usual dose	Precautions for use	Significant adverse effects	Advantages
Propofol	1–2 min	Short term: 0.5–1 hour Variable: 25–50 hours (depends on dose and time of sedation)	5–50 mcg/kg/min; consider dose adjustment for obese patient	Hypotension, bradycardia, hepatic failure, pancreatitis	Hypotension, respiratory depression, bradycardia, PRIS, hypertriglyceridemia, pancreatitis	No significant drug interactions
Midazolam	2–5 min (IV)	2–6 hours (prolonged with CI)	1–2 mg q2–4 hours OR 1–5 mg/hour (0.02–0.1 mg/kg/hour)	Hepatic failure, end-stage renal failure or dialysis, delirium	Oversedation, delirium, respiratory depression	Less hemodynamic instability than propofol
Dexmedetomidine	5–10 min (with LD) 1–2 hours (without LD)	1–2 hours	LD: 1 mcg/kg (optional) MD: 0.2–0.7 mcg/kg/ hour (up to 1.5 mcg/ kg/hour)	Hepatic failure, symptomatic bradycardia	Hypo/hypertension, bradycardia, dry mouth	Minimal respiratory depression Lowers shivering threshold
Fentanyl	1–2 min peak: 5–10 min	0.5–1 hour	LD: 50–100 mcg (0.35–0.5 mcg/kg) MD: 25–100 mcg/ hour (0.7–10 mcg/kg/ hour) consider dose adjustment for obese patients	Potential drug interactions if used with CYP3A4 inhibitors or inducers	Muscle rigidity with high bolus doses, gastric dysmotility, hypotension, respiratory depression	Rapid onset

Table 15.2 (*Continued*) Pharmacological properties of sedative agents

Drug	Onset	Duration	Usual dose	Precautions for use	Significant adverse effects	Advantages
Ketamine	30 sec IV	Alpha phase—anesthetic effect duration 45 min Beta phase—analgesic effect duration 2.5 hours	**Dosing protocols vary: Anesthesia** LD: 1–4.5 mg/kg if solo agent 0.5–2 mg/kg if adjuvant drug over 1 min MD: 0.1–0.5 mg/min No dosing recommendations for off-label use	Nystagmus, increase in muscle, transient increase in blood pressure; requires continuous cardiac monitoring for duration of use	Tachyarrhythmias, delirium, hallucinations/emergence psychosis, increased ICP, severe respiratory depression/apnea can occur with rapid IV bolus of large dose	No respiratory compromise due to preserved pharyngeal and laryngeal reflexes (unless rapid loading dose given), no dose adjustment for obesity

Abbreviations: CI, continuous infusion; ICP, intracranial pressure; IV, intravenous; LD, loading dose; MD, maintenance dose; PRIS = propofol infusion syndrome.

Table 15.3 Studies of the agents for sedation in critically ill patients

Study	Design	Patients	Intervention	Significant results
Chamorro 1996[7]	Multicenter, prospective, randomized, unblinded	98 patients from nine Spanish ICUs (14 were neurological or neurotrauma patients)	Propofol ($n = 50$) vs. midazolam ($n = 48$)	No significant difference regarding effectiveness of sedation between the groups. Propofol time to waking 23 ± 16 minutes vs. midazolam 137 ± 185 minutes
Kelly 1999[8]	Multicenter, prospective, randomized, double-blind, pilot	42 neurotrauma patients from 11 ICUs	Propofol 2% plus NS ($n = 23$) vs. morphine plus intralipid ($n = 19$) All patients received low-dose (1–3 mg/hour) morphine for analgesia	Propofol group injury severity score was greater than the morphine group No significant difference in adverse events Propofol group required less adjunctive ICP therapy but more vasopressors
Sandiumenge Camps 2000[9]	Prospective, randomized, unblinded	63 patients from one Spanish ICU (43 were neurotrauma patients)	Propofol 2% ($n = 32$) vs. midazolam ($n = 31$)	Increased rate of failure in the propofol group attributed to inexperience with new formulation (as compared to historical data using the 1% formulation) No significant hemodynamic differences between the groups
Jakob 2012[10]	Two, multicenter, randomized, double-blind, phase 3	31 ICUs in 8 countries 44 ICUs in 9 countries	**PRODEX:** Propofol ($n = 247$) vs. dexmedetomidine ($n = 251$) **MIDEX:** Midazolam ($n = 251$) vs. dexmedetomidine ($n = 249$)	Dexmedetomidine was shown to be non-inferior to the standard in both groups Patients in the dexmedetomidine group were more arousable and better able to communicate discomfort or pain
Erdman 2014[11]	Multicenter, retrospective, cohort	190 patients from two neuro-ICUs	Propofol ($n = 95$) vs. dexmedetomidine ($n = 95$)	The frequency of severe bradycardia and hypotension were similar in both groups

Abbreviations: Dex, dexmedetomidine; ICP, intracranial pressure; ICU, intensive care unit; NS, normal saline; RASS, Richmond Agitation Sedation Scale.

15.5.1 Propofol (Diprivan)

Mechanism of Action

It is a short-acting GABA$_A$ receptor agonist with lipophilic properties.[12]

Pharmacokinetics

- Metabolism occurs in the liver by conjugation to inactive metabolites, which are eliminated through the kidneys.
- Clearance is not affected by renal disease but patients with hepatic dysfunction may have a longer elimination half-life as it redistributes from fat and muscle to plasma.[13,14]
- There is no dose adjustment required for renal failure or hepatic insufficiency.
- It has a rapid onset and short duration of action.[12]
- Even after a continuous infusion, rapid clearance results in prompt awakening.[5]
- It has a dose-dependent effect on cerebral metabolism and is also useful for the control of seizures.[5]

Formulation Considerations

- Standard propofol is a 1% (10 mg/mL) lipid emulsion containing 1.1 kcal/mL (0.1 gram of fat per 1 mL of propofol).[1,2]
- It also contains 0.005% disodium edetate (ethylenediaminetetraacetic acid [EDTA]) to decrease the rate of microorganism growth, which is known to chelate trace metals, including zinc.
- Zinc supplementation may be considered in patients at high risk of zinc deficiency (sepsis, burns, large-volume diarrhea) if propofol is used for more than 5 days.
- Manufacturers recommend discarding propofol bottles and changing intravenous tubing every 12 hours to decrease the risk of contamination.

PRIS

Highly lethal syndrome known as propofol infusion syndrome
- Mechanism of action
  - May include alterations in the liver metabolism of the lipid emulsion, leading to an accumulation of ketone bodies and lactate and/or disruptions in the mitochondrial respiratory chain.[13,14]
- Clinical characteristics of PRIS

- o Rhabdomyolysis, increased creatine kinase, acute renal failure, severe metabolic acidosis, hyperkalemia, arrhythmias, cardiac arrest, dyslipidemias (particularly hypertriglyceridemia), and hypotension.[13,14]
- Risk factors for PRIS
  - o Propofol doses higher than 5 mg/kg/hour and a duration of therapy of more than 48 hours.[13,14,15]
- The successful management of PRIS relies on prompt recognition as it carries a high mortality rate.
  - o Propofol infusion should be stopped immediately and an alternative sedative agent should be used.
  - o Consider avoiding in patients with acute liver failure or pancreatitis, because the symptoms of PRIS may be difficult to distinguish from the underlying disease state abnormalities.
  - o Recommend monitoring triglycerides at baseline and then every 3 to 5 days.
    - – Liver function tests should also be monitored but not as frequently.

15.5.2 Midazolam (Versed)

Pharmacokinetics

- A highly lipophilic agent that is used for its rapid onset and short duration of action.
- Its short-acting properties become long acting in a continuous infusion for more than 24 hours.
- Benzodiazepines bind to the postsynaptic $GABA_A$ receptor and undergo phase-I hepatic metabolism to an active glucuronidated metabolite, α-hydroxymidazolam, which is then renally excreted.[2,5]
- Clearance of midazolam or its metabolite is significantly altered if either hepatic (primary drug accumulation) or renal (active metabolite α-hydroxymidazolam accumulation) functions are significantly impaired.[2]
  - o High lipophilicity and a large volume of distribution may lead to significant drug accumulation and a depot effect in the ICU patient.[2]
  - o The routine use of a benzodiazepine antagonist, such as flumazenil, is not recommended after prolonged benzodiazepine therapy because of the risks of inducing withdrawal symptoms and increasing myocardial oxygen consumption.[2]

Adverse Effects

- Hypotension and respiratory depression occur at high doses.[16]
- Oversedation is the most common unintended effect of midazolam.
- Another common unintended adverse effect is potentiating delirium.[16]

- The SEDCOM study compared the sedative effects of midazolam with those of dexmedetomidine in medical and surgical adult ICU patients.[17]
- The prevalence of delirium was lower in the dexmedetomidine group (54%) than in the midazolam group (76.6%), $p < 0.001$.[17]

15.5.3 Dexmedetomidine (Precedex)

Mechanism of Action

It is a highly selective α2 adrenergic agonist in the central nervous system (CNS) that produces dose-dependent sedation and anxiolysis while maintaining patient arousability without significant respiratory depression.

- It has roughly eight times the affinity for α2 receptors as compared to clonidine.[16]
- It provides a hypnotic and sedative effect by inhibition of norepinephrine release from the locus coeruleus.[18,19]

Pharmacokinetics

- Metabolism occurs in the liver by glucuronidation to inactive metabolites, which are eliminated through the kidneys.
- Its clearance is not affected by renal disease but patients with hepatic dysfunction may have a longer elimination half-life.

Dosing for ICU Sedation

- Loading dose (LD) of 1 mcg/kg intravenously over 10 minutes, followed by 0.2 to 0.7 mcg/kg/hour.
  - The LD may initially cause severe tachycardia and hypertension, but it can then quickly lead to significant bradycardia and/or hypotension secondary to receptor saturation.[18]
    – The LD is rarely administered in clinical ICU practice.[18]
- For the maintenance infusion dose, randomized trials have safely used dexmedetomidine at higher than manufacturer-recommended doses, up to 1.5 mcg/kg/hour.
  - Clinical efficacy with doses greater than 1.5 mcg/kg/hour remains unclear.[18,19,20]

Duration of Use

Although the package insert recommends a therapy of 24 hours or less, longer use for up to 7 days has been found safe in large randomized trials.[21]

Withdrawal Symptoms

- Case reports have been published describing the symptoms of withdrawal when used beyond 7 days at higher-than-recommended doses (e.g., tachycardia, hypertension, anxiety, and general discomfort).
  - A slow taper may be necessary, or the addition of clonidine has been used in some cases to help decrease withdrawal symptoms.[22]
- Other Considerations: It is considered a weak sedative and would not be appropriate if deep sedation is required (i.e., in a patient requiring neuromuscular blockade).

15.5.4 Fentanyl (Sublimaze)

The opiate analgesic is commonly used in the neuro-ICU for sedation because it has a rapid onset and a short duration of action.

Mechanism of Action

- It acts by binding to the μ-receptor in the CNS just like morphine but is roughly 100-times more potent than morphine.[16]
- Prolonged effects are seen after continuous infusions or repeated bolus doses as the drug accumulates in fatty tissue.[2,5]

Pharmacokinetics

Fentanyl is highly lipophilic, hepatically metabolized by the cytochrome P450 system to inactive metabolites that are renally excreted.[5,16]

Adverse Effects

- Respiratory depression, decreased gastric motility, constipation, hypotension, and muscle rigidity are some of the commonly seen.[2]
  - A bowel regimen should be initiated on day 1 unless contraindicated, with assessment for adequacy every 24 to 48 hours.

Dosage Forms

When converting from one dosage form to another, specific manufacturer recommendations should be used rather than converting on a 1:1 mcg basis.
- Injectable form of fentanyl is most commonly used in the ICU setting.
- The fentanyl patch is not generally appropriate for use in the ICU because of its latent onset (about 12 hours) and erratic/increased absorption in febrile patients unless chronic pain issues are present.[2,5]

15.5.5 Ketamine (Ketalar)

It is a nonbarbiturate anesthetic and analgesic agent. Its indications include: a sole anesthetic agent for diagnostic or surgical procedures that do not require skeletal muscle relaxation or as adjuvant anesthetic agent. It produces a dissociative sedation state with profound analgesia and amnesia without compromising the patient's airway.[23] It has been used off-label for the management of acute and chronic pain, procedural sedation, and analgesia and refractory status epilepticus.

Mechanism of Action

Rapid-acting noncompetitive N-methyl-D-aspartic acid (NMDA) receptor antagonist and sigma opioid receptor

Pharmakokinetics

Metabolism in the liver via N-dealkylation CYP3A4

Adverse Effects

- Emergence reactions including hallucination, delirium, or psychosis, and nausea and vomiting
- Increased intracranial pressure (ICP) is controversial and newer evidence suggests it can be safely used in patients with neurologic injury[24]

Dosing

Anesthetic Dosing

- **Induction**: 1 to 4.5 mg/kg as solo agent, slow IV push over 1 min (1/2 dose is recommended for adjuvant treatment with benzodiazepine)
- **Maintenance**: 0.5 to 2.5 mg/kg repeated as needed to maintain proper anesthetic level. Infusion dosing at 0.1 to 0.5 mg/min can be used along with benzodiazepines.

References

[1] Barr J, Fraser GL, Puntillo K, et al. American College of Critical Care Medicine. Clinical practice guidelines for the management of pain, agitation, and delirium in adult patients in the intensive care unit. Crit Care Med. 2013; 41(1):263–306

[2] Jacobi J, Fraser GL, Coursin DB, et al. Task Force of the American College of Critical Care Medicine (ACCM) of the Society of Critical Care Medicine (SCCM), American Society of Health-System Pharmacists (ASHP), American College of Chest Physicians. Clinical practice guidelines for the sustained use of sedatives and analgesics in the critically ill adult. Crit Care Med. 2002; 30(1):119–141

[3] Sessler CN, Gosnell MS, Grap MJ, et al. The Richmond Agitation-Sedation Scale: validity and reliability in adult intensive care unit patients. Am J Respir Crit Care Med. 2002; 166(10):1338–1344

[4] Ely EW, Truman B, Shintani A, et al. Monitoring sedation status over time in ICU patients: reliability and validity of the Richmond Agitation-Sedation Scale (RASS). JAMA. 2003; 289(22):2983–2991

[5] Keegan MT. Sedation in the neurologic intensive care unit. Curr Treat Options Neurol. 2008; 10 (2):111–125

[6] Kress JP, Pohlman AS, O'Connor MF, Hall JB. Daily interruption of sedative infusions in critically ill patients undergoing mechanical ventilation. N Engl J Med. 2000; 342(20):1471–1477

[7] Chamorro C, de Latorre FJ, Montero A, et al. Comparative study of propofol versus midazolam in the sedation of critically ill patients: results of a prospective, randomized, multicenter trial. Crit Care Med. 1996; 24(6):932–939

[8] Kelly DF, Goodale DB, Williams J, et al. Propofol in the treatment of moderate and severe head injury: a randomized, prospective double-blinded pilot trial. J Neurosurg. 1999; 90(6):1042–1052

[9] Sandiumenge Camps A, Sanchez-Izquierdo Riera JA, Toral Vazquez D, Sa Borges M, Peinado Rodriguez J, Alted Lopez E. Midazolam and 2% propofol in long-term sedation of traumatized critically ill patients: efficacy and safety comparison. Crit Care Med. 2000; 28(11):3612–3619

[10] Jakob SM, Ruokonen E, Grounds RM, et al. Dexmedetomidine for Long-Term Sedation Investigators. Dexmedetomidine vs midazolam or propofol for sedation during prolonged mechanical ventilation: two randomized controlled trials. JAMA. 2012; 307(11):1151–1160

[11] Erdman MJ, Doepker BA, Gerlach AT, Phillips GS, Elijovich L, Jones GM. A comparison of severe hemodynamic disturbances between dexmedetomidine and propofol for sedation in neurocritical care patients. Crit Care Med. 2014; 42(7):1696–1702

[12] Beretta L, De Vitis A, Grandi E. Sedation in neurocritical patients: is it useful? Minerva Anestesiol. 2011; 77(8):828–834

[13] Hutchens MP, Memtsoudis S, Sadovnikoff N. Propofol for sedation in neuro-intensive care. Neurocrit Care. 2006; 4(1):54–62

[14] Kam PCA, Cardone D. Propofol infusion syndrome. Anaesthesia. 2007; 62(7):690–701

[15] Oddo M, Crippa IA, Mehta S, et al. Optimizing sedation in patients with acute brain injury. Crit Care. 2016; 20(1):128–138

[16] Makii JM, Mirski MA, Lewin JJ, III. Sedation and analgesia in critically ill neurologic patients. J Pharm Pract. 2010; 23(5):455–469

[17] Riker RR, Shehabi Y, Bokesch PM, et al. SEDCOM (Safety and Efficacy of Dexmedetomidine Compared with Midazolam) Study Group. Dexmedetomidine vs midazolam for sedation of critically ill patients: a randomized trial. JAMA. 2009; 301(5):489–499

[18] Grof TM, Bledsoe KA. Evaluating the use of dexmedetomidine in neurocritical care patients. Neurocrit Care. 2010; 12(3):356–361

[19] Gerlach AT, Dasta JF. Dexmedetomidine: an updated review. Ann Pharmacother. 2007; 41 (2):245–2

[20] Venn M, Newman J, Grounds M. A phase II study to evaluate the efficacy of dexmedetomidine for sedation in the medical intensive care unit. Intensive Care Med. 2003; 29(2):201–207

[21] Shehabi Y, Ruettimann U, Adamson H, Innes R, Ickeringill M. Dexmedetomidine infusion for more than 24 hours in critically ill patients: sedative and cardiovascular effects. Intensive Care Med. 2004; 30(12):2188–2196

[22] Kukoyi A, Coker S, Lewis L, Nierenberg D. Two cases of acute dexmedetomidine withdrawal syndrome following prolonged infusion in the intensive care unit: report of cases and review of the literature. Hum Exp Toxicol. 2013; 32(1):107–110

[23] Green SM, Roback MG, Kennedy RM, Krauss B. Clinical practice guideline for emergency department ketamine dissociative sedation: 2011 update. Ann Emerg Med. 2011; 57(5):449–461

[24] Himmelseher S, Durieux ME. Revising a dogma: ketamine for patients with neurological injury? Anesth Analg. 2005; 101(2):524–534

16 Pain Management in the Neuro-Intensive Care Unit (ICU)

Amy Shah, David A. Wyler, and Andrew Ng

Abstract

Pain, an unpleasant sensory and emotional experience, presents unique challenges in the neuro-intensive care unit. A recent shift in strategy to address pain has evolved in the general ICU. Providers aim toward maintaining patient arousal while treating their patient's pain. The ICU liberation collaborative focuses on analgosedation or treating pain first and utilizing numerous tools for continued assessment in distinguishing pain from agitation and delirium (PAD). The endpoint is earlier liberation from ICU and mechanical ventilation by reducing sedative medications and supporting early mobility. This chapter aims to highlight the challenges of managing pain in the neuro-ICU while practicing within the framework of the current ICU liberation movement. Tools for assessment, individualized therapy, patients with neurodegenerative diseases at risk for pain, and special cases that make management of pain in the neuro-ICU particularly difficult will be discussed in this chapter.

Keywords: ICU liberation collaborative, ABCDEF bundle, ongoing assessment, individualized pain therapies, opioid therapy, adjunct medication, regional blocks, nonpharmacologic therapy

16.1 Introduction

Pain, an unpleasant sensory and emotional experience, presents unique challenges to care providers in the neuro-intensive care unit (neuro-ICU). Over the last decade, convincing data has driven a paradigm shift in the general ICU toward maintaining patient arousal while treating pain.[1] The ICU liberation collaborative focuses on treating pain first and utilizing numerous tools for continued assessment in distinguishing pain from agitation and delirium (PAD). The endpoint is earlier liberation from ICU and mechanical ventilation by reducing sedative medications and supporting early mobility.[1,2] The Critical Care Medicine (CCM) collaborative created the ABCDEF bundle to accomplish this purpose which stands for:

- Assess, Prevent, and Manage Pain
- Both spontaneous awakening trials (SATs) and spontaneous breathing trials (SBTs)
- Choice of Sedation

- Delirium: Assess, Prevent, and Manage
- Early Mobility and Exercise
- Family Engagement and Empowerment[1,2,3]

Several risks limit these strategies of caring for neurologically injured patients, and there is a paucity of data to validate the current trend in the neuro-ICU population.[4,5] Nonetheless, guidelines recommend whenever it is safe, treat pain judiciously and preserve the neurologic examination, the gold standard monitor for the central nervous system (CNS).[1,4]

This chapter aims to highlight the challenges of managing pain in the neuro-ICU while practicing within the framework of the current ICU liberation movement. Individualized therapy will be discussed for postoperative patients, patients with neurodegenerative diseases at risk for pain, and special cases that make management of pain in the neuro-ICU particularly difficult. Although opioid therapy is the mainstay for pain management historically, these medications often over-sedate frail neurologically susceptible patients.[4] Thus, opioid-sparing therapies such regional anesthesia, adjunct pain medications, and various relaxation techniques are discussed in detail. This chapter intends to provide a quick guide for the A component (assess, prevent, and manage pain) of the ABCDEF bundle in the neuro-ICU.

16.2 Modern Strategy of Pain Management in ICU Liberation

- Joint Commission on Accreditation of Healthcare Organization (JCAHO) mandated in 2002 "implementation of standards" in pain assessment, prevention, and treatment which was termed the "5th vital sign" in the ICU.[1,4]
- Studies supported reducing sedation and mobilizing patients improved ICU outcomes.[1,2,3,6]
- ABCDEF bundle implemented liberation strategy to address CCM Guideline 2012.[1,2]
- CCM guidelines excluded neurologically injured patients for safety reasons.[1]
- Addressing the A component (assess, prevent, and treat pain) of the ABCDEF bundle first was recommended since pain confounds delirium and agitation.[1,2]
- The use of different pain scales for continuous ongoing assessment was recommended.[1,6,7]
- Prevent/anticipate pain prior to surgery and painful procedures in ICU.[1]
- Opioid adjuncts reduce dose and ultimately neuro-confounding and neuro-toxic effects.[3,5,6]

16.3 Challenges of Pain Management in Neuro-ICU[1,4,5,7]

- Balance maintaining neurologic examination versus providing comfort.
- Balance neurologic examination versus offering enough sedation for "neuro-specific" issues such as reducing cerebral blood volume (CBV), intracranial pressure (ICP), and cerebral metabolic rate for oxygen (CMRO2) and seizure control.[4,5,8]
- Severity of brain injury dictates, and ICP and other multimodality monitoring may be helpful.[4]
- Balance neurologic examination versus offering enough sedation to provide endotracheal tolerance, ventilator synchrony, and shivering control.[7]
- Early mobilization recommended only if neuro-specific issues are well controlled.

16.4 Individualizing Therapy in NICU

16.4.1 Pharmacologic Interventions of Pain (▶ Table 16.1)

Specific comorbidities that require special considerations for pain management (▶ Table 16.2)

Nonopioid Analgesics (Primarily for Mild Pain)[5]

- Acetaminophen[10,11]
  - ○ Useful in patients unable to receive oral medications
  - ○ Intravenous (IV) dose may reduce opioid requirements[11]
- Nonsteroidal anti-inflammatory drugs (NSAIDs)[12]
  - ○ Avoid in neurosurgical population for platelet inhibition
  - ○ May lead to kidney injury with chronic use and risk aseptic meningitis

Opioid Analgesics (see ▶ Table 16.1)[9]

- Indicated in NICU for severe pain (patient reported or assessed by ICU tool) or patient–ventilator dyssynchrony[4,13,14]
- Side effects include CNS depression, respiratory depression, bradycardia, nausea, vomiting, constipation, urinary retention, and pruritus

Patient-Controlled Analgesia (PCA)[15]

- Better patient satisfaction if alert, awake, and capable of self-administering

Table 16.1 Properties of commonly used analgesics in critical care

Drug/Class	Mechanism of action	Dose	Advantages	Disadvantages	Metabolism	Notes
Acetaminophen	Exact mechanism unknown; antipyretic effect on hypothalamus; prostaglandin synthesis inhibition	IV: 1,000 mg every 6 hours PO: 650–1,000 mg every 4–6 hours (≤4,000 mg/day)	Has analgesic and antipyretic properties IV formulation rapid acting	No anti-inflammatory property	Hepatic	Available in IV formulation, may mask an infectious process IV formulation is costly and may be restricted Caution use with liver failure
Nonsteroidal anti-inflammatory drug[a]						
Ketorolac	COX-1 and 2 inhibitor	IV: 15–30 mg every 6 hours up to 5 days	Potent analgesia, no respiratory depression Good anti-inflammatory property	Risk of bleeding and renal dysfunction	Hepatic (with renal clearance)	Available in IV formulation, use is limited to 5 days, avoid in renal failure Infrequently used in neuro-ICU due to bleeding risk
Ibuprofen	COX-1 and 2 inhibitor	IV: 400–800 mg every 4–6 hours (<3,200 mg/day)	No respiratory depression	Risk of bleeding and renal dysfunction	Renal	Avoid in renal failure, available in IV formulation

Table 16.1 (*Continued*) Properties of commonly used analgesics in critical care

Drug/Class	Mechanism of action	Dose	Advantages	Disadvantages	Metabolism	Notes
Naproxen Sodium	COX-1 and 2 inhibitor	PO: 500 mg every 12 hours (Max 1,250 mg. day)	No respiratory depression Used for arthritic pain, migraines, gout	Risk of bleeding and renal dysfunction	Hepatic	Not recommended with CrCl < 30 mL/ minute Delayed-release not recommended for acute pain
Celecoxib	COX-2 inhibitor	200 mg twice a day	No respiratory depression, reduce risk gastric bleeding	Some risk of bleeding	Hepatic	Not commonly used in ICU setting
Opioids						
Tramadol	Partially binding opioid μ receptor Inhibits reuptake of norepinephrine and serotonin	Immediate release: 50–100 every 4–6 hours (max 400 mg/ day)	Good for moderate to moderate-severe pain	CNS and respiratory depression Increased risk of seizures Serotonin syndrome in patients on SSRI, SNRIs, TCAs, and neuroleptics	Hepatic	Titrating may improve tolerability Active metabolite has 200-fold greater affinity for opioid receptor Max dose for renal failure is 200 mg/day Max dose for patients with cirrhosis 50 mg/ 12 hours Toxicity may be due to monoamine effect rather than opioid effect[28]

(*Continued*)

Table 16.1 (*Continued*) Properties of commonly used analgesics in critical care

Drug/Class	Mechanism of action	Dose	Advantages	Disadvantages	Metabolism	Notes
Morphine	Opioid receptor agonist	IV: 2–5 mg every 2–4 hours Initial continuous infusion: 1–2 mg/hour PO: 10–30 mg every 3–4 hours	Easy titration	Risk of respiratory depression, active metabolites in renal failure	Hepatic (renal clearance)	Avoid in renal failure, pruritus related to histamine release
Fentanyl	Opioid receptor agonist	IV: 25–50 mcg every 5–15 minutes Initial continuous infusion: 10–20 mcg/hour	Easy titration, available in several formulations; rapid onset	Risk of respiratory depression, chest wall rigidity at high doses	Hepatic	Short half-life, significant increase in context-sensitive half-life with prolonged infusion
Hydromorphone	Opioid receptor agonist	PO: 1–2 mg every 3–4 hours IV: 0.5–1 mg every 3–4 hour Initial continuous infusion: 0.2–0.3 mg/hour	Easy titration	Risk of respiratory depression	Hepatic	Shorter duration of action compared to morphine, may require frequent dosing in opioid tolerant, less pruritic than morphine

Table 16.1 (Continued) Properties of commonly used analgesics in critical care

Drug/Class	Mechanism of action	Dose	Advantages	Disadvantages	Metabolism	Notes
Remifentanil	Opioid receptor agonist	Loading dose: 1.5 mcg/kg Continuous infusion: 0.5–15 mcg/kg/hour	Easy titration, ultra-rapid onset and elimination	Risk of respiratory depression, rebound hyperalgesia	Plasma esterases	Consider longer acting opioid before discontinuation
Oxycodone	Opioid receptor agonist	Initial PO: 5–10 mg every 3–4 hour	Intermediate duration of action	Respiratory depression	Hepatic	Available in combination with acetaminophen, caution with patients with simultaneous use of acetaminophen
Membrane channel stabilizers						
Gabapentin	Analgesic mechanism is unknown: GABA analogue (no effect on GABA receptor)	100 mg three times a day can titrate up to 1,800 mg/day	Effective in neuropathic pain and partial seizures Reduction in opioid requirement when used as part of multi-modal therapy	Sedation	Negligible (renal excretion)	Rapid discontinuation may precipitate seizure, gradual titration Adjust dose for renal impairment based on CrCl

(Continued)

Individualizing Therapy in NICU

Table 16.1 (*Continued*) Properties of commonly used analgesics in critical care

Drug/Class	Mechanism of action	Dose	Advantages	Disadvantages	Metabolism	Notes
Pregabalin	Exact mechanism unknown: GABA analogue that binds to voltage gated calcium channel	50 mg three times a day, may increase to 100 mg three times a day	Effective in neuropathic pain, fibromyalgia and epilepsy Reduction in opioid requirement when used as part of multi-modal therapy	Dose-dependent symptoms of dizziness and sedation Requires titration	Negligible (renal excretion)	Gradual titration Adjust dose for renal failure based on CrCl No effect on opiate receptor
Anesthetics						
Ketamine	NMDA antagonist	Loading dose: 0.1–0.5 mg/kg Infusion dose: 0.05–0.4 mg/kg/ hour	Minimal respiratory depression, prevention in pain chronicization	Psychomimetic reactions	Hepatic	Minimal effect on ICP at subanesthetic dose, useful with opioid tolerant patients
Dexmedetomidine	Central α₂-receptor agonist	Loading dose: 1 mcg/kg over 10 minutes Infusion dose: 0.2–0.7 mcg/kg/ hour	Easy titration, no respiratory depression, mild analgesic property, minimal effect on ICP	Hypotension, bradycardia at high doses	Hepatic	Useful with mechanical ventilation weaning process, cooperative sedation Loading dose not commonly used due to rapid decrease in BP Extended use up to 5–7 days feasible in appropriate patient selection

Table 16.1 (*Continued*) Properties of commonly used analgesics in critical care

Drug/Class	Mechanism of action	Dose	Advantages	Disadvantages	Metabolism	Notes
Lidocaine[30]	Sodium channel blocker	Loading dose: 1–2 mg/kg Infusion dose: 1–2 mg/kg/hour optimal dose	Effective in treatment of acute pain Anti-inflammatory properties Reduction in opioid requirement when used as part of multi-modal therapy	Cardiac toxicity at high dose Seizures Prolonged time to reach steady state without bolus	Hepatic	Avoid in chronic liver failure Therapeutic plasma level 2.5–3. 5 μg/mL CNS toxicity can occur at levels of > 5 μg/mL. CNS toxicity signs: numbness of tongue, metallic taste, light headedness, tinnitus, drowsiness, muscle twitching, unconsciousness, coma, and death

Note: ᵃNSAIDs are contraindicated for perioperative pain in the setting of coronary artery bypass graft surgery.
Abbreviations: BP, blood pressure; CNS, central nervous system; GABA, gamma aminobutyric acid; ICP, intracranial pressure; ICU, intensive care unit; IV, intravenous; NMDA, N-methyl-D-aspartate; NSAIDs, nonsteroidal anti-inflammatory drugs; SNRIs, serotonin–norepinephrine reuptake inhibitor; SSRI, selective serotonin reuptake inhibitor; TCAs, tricyclic antidepressants.

Table 16.2 Pain management in specific patient populations

Pathophysiology	Notes
Elderly	Decreased GFR, drug doses adjusted based on creatinine clearance Decreased respiratory center sensitivity, opioids started at lower dose Decreased receptors in CNS (5HT, AcH, and Dop); therefore, side effects of buprenorphine, tramadol, and tapentadol are potentiated
End-stage renal disease	Decreased GFR and increased volume of distribution, renal dosing
Chronic liver disease	Decreased hepatic blood flow and drug metabolism, doses should be decreased
Cardiac disease	Caution drugs that may cause bradycardia or hypotension (e.g., high doses of opioids, dexmedetomidine) or hypertension or arrhythmias (e.g., ketamine)
Pulmonary disease	Obese patients have obstructive sleep apnea and decreased FRC Supplemental oxygenation or CPAP use may be helpful Minimize opioid use and maximize adjuncts
Dementia	Avoid drugs that potentiate cognitive impairment (e.g., opioids, membrane channel stabilizers) Avoid polypharmacy PCA less suitable
Opioid tolerant	Exhibit opioid-induced hyperalgesia; therefore, higher doses of opioids required Respiratory depression less common Variable opioid cross-tolerance Ketamine helpful in opioid tolerance Maximize use of adjuvants
Substance use disorder	Methadone maintenance therapy should continue with addition of opioids to manage acute pain Should discontinue the use of buprenorphine; intravenous opioids which exhibit high μ-receptor affinity should be used to manage pain Maximize use of adjunct agents PCA to maintain a more stable plasma concentration compared to intermittent intravenous boluses
Alcoholism	Acute ingestion has depressive effect on CNS and increases sensitivity to sedatives Alcohol increases endogenous opioid levels Chronic alcohol ingestion causes chronic liver disease which decreases drug metabolism

(Continued)

Table 16.2 (*Continued*) Pain management in specific patient populations

Pathophysiology	Notes
Postoperative spine	NSAIDs may inhibit bone healing Membrane channel stabilizers help with neuropathic pain Treat muscle spasms with muscle relaxants (e.g., diazepam, cyclobenzaprine, tizanidine, baclofen)
Craniotomy	Frequent neurologic assessments; thus, easily titratable drugs preferred Avoid drugs that sedate and decrease respiratory function Opioids decrease ICP in adequately ventilated patients Dexmedetomidine and subanesthetic ketamine have minimal effect on ICP Scalp blocks reduce opioid requirements

Abbreviations: CNS, central nervous system; CPAP, continuous positive airway pressure; FRC, functional residual capacity; GFR, glomerular filtration rate; ICP, intracranial pressure; NSAIDs, nonsteroidal anti-inflammatory drugs; PCA, patient-controlled analgesia.

Table 16.3 PCA dosing guidelines

	Moderate pain	Moderate-severe pain	Severe pain
Drug/Concentration	Dose/Lockout interval/Hourly max/Nursing PRN dose		
Morphine (1 mg/mL) Fentanyl (10 mcg/mL) Hydromorphone (0.2 mg/mL)	1 mL/6 minutes/ 10 mL/1–2 mL every 1–2 hours	1–1.5 mL/6 minutes/ 10–15 mL/2–3 mL every 1–2 hours	1–2 mL/6 minutes/ 10–20 mL/2–4 mL every 1–2 hours

Note: Concomitant basal infusion has been associated with respiratory depression.
Abbreviation: PCA, patient-controlled analgesia.

- Fentanyl or hydromorphone for opioid tolerant patients (▶ Table 16.3)
- Pumps record total daily opioid and can be used in conversion to oral regimen

Membrane Stabilizing Agents (Gabapentin and Pregabalin)[16,17]

- Effective in neuropathic pain and offer reduction in opioid requirements
- May also be effective in reducing opioid doses in subarachnoid hemorrhage (SAH) and other forms of meningismus[17]
- Adjusted in patients with renal insufficiency

Ketamine[5,18,19]

- Adjunct to reduce opioid requirements, opioid tolerance, and opioid-induced hyperalgesia
- Believed to increase ICP, although newer evidence contests the notion[19]
- Minimal side effects at subanesthetic doses (less than 1 mg/kg): Increased salivation, hypertension, tachycardia, hallucinations of visual, tactile, and auditory perception

Dexmedetomidine[4,5,20]

- α_2-adrenegic receptor agonist in CNS
- Avoid loading dose in NICU patients due to profound but transient hypotension which can occur
- Higher doses limited by the hypotensive and bradycardic response
- Currently FDA approved for continuous ICU sedation at doses 0.2 to 0.7 mcg/kg/hour up to 24 hours (growing evidence supports safe use of up to 1.5 mcg/kg/hour for up to 28 days)

16.4.2 Nonpharmacologic Approach

It may reduce analgesic dose and associated adverse reactions[6]
- Music therapy
- Acupuncture
- Meditation
- Heat and cold application

16.5 Neuro-specific Diseases at Risk for Pain

16.5.1 Pain with SAH

- Sudden onset of severe headache ("worst headache of my life")
- Headache after SAH can last for at least 2 weeks and may be associated with the volume of blood in the subarachnoid space on the initial head CT[29]
- Treatment: Opioids, membrane stabilizers, and dexamethasone

16.5.2 Spondylosis and Disk Herniation[21,22]

- Pain usually occurs in the lower back and may have radiculopathy
  - Lifetime prevalence is 3 to 5% in adults
- Mechanism
  - Chronic micro-trauma leading to stress-type fracture
  - Degenerative age-related change in the nucleus pulposus of the disk

- **Treatment**: Pharmacologic, physical therapy, and epidural steroid injection may provide modest transient pain relief, or surgery

16.5.3 Spasticity

Central Poststroke Pain[23,24]

- Mechanism
  - Pain is a direct consequence of ischemic damage
- Risk factors for chronic pain
  - Increased stroke severity
  - Premorbid depressive symptoms
- Increased stroke severity strongly associated with pain attributable to spasticity and subluxation
- Treatment
  - Tricyclic antidepressants (TCAs) (first line)—amitriptyline
  - Gabapentin/pregabalin (first line if TCA contraindicated)
  - Opioids

Movement Disorders

- Parkinson's disease[25]
  - Different causes of pain: Musculoskeletal, radicular, dystonia-associated, central, and discomfort from akathisia
  - Approximately 30 to 50% of patients experience pain
  - Treatment: Pain-specific and treat underlying cause

Transverse Myelitis[26,27]

- Begins with back or radicular pain, paresthesia, an ascending sensory level, and often progresses to paraplegia
- Spasticity is an adaptive response to facilitate ambulation; painful when excessive
- **Mechanism**: Direct neural injury or spasticity
- **Treatment**: NSAIDs, TCA, and anticonvulsants such as gabapentin, carbamazepine, and opioids

16.6 Ongoing Continuous Pain Monitoring in NICU[7,13,14]

16.6.1 Pain Scales

Based on patient's ability to self-report:
- **Numerical rating scale**: preferred approach in alert patients (▶ Fig. 16.1)

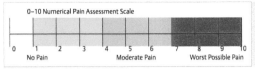

Fig. 16.1 Numerical rating scale.

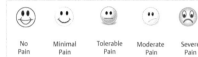

Fig. 16.2 Faces Pain Scale.

Table 16.4 Critical care pain observation tool

Indicator	Description	Score
Facial expression	Relaxed, Neutral	0
	Tens	1
	Grimacing	2
Body movements	Absence of Movements	0
	Protection	1
	Restlessness	2
Muscle tension	Relaxed	0
	Tense or rigid	1
	Very tense or rigid	2
Compliance with ventilation OR Vocalization (Extubated patients)	Tolerating ventilator or movement	0
	Coughing but tolerating	1
	Fighting ventilator	2
	Talking in normal Tone or no sound	0
	Sighing, moaning	1
	Crying, sobbing	2

- **Faces scale (▶ Fig. 16.2) or behavior pain scale**: can be used in nonverbal patient
- Critical Care Pain Observation Tool (CPOT) or Behavioral Pain Score (BPS) based on behavior when non-self-reporting (▶ Table 16.4)
- Family engagement may help with assessment

References

[1] Barr J, Fraser GL, Puntillo K, et al. American College of Critical Care. Clinical practice guidelines for the management of pain, agitation, and delirium in adult patients in the intensive care unit. Crit Care Med. 2013; 41(1):263–306

[2] Balas MC, Vasilevskis EE, Olsen KM, et al. Effectiveness and safety of the awakening and breathing coordination, delirium monitoring/management, and early exercise/mobility bundle. Crit Care Med. 2014; 42(5):1024–1036

[3] Ely EW. The ABCDEF bundle: science and philosophy of how ICU liberation serves patients and families. Crit Care Med. 2017; 45(2):321–330

[4] Makii JM, Mirski MA, Lewin JJ, III. Sedation and analgesia in critically ill neurologic patients. J Pharm Pract. 2010; 23(5):455–469

[5] Dunn LK, Naik BI, Nemergut EC, Durieux ME. Post-craniotomy pain management: beyond opioids. Curr Neurol Neurosci Rep. 2016; 16(10):93

[6] Erstad BL, Puntillo K, Gilbert HC, et al. Pain management principles in the critically ill. Chest. 2009; 135(4):1075–1086

[7] Payen JF, Bru O, Bosson JL, et al. Assessing pain in critically ill sedated patients by using a behavioral pain scale. Crit Care Med. 2001; 29(12):2258–2263

[8] Costello TG, Cormack JR. Anaesthesia for awake craniotomy: a modern approach. J Clin Neurosci. 2004; 11(1):16–19

[9] Trescot AM, Datta S, Lee M, Hansen H. Opioid pharmacology. Pain Physician. 2008; 11(2) Suppl: S133–S153

[10] Yeh YC, Reddy P. Clinical and economic evidence for intravenous acetaminophen. Pharmacotherapy. 2012; 32(6):559–579

[11] Memis D, Inal MT, Kavalci G, Sezer A, Sut N. Intravenous paracetamol reduced the use of opioids, extubation time, and opioid-related adverse effects after major surgery in intensive care unit. J Crit Care. 2010; 25(3):458–462

[12] Scott WW, Levy M, Rickert KL, Madden CJ, Beshay JE, Sarode R. Assessment of common nonsteroidal anti-inflammatory medications by whole blood aggregometry: a clinical evaluation for the perioperative setting. World Neurosurg. 2014; 82(5):e633–e638

[13] Puntillo K, Pasero C, Li D, et al. Evaluation of pain in ICU patients. Chest. 2009; 135(4):1069–1074

[14] Puntillo KA, Neuhaus J, Arai S, et al. Challenge of assessing symptoms in seriously ill intensive care unit patients: can proxy reporters help? Crit Care Med. 2012; 40(10):2760–2767

[15] Macintyre PE. Safety and efficacy of patient-controlled analgesia. Br J Anaesth. 2001; 87(1):36–46

[16] Ruts L, Drenthen J, Jongen JL, et al. Dutch GBS Study Group. Pain in Guillain-Barre syndrome: a long-term follow-up study. Neurology. 2010; 75(16):1439–1447

[17] Dhakal LP, Hodge DO, Nagel J, et al. Safety and tolerability of gabapentin for aneurysmal subarachnoid hemorrhage (SAH) headache and meningismus. Neurocrit Care. 2015; 22(3):414–421

[18] Loftus RW, Yeager MP, Clark JA, et al. Intraoperative ketamine reduces perioperative opiate consumption in opiate-dependent patients with chronic back pain undergoing back surgery. Anesthesiology. 2010; 113(3):639–646

[19] Zeiler FA, Teitelbaum J, West M, Gillman LM. The ketamine effect on intracranial pressure in nontraumatic neurological illness. J Crit Care. 2014; 29(6):1096–1106

[20] Tan JA, Ho KM. Use of dexmedetomidine as a sedative and analgesic agent in critically ill adult patients: a meta-analysis. Intensive Care Med. 2010; 36(6):926–939

[21] Kreiner DS, Hwang SW, Easa JE, et al. North American Spine Society. An evidence-based clinical guideline for the diagnosis and treatment of lumbar disc herniation with radiculopathy. Spine J. 2014; 14(1):180–191

[22] Tarulli AW, Raynor EM. Lumbosacral radiculopathy. Neurol Clin. 2007; 25(2):387–405

[23] O'Donnell MJ, Diener HC, Sacco RL, Panju AA, Vinisko R, Yusuf S, PRoFESS Investigators. Chronic pain syndromes after ischemic stroke: PRoFESS trial. Stroke. 2013; 44(5):1238–1243

[24] Flaster M, Meresh E, Rao M, Biller J. Central poststroke pain: current diagnosis and treatment. Top Stroke Rehabil. 2013; 20(2):116–123

[25] Truini A, Frontoni M, Cruccu G. Parkinson's disease related pain: a review of recent findings. J Neurol. 2013; 260(1):330–334

[26] Frohman EM, Wingerchuk DM. Clinical practice: transverse myelitis. N Engl J Med. 2010; 363 (6):564–572

[27] Krishnan C, Kaplin AI, Deshpande DM, Pardo CA, Kerr DA. Transverse myelitis: pathogenesis, diagnosis and treatment. Front Biosci. 2004; 9:1483–1499

[28] Sansone RA, Sansone LA. Tramadol: seizures, serotonin syndrome, and coadministered antidepressants. Psychiatry (Edgmont Pa). 2009; 6(4):17–21

[29] Glisic EK, Gardiner L, Josti L, et al. Inadequacy of headache management after subarachnoid hemorrhage. Am J Crit Care. 2016; 25(2):136–143

[30] Eipe N, Gupta S, Penning J. Intravenous Lidocaine for acute pain: an evidence based clinical update. BJA Educ. 2016; 16(9):292–298

17 Advanced Hemodynamic and Neurological Monitoring in the Neuro-ICU

David F. Slottje and John W. Liang

Abstract

Hemodynamic instability is a common issue faced in the neurological intensive care unit (neuro-ICU). Practitioners often find themselves pondering about the patient's volume status and whether to give or to withhold fluids in order to optimize cerebral blood flow and brain tissue oxygen delivery. The physical examination, a vital component of care, is often limited in this patient population. Each patient has a different and unique combination of cardiac function, systemic and pulmonary vascular resistance, concurrent infections, and confounding medications, which vary hour by hour. It is not surprising that simple bedside vital signs and urine output measurements are often inadequate estimates of volume status. In this chapter we will discuss advanced hemodynamic monitoring and neuromonitoring techniques that are available, along with respective advantages and limitations.

Keywords: hemodynamic monitoring, cardiovascular function, thermodilution, minimally invasive, monitoring

17.1 Hemodynamic Monitoring

Patients who are critically ill in the neurological intensive care unit (neuro-ICU) can quickly become hemodynamically unstable. Having the appropriate tools to adequately assess hemodynamics beyond basic vital signs is imperative in preventing organ failure or death. It is not uncommon for patients to require continuous blood pressure monitoring or vasopressors which require arterial lines and central venous catheters. When initial resuscitation efforts fail, advanced hemodynamic monitors are implemented to provide additional information to further guide treatment. The choice of monitor is dependent on what specific information is needed, what system is available, and the experience of the practitioner (▶ Table 17.1). Regardless of the monitor, the practitioner must have a strong understanding of physiology and knowledge of normal hemodynamic values (▶ Table 17.2) in order to interpret the data provided effectively.

Table 17.1 Advantage and disadvantages of hemodynamic monitors

Monitor	Advantages	Disadvantages/Risks
Arterial line	Measures continuous BP Easy access to blood draws	Hemorrhage Hematoma Thrombosis Damage to surrounding tissue or nerves Pseudoaneurysm Infection Embolization
Central venous catheter	Measures: • RAP • CVP • SCVO$_2$	Limited by respiratory variation and PEEP Pneumothorax Hemothorax Infection
Pulmonary artery catheter	Measures: • CVP • PAP • PAOP • CI • SVO$_2$	Pneumothorax Hemothorax Arrhythmias Pulmonary artery rupture Typically needs to be removed in 72 hours
Pulse contour analysis	Measures: • CO • SVR (needs CVP) • SVV Minimally invasive Not affected by hypothermia Not labor intensive Well validated (in ideal setting)	Uses a proprietary algorithm that is not published Higher potential for error Does not provide as much information as other more invasive monitors Inaccurate with tachyarrhythmias
PiCCO	Less invasive than PAC Measures: • CO • SVR • ELWI • GEDI • SVV • PPV	Can be labor intensive Requires frequent calibration Data may not be accurate or obtainable in patients with: • Intracardiac shunts • Aortic aneurysm • Aortic stenosis • Pneumonectomy • PE
Volume view/ EV 1000	Measures: • CO • SV • SVV • SVR • EVWI • GEDV • GEF	Has similar limitations as the PiCCO monitor

(Continued)

Table 17.1 (*Continued*) Advantage and disadvantages of hemodynamic monitors

Monitor	Advantages	Disadvantages/Risks
LiDCO	Less invasive than PAC Measures: • CO • SV • SVV • SVR Does not require a central line	Does not offer volumetric measures such as: • GEDI • ELWI Cannot be used in: • Patients < 40 kg • Patients on muscle relaxants Ion selected electrode needs to be replaced every 3 days Expensive

Abbreviations: BP, blood pressure; CI, cardiac index; CO, cardiac output; CVP, central venous pressure; ELWI, extravascular lung water index; EVWI, extravascular water index; GEDI, global end diastolic volume index; GEDV, global end diastolic volume; GEF, global ejection fraction; PAC, pulmonary artery catheter; PAOP, pulmonary artery occlusion pressure; PAP, pulmonary artery pressure; PE, pulmonary embolism; PEEP, positive end-expiratory pressure; PPV, pulse pressure variation; RAP, right atrial pressure; SCVO2, central venous O2 saturation; SV, stroke volume; SVO2, mixed venous O2 saturation; SVR, systemic vascular resistance; SVV, stroke volume variation.

17.1.1 Invasive Monitoring: Pulmonary Thermodilution

Pulmonary Artery Catheter

The pulmonary artery catheter (PAC) or Swan-Ganz catheter was considered the goal standard for hemodynamic monitoring for decades but has lost favor with intensivists with the advent of newer minimally invasive monitors. The PAC is inserted through the jugular or subclavian vein into the right heart and placed directly into the pulmonary artery. This allows measurements of the right atrial pressure (CVP), pulmonary artery pressure, and pulmonary artery occlusion pressure or wedge pressure, which is a reflection of the left atrial filling pressure. There are disadvantages to using a PAC. First, it is invasive and technically difficult. It requires a high degree of expertise to properly interpret the arterial waveform tracings as it advances into the pulmonary artery. In a survey of 534 critical care physicians working in 86 European ICUs, a significant portion felt knowledge was less than adequate.[1] A Cochrane review of randomized trials from 1954 to 2012 demonstrated that there was no alteration in mortality, length of stay, or cost saving associated with PAC usage.[2] The best indication for PAC remains right ventricular heart failure or pulmonary hypertension because there is currently no other method capable of direct measurements of right heart or pulmonary pressures.

Table 17.2 Normal hemodynamic values

Mean arterial blood pressure (MAP)	70–100 mm Hg
Mixed venous O_2 saturation (SVO$_2$)	60–75%
Central venous O_2 saturation (SCVO$_2$)	70%
Right atrial pressure (RAP) Central venous pressure (CVP)	2–6 mm Hg
Stroke volume (SV)	50–100 mL
Cardiac output (CO)	4–8 L/min
Cardiac index (CI)	2.5–4 L/min/m^2
Systemic vascular resistance (SVR)	800–1,200 dynes·sec/cm^{-5}
Pulmonary artery pressure (PAP) Systolic Diastolic Mean	15–30 mm Hg 8–15 mm Hg 9–18 mm Hg
Pulmonary artery occlusion pressure (PAOP)	8–12 mm Hg
Oxygen delivery (DO$_2$)	950–1,150 mL/min
Oxygen consumption (VO$_2$)	200–250 mL/min
Extravascular lung water index (ELWI)	0–7 mL/kg
Global end diastolic volume index (GEDI)	650–800 mL/kg

17.1.2 Less Invasive: Transpulmonary Thermodilution

Transpulmonary thermodilution (TPTD) is a way to measure cardiac output (CO) that is less invasive and modified from the pulmonary artery catheter (PAC) right-heart thermodilution method introduced by Drs. Swan and Ganz in the early 1970s. A known amount of solution with known temperature, typically 15 to 20 cc of cold saline, is bolus into the central venous circulation where it travels through the right heart, the lungs, the left heart, and ultimately into the central arterial circulation where a thermostat, at the tip of a femoral or axillary arterial catheter, depending on the manufacturer, measures the rate and degree of temperature change. The CO is inversely proportional to the area under the thermodilution curve. This method has been compared to pulmonary artery thermodilution with clinically acceptable accuracy.[7,8]

Because the injector solution passes through all four chambers of the heart and the pulmonary vasculature, it is possible to calculate several additional volumetric parameters as well as fluid status in the lungs:

- Global end diastolic volume (GEDV) and global end diastolic volume index (GEDI)
  - These are related to the volume in all four chambers of the heart at the end of diastole and serves as a proxy of preload.
  - A low GEDV or GEDI may suggest responsiveness to preload resuscitation.
- Global ejection fraction (GEF) and cardiac function index (CFI)
  - GEF is a marker of cardiac contractility with normal ranges between 25 and 35%.
  - CFI is another marker of cardiac contractility and is mathematically calculated by dividing CO by GEDV.
  - A low GEF and CFI suggests that poor ventricular performance is the cause for a low stroke volume (SV) or CO; this may prompt addition of inotropic support.
- Extravascular lung water (EVLW) and extravascular lung water index (EVLWI) and pulmonary vascular permeability index (PVPI)
  - Fluid build-up in the lung can affect oxygenation. EVLW and EVLWI assess pulmonary edema and can be helpful in monitoring disease progression.
  - Elevated EVLW or EVLWI may be seen in heart failure, volume overload, or lung injury.
  - Pulmonary vascular permeability index (PVPI) can be used to differentiate the mechanism for elevated EVLW: high PVPI is seen in pulmonary edema as a result of lung injury, such as in acute respiratory distress syndrome (ARDS), whereas normal PVPI is seen in hydrostatic and cardiogenic pulmonary edema.

In general, TPTD is useful in patients with unstable hemodynamics, unclear volume status, or impairment in tissue oxygen delivery and demand. Typical conditions include septic shock, cardiogenic shock, pulmonary edema, and ARDS. It can also be considered if strict maintenance of hemodynamic parameters (i.e., euvolemia for subarachnoid vasospasm) is critical. The additional volumetric data is helpful to guide intervention selection such as fluid resuscitation, diuresis, inotropic or vasopressor support, etc.

Pulse Contour Cardiac Output (PiCCO)

PiCCO is a system which combines the principles of arterial pulse contour analysis with transpulmonary thermodilution to measure CO.

Access Requirements

- Central venous catheter
- Femoral, brachial, or axillary arterial line

Technology

Similar to VolumeView, the pulse contour analysis provides continuous hemo-dynamic information while calibration with thermodilution provides intermittent volumetric parameters.

Data Output

- Hemodynamics (CO, SV, systemic vascular resistance [SVR], stroke volume index [SVI])
- Preload (GEDV, GEDI)
- Contractility (GEF)
- Volume (pulse pressure variation [PPV], stroke volume variation [SVV])
- Lung water (EVLW, EVLWI)
- Afterload (SVR, systemic vascular resistance index [SVRI])
- Intrathoracic blood volume index

Limitations

- Need to be on controlled mechanical ventilation; no spontaneous breathing
- Requires regular calibration three to four times a day
- Maximum duration of 10 days
- Not recommended with intracardiac shunts
- Data may be inaccurate with severe tachyarrhythmias, valvular insufficiency, pulmonary embolism, partial lung resection, and possibly with aortic aneurysms

VolumeView/EV1000

The VolumeView system consists of the VolumeView sensor and the EV1000 Clinical Platform monitor. It combines the concept of pulse contour analysis and TPTD into one system.

Access Requirements

- Central venous catheter, in the subclavian or internal jugular vein
- Femoral arterial line

Technology

TPTD is used to measure a calibrated cardiac output (CO_{TT}). The CO_{TT} is then used in the calibration of a proprietary algorithm to estimate a continuous CO (CO_{Cont}) via pulse contour analysis, similar to FloTrac.

Data Output

Hemodynamics (CO_{Cont}, SV, SVI, and SVV)
- Preload (GEDV/GEDI)
- Afterload (SVR/SVRI)
- Contractility (GEF/CFI)
- Lung water (EVLW/EVLWI and PVPI)

Advantages

- Unlike FloTrac, TPTD is not affected by the mode of ventilation and it is more accurate in patients suffering from septic shock.[10]
- Demonstrated to have no significant difference compared to PAC-thermodilution when used in cardiogenic shock patients, irrespective of mitral or tricuspid regurgitation, intra-aortic balloon pump, or therapeutic hypothermia.[11]

Limitations

- It requires both a central venous and central arterial line.
- Calibrations must be done at least every 8 hours in order for the continuous pulse contour derived estimation of CO_{Cont} to be reliable.
- The error between CO_{Cont} and CO_{TT} was shown to be lower with shorter recalibration intervals, 1 and 2 hours, compared to the standard 8 hours.[12] This suggests that recalibration should be done more frequently in unstable patients and after any significant clinical intervention.

Dilution Cardiac Output (LiDCO)

It is operator-dependent system that combines the concepts of pulse power analysis (rather than pulse contour analysis) with lithium dilution to measure CO. It has been shown to be at least as accurate as bolus thermodilution via pulmonary artery catheter.[9]

Access Requirements

Radial arterial line as well as a venous (central or peripheral) line.

Technology

- A bolus of lithium chloride is flushed through the venous line and a lithium sensor, attached to the arterial line, detects the concentration of lithium in the blood.

- The lithium concentration "wash-out" time is used to calibrate the arterial waveform analysis providing continuous readings for SV, SVV, and CO.

Data Output

SV, SVV, PPV, and CO are obtained.

Advantages

- Similar to other TDTP, more accurate than pulse contour analysis especially in patients with unstable hemodynamics
- CO correlates well with PAC
- Injectate can be given via central or peripheral venous line

Limitations

- It does not provide any advanced volumetric variables such as GEDV, GEF, CFI, or EVLW.
- It requires calibration every 8 hours with approximately 5 mL sample of blood each time. Hemoglobin and sodium levels need to be entered for the software calculations.
- For proper calibration the dose of lithium chloride may require adjustment based on patient size.
- Although the typical lithium dose (0.15–0.30 mmol/dose for average adult) is small and toxicity is unlikely, the risk remains higher than cold saline injection.
- LiDCO cannot be used in patients on lithium therapy (i.e., bipolar).

17.1.3 Minimally Invasive Monitoring: Pulse Contour Analysis

Pulse contour analysis is based on the concept that the SV is proportional to the area under the arterial pressure waveform. Once the SV is obtained, the CO can be easily calculated using CO = SV × HR. Various companies have developed methods of analyzing the waveform and calculating CO via proprietary algorithms. One of the main disadvantages of pulse contour analysis is that it becomes more inaccurate when a patient is unstable on pressors.

FloTrac/Vigileo

Uncalibrated, minimally invasive pulse contour analysis sensor. The FloTrac sensor is connected to the Vigileo monitor but is also compatible with the newer EV1000 Clinical Platform monitor.

Access Requirements

Peripheral or central arterial line, typically radial.

Technology

The sensor measures the arterial pulse rate (PR) instead of the HR; therefore, it captures perfusing beats. SV is calculated and updated every 20 seconds utilizing a proprietary formula which incorporates: age, gender, body surface area, waveform skewness and kurtosis, and standard deviation of arterial pulse pressure. The PR is multiplied by the calculated SV to return CO.

Data Output

- CO, SV, stroke volume variation (SVV), and stroke volume index (SVI)
- SVR (if combined with CVP reading from central venous catheter)

Stroke Volume Variation (SVV)

- SVV is determined by assessing the arterial pulse pressure changes during the respiratory cycle.
- SVV above 10 is associated with an increase in SV after fluid bolus.
- **Note:** SVV is not a measure of volume status but rather preload responsiveness. A patient with SVV below 10% suggests low likelihood of fluid responsiveness but does not discern between euvolemia versus hypervolemia.
- SVV has only been validated for use in patients that are on controlled mechanical ventilation with fixed respiratory rates and tidal volume of > 8 cc/kg. SVV is not reliable in spontaneous breathing due to the natural fluctuating rates and tidal volumes.

Advantages

- It is quick and simple to set up.
- It does not require central vascular access (unless SVR is desired).
- The output is well validated in hemodynamically stable patients[3,4] and not affected in patients undergoing therapeutic hypothermia.
- The sensor monitors arterial vascular changes continuously and calibrates automatically, making the system operator-independent.

Limitations

- Multiple variables in calculating SV makes this method the most mathematically complex and therefore greater potential for sources of error. Accuracy of input parameters (age, gender, height, weight) as well as a good arterial pressure waveform is vital to the algorithm's calculation of SV and CO.

- Accuracy may be compromised in severe shock states due to peripheral vaso-constriction[5,6] dampening the arterial waveform leading to a falsely low CO. It is recommended to use a central arterial access, such as femoral artery, in these situations.
- Arrhythmia will affect the accuracy of SVV; CO and SV are not affected.

17.1.4 Noninvasive Hemodynamic Monitoring

These products are completely noninvasive with no venous or arterial access required.

ClearSight System

ClearSight utilizes the volume clamp method to provide real-time, noninvasive, continuous monitoring of key hemodynamic parameters. It consists of a finger blood pressure cuff outfitted with infrared sensing technology. The blood pressure cuff deflates and inflates while the infrared sensors continuously monitor finger arterial volume and pulsations. This occurs 1,000 times per second and arterial variations are displayed as a waveform similar to that obtained by a traditional arterial line. The system then uses a proprietary algorithm to analyze the arterial waveform to return hemodynamic variables.

The ClearSight system can utilize one finger cuff for up to 8 hours, or two finger cuffs for up to 72 hours by alternating between each finger hourly. Movement of the patient's hand above or below the heart level is automatically adjusted for without affecting the waveform measurements.

Data Output

Blood pressure, PR, SV, SVV, SVR, and CO are obtained.

Advantages

- CO measurement comparable to PiCCO TPTD in stable patients undergoing elective coronary artery bypass grafting (CABG).[13]
- Noninvasiveness and easy installation make this an attractive method for continuous perioperative CO monitoring in hemodynamically stable patients.

Limitations

- Reliability of this method during times of hemodynamic instability or significant changes in peripheral vascular resistance is limited due to finger hypoperfusion.[14]

- Compared to PiCCO TPTD in critically ill patients, there was poor estimations of cardiac function and unreliable detection of CO change in response to volume expansion.[15]
- Reliability during therapeutic hypothermia is unknown.

Cheetah NICOM

Cheetah NICOM is a noninvasive monitoring system consisting of four sensor pads applied to the thorax utilizing the concept of bioreactance. An electrical current is applied across the thorax by the transmitting sensors, blood flow in the thorax leads to a time delay in the current, and the signal is detected by the recorded sensors. The signal recorded is analyzed using a proprietary algorithm and converted into the aortic waveform. SV is obtained by calculating the area under the systolic portion of the waveform. Electrical propagation in the thoracic cavity is influenced by body surface area. Therefore, CO calculation incorporates SV and HR, as well as age, weight, and height.

Data Output

CO, cardiac index (CI), SV, SVI, and SVV

Advantages

- Easy to set up
- Works on spontaneously breathing or mechanically ventilated patients
- Provides changes in SV in response to fluid challenge or passive leg raise
- Studies performed on relatively stable post-cardiac surgery patients have shown good correlation when Cheetah NICOM was compared to PAC-thermodilution[16] or FloTrac.[17]

Limitations

- Certain conditions may affect the accuracy of the monitor. These include severe aortic insufficiency, severe anatomic abnormalities of the thoracic aorta (i.e., aortic graft, large aortic aneurysm, or aortic dissection), left ventricular assist devices, and external and some older models of internal pacemakers.
- Because the system relies on electrical currents passing through the thorax, it may be affected by conditions that increases the thoracic volume (i.e., obesity, chronic obstructive pulmonary disease, pulmonary edema, or pleural effusion) and studies on this are limited.
- Current data regarding the accuracy of Cheetah NICOM in the critically ill shows poor correlation when compared to PAC-thermodilution[18] or PiCCO-TPTD.[19]

17.2 Neurological Monitoring

The critical care management of neurologically injured patients extends beyond the initial stabilization. It is well known that these patients are at risk of a secondary brain injury which contributes to an increase in morbidity and mortality. Neuromonitoring has a key role in the early recognition and management/prevention of secondary brain injury. Often referred to as multimodality monitoring, advanced hemodynamic monitoring is utilized along with invasive and noninvasive neuromonitoring (▶ Table 17.3) to optimally manage a patient.

17.2.1 Noninvasive Monitors

Transcranial Doppler

Transcranial Doppler (TCD) (▶ Fig. 17.1) is an important bedside tool in the neuro-ICU. Details on the use have been described in Chapter 18.

Uses

- Detection of vasospasm in subarachnoid hemorrhage (SAH)
- Prediction of stroke risk in sickle cell patients
- Ancillary test to support the diagnosis of death by neurologic criteria

Advantages

Convenient noninvasive test that can be performed regularly on SAH patients to help detect vasospasm. The sensitivity of this test is highest among anterior circulation vessels, especially the middle cerebral artery (MCA) and internal carotid artery (ICA).

Limitations

- Provides no useful information on distal vasculature
- Reliability of TCD results are operator-dependent
- Quality may be limited due to poor insonation bone windows typically seen in African Americans, females, and elderly patients
- Elevated velocities do not always correlate with delayed cerebral ischemia[21]

Continuous Electroencephalogram (cEEG)

Continuous EEG has traditionally been used in the management of status epilepticus as well as nonconvulsive status epilepticus (NCSE). In addition to seizure monitoring and management, cEEG is commonly used intraoperatively as well as in the ICU for titration of medications (sedatives, barbiturates), neuro-

Table 17.3 Neuromonitors

Monitor	Advantage	Disadvantage
Noninvasive		
TCD	Bedside Inexpensive	Isolated point in time—not continuous Poor or no windows
EEG	Continuous monitoring	Should be removed for imaging due to artifact
NIRS	Continuous monitoring	Not well validated (in adults) Not effective with deep injury Variable penetrance with increased skull thickness Can be affected by thick forehead muscles Not reliable with underlying scalp hematoma or fluid collection
Invasive		
External ventricular drain	Gold standard Continuous monitoring Allows CSF drainage Waveforms provide information on brain compliance Allows for in vivo calibration	Risk of pericatheter hemorrhage Risk of overdrainage causing subdural High clot burden increases its risk of failure Catheter occlusion from blood or tissue can require frequent flushing (proximal and distal) Pressure transducer may require frequent "zeroing" depending on patient positioning Risk of infection CSF leak may cause falsely low ICP and increase risk of ventriculitis
Intracranial pressure monitor (microsensors)	Intraparenchymal or subdural placement Easier to place than external ventricular drain (EVD) Less complication risk	Unable to drain CSF Measures only local area pressure; not good for global injury Tend to drift over time leading to inaccurate numbers

(*Continued*)

Table 17.3 (*Continued*) Neuromonitors

Monitor	Advantage	Disadvantage
Invasive		
Jugular venous oximetry	Ideal for a wide variety of patients: TBI, SAH with vasospasm, surgical patients, cardiac arrest patients Assesses global cerebral oxygen delivery and metabolic demand	Mechanical or technical complications during placement Increased risk of thrombosis with prolonged placement Values can be altered based on the oxyhemoglobin dissociation curve Not ideal in patients with infratentorial lesion (brainstem or cerebellum) Contraindicated with coagulopathy SjvO2 may be affected by placement site (dominant vs. nondominant) Should not be used in patients with uncontrolled ICP Unable to detect regional ischemia
Brain tissue oxygen tension monitor (PbtO$_2$)	Gold standard Real-time monitoring of cerebral oxygenation Assists in determining optimal CPP for patients Well-defined ranges have been established	Expensive Contraindicated if coagulopathic Can require frequent troubleshooting Measures PBtO2 regionally making placement important Takes 2 hours to equilibrate
Thermal diffusion and laser doppler flowmetry	Real-time assessment of regional cerebral blood flow Thermal flow is invasive while laser flow is noninvasive	Not ideal with global injury Affected by artifact Limited clinical use of laser doppler flowmetry
Microdialysis	Can aid in the early detection of ischemia	Expensive Labor intensive Requires frequent troubleshooting

Abbreviations: CPP, cerebral perfusion pressure; CSF, cerebrospinal fluid; EEG, electroencephalogram; EVD, external ventricular drain; ICP, intracranial pressure; NIRS, near-infrared spectroscopy; SAH, subarachnoid hemorrhage; TBI, traumatic brain injury; TCD, Transcranial Doppler.

prognostication after cardiac arrest, and the diagnosis of death by neurologic criteria.[22] cEEG has also shown to be useful in SAH patients in early detection of vasospasm and cerebral ischemia.[23,25]

Quantitative EEG (qEEG) has become a power tool in critical care EEG (▶ Fig. 17.2). By applying various computer algorithms, the digitized EEG is able to condense hours of raw data into color maps of brain functioning.[22] Several

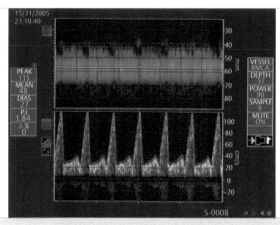

Fig. 17.1 Transcranial Doppler (TCD) of the right middle cerebral artery (MCA) of a 65-year-old man with severe traumatic brain injury (TBI). He became progressively encephalopathic by day 12 post-injury without clear explanation. The family considered withdrawal of care. His TCD pulsatility index (PI) of 1.84 suggested increased intracranial pressure, prompting a lumbar puncture with opening pressure of 52-cm H_2O. A repeat head computed tomography (CT) revealed the presence of bilateral subdural hygromas. He was taken to the operating room (OR) for subdural evacuation and subsequently regained consciousness and was eventually discharged to a rehabilitation facility.

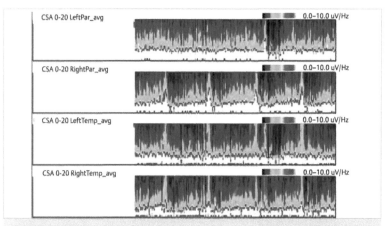

Fig. 17.2 Quantitative EEG (qEEG) analysis of a compressed spectral array, showing cyclic seizures manifesting as spikes in the power spectrum in the right parietal region. (Courtesy of Larry Hirsch, Department of Neurology, Columbia University). Reproduced with permission from Jallo J, Loftus C, eds. Neurotrauma and Critical Care of the Brain. 1st ed. Thieme; 2009.

studies on qEEG in SAH patients demonstrated high sensitivity for detecting vasospasm and infarct.[22,23,24,25] Despite showing promise, there is a lack of consensus regarding which parameters should be monitored when applied.

Advantages

- Noninvasive
- Continuous EEG can offer long-term, noninvasive, real-time detection of secondary neurological insults as they occurs in patients with limited neurological examinations to follow reliably.
- Quantitative EEG, in contrast to cEEG, is less time consuming and can be incorporated into existing multi-modal monitoring programs although it is not universally applied.

Disadvantages

- Labor intensive
- Time consuming
- Should be removed for intracranial imaging due to causing streak artifact
- Limited availability
- Requires high level of expertise to interpret data appropriately in the critically ill population

Near-infrared Spectroscopy Measurement of Regional Brain Tissue Oxygen Saturation (NIRS)

Near-infrared spectroscopy (NIRS) offers continuous noninvasive monitoring of regional oxygenation of tissues. The device, which is applied to the skin, consists of a near-infrared light (700–1,000 nm wavelength) emitter and two photodetectors (▶ Fig. 17.3). The light is absorbed into the brain tissue between 2 and 3 mm. The absorption of light is proportional to the concentration of iron in hemoglobin. Although used frequently in the cardiothoracic population, NIRS has not been widely used in traumatic brain injury (TBI) or following cranial surgery. Soft tissue swelling, hematoma, and craniectomy have created significant challenges to its use in trauma or postsurgical patients.[26]

Use

- Extracorporeal membrane oxygenation (ECMO) patients
- Coronary artery bypass graft surgery

Advantages

- Convenient noninvasive test that can be performed continuously

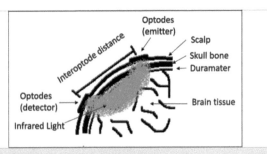

Fig. 17.3 The placement of near-infrared spectroscopy sensors over the forehead and the path of near-infrared light from emitter to 2 detectors. Reproduced with permission from Singh G P. Near-infrared spectroscopy—current status. Journal of Neuroanaesthesiology and Critical Care 2016; 03(04): 66–69.

Limitations

- Measurements may be inaccurate in the setting of hematoma or other mass lesion
- Measurements may be inaccurate in the setting of scalp swelling, hematoma, or craniectomy
- Scatter artifact
- Use is limited to superficial or cortical injury
- Cross contamination with intra- and extracranial oxygen sources can create situations where the flow appears normal in a true low-flow state

17.2.2 Invasive Monitors: Cerebral Oximetry

Several techniques exist for assessing the adequacy of oxygen delivery to the injured brain. These include direct brain tissue oxygen ($PbtO_2$) monitoring, jugular bulb monitoring of arteriovenous oxygen content difference ($AVDO_2$), microdialysis monitoring of extracellular glutamate and other molecules, and NIRS measurement of regional brain tissue oxygen saturation. Of these techniques, only $AVDO_2$ monitoring is recommended by current professional guidelines,[26] although $PbtO_2$ monitoring has gained some traction in clinical practice. Significant interest exists in the study of all of these modalities, as there is mounting evidence that secondary brain injury may occur even in the setting of normal intracranial pressure (ICP) and normal cerebral perfusion pressure.[27] Theoretically, cerebral oximetry can serve as the basis for goal-directed therapy to ensure adequate delivery of oxygen to meet the high metabolic demand of jeopardized brain tissue.

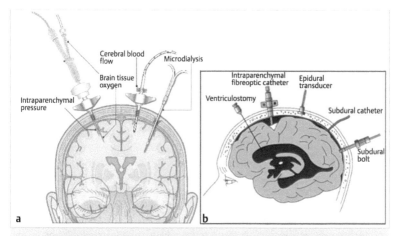

Fig. 17.4 Showing various intracranial monitors. Brain tissue oxygen monitor which can also measure intraparenchymal pressure. (**a**) Microdialysis catheter. (**b**) Cerebral blood flow catheter.

Direct Brain Tissue Oxygen (PbtO$_2$) Monitoring

There are several commercially available PbtO$_2$ monitoring devices, including the Licox (Integra, Plainsboro, NJ, USA) and the Neurovent (Raumedic, Mills River, NC, USA) (► Fig. 17.4). These devices require insertion of a probe into the white matter of the brain through a twist-drill burr hole. The Licox probe contains a Clark polarographic electrode in which an adjacent cathode and anode are immersed in an electrolyte solution separated from the brain tissue by an oxygen-permeable membrane. Following insertion into the brain, oxygen diffuses into the electrolyte solution housing the electrode. The pO$_2$ of the solution affects the current passed between anode and cathode. The probe monitors this current, allowing for the continuous measurement of PbtO$_2$.[28] The Neurovent probe contains luminescent ruthenium which emits light that is detected by a photodetector. The ruthenium luminophore is deactivated by oxygen, a process known as luminescence quenching. As a result, the PbtO$_2$ can be deduced from the amount of light detected.[29]

A large body of evidence from observational studies suggests that low PbtO$_2$ correlates with increased risk of death and poor outcome following brain injury. Although the optimal value for PbtO$_2$ has not been established, it seems that values less than 20 mm Hg are deleterious.[30],[31],[32],[33],[34],[35] Although the correlation between low PbtO$_2$ and adverse outcome has been well established, the question of whether treatment protocols aimed at improving PbtO$_2$ can avert these poor outcomes remains a matter of controversy. Cohort studies comparing treatment protocols based on monitoring of ICP in conjunction with PbtO$_2$ as compared to monitoring of ICP alone have shown mixed results. Several studies have shown improved outcomes with the addition of PbtO$_2$ monitoring,[36,37] one study demonstrated worse neurologic outcomes with the addition of PbtO$_2$ monitoring,[38] and others have shown no difference.[39,40]

The BOOST Trial, a phase 2 randomized clinical trial, compared a TBI treatment protocol based upon solely ICP control with a protocol based upon ICP and PbtO2 goal-directed interventions. In this study PbtO$_2$ was measured using the Licox device (Integra, Plainsboro, NJ, USA). The PbtO$_2$ group had statistically significant reduction in duration of brain tissue hypoxia (defined as PbtO$_2$ < 20 mm Hg) and a nonstatistically significant trend toward decreased mortality. At the time of writing of this manual, a phase 3 study is planned to better evaluate this question.[41]

In clinical practice, PbtO$_2$ monitoring is used most commonly in the setting of TBI. In cases of focal brain injury, the insertion site of the monitor is a subject of controversy. Placement in the frontal white matter contralateral to the injury allows for a measurement of global brain oxygenation, whereas placement adjacent to the injured tissue theoretically allows for metabolic assessment of the "penumbral" region. There is no clear evidence suggesting that one approach is superior. In theory, PbtO$_2$ monitoring may be particularly useful in poly-trauma patients with concurrent brain and lung injuries in whom neurologic—and pulmonary—protective strategies may need to be balanced against one another. PbtO$_2$ monitoring has also been used to detect vasospasm in subarachnoid hemorrhage, although a prospective observational study concluded that this practice did not detect ischemic events rapidly enough to allow for corrective measures to be taken.[42]

Advantages

It provides regional assessment of brain oxygenation.

Limitations

- Requires insertion of intracranial probe
- Oxygen must diffuse into Clark electrode to provide accurate information; may take up to an hour
- Provides regional assessment of brain oxygenation which may not reflect global brain oxygenation or oxygenation of penumbral brain tissue remote to the monitor
- Evidence-based treatment protocols for PbtO$_2$ directed interventions have yet to be rigorously established

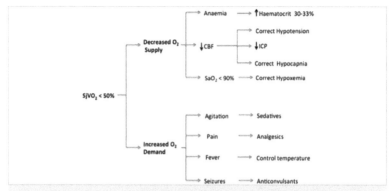

Fig. 17.5 Schematic diagram of strategies to correct low jugular venous oxygen saturation. Reproduced with permission from Bhardwaj A, Bhagat H, Grover V K. Jugular venous oximetry. Journal of Neuroanaesthesiology and Critical Care 2015; 02(03): 225–231.

Jugular Bulb Monitoring of Arteriovenous Oxygen Content Difference ($AVDO_2$)

Jugular bulb oxygen monitoring provides an indirect measurement of cerebral oxygen use. The catheter is placed in a retrograde fashion using the Seldinger technique in the dominant jugular vein (usually the right).[46] The easiest way to understand how it measures oxygen use is by thinking of the concept of supply and demand (▶ Fig. 17.5). An injured brain may increase the amount of oxygen extracted causing the jugular venous oxygenation to be lower than normal; demand is greater than supply. Likewise, when the supply exceeds demand, the amount of oxygen returned will be higher than normal.

Another way to understand this is mathematically. The supply is cerebral oxygen delivery (DO_2) which is dependent on cerebral blood flow (CBF) and arterial oxygen content (CaO_2).

$$DO_2 = CBF \times CaO_2$$

The demand (consumption) by the brain is the cerebral metabolic rate (CMRO2). This is affected by the CBF and by the difference in arterial and jugular venous oxygen content $AjvDO_2$ which is the same as $CaO_2 - CjvO_2$.

$CMRO_2 = CBF \times (AjvDO_2)$, which can berearranged as $AjvO_2 = CMRO_2/CBF$

If $CMRO_2$ is relatively constant then changes in the difference in oxygen content are compensated by the CBF (▶ Fig. 17.5). Low $SjvO_2$ can be caused by either decreased O_2 supply, from hypotension, vasospasm, increased ICP, hypoxia, anemia, sepsis, or hyopcapnea or increased O_2 demand, from increased

Table 17.4 Management of low and high jugular venous oxygen saturation

Low SjvO$_2$ (<50%)	
Decreased O$_2$ supply	**Increased O$_2$ demand**
Transfuse to increase hemoglobin	Sedate if agitated
Increase blood pressure	Treat pain
Drain CSF	Maintain normothermia
Decrease respiratory rate or sedate	Treat shivering
Inotropes if indicated	Treat seizures
High SjvO2 (>75%)	
Increase O$_2$ supply	**Decrease in consumption**
Treat hypertension	Decrease sedation
Increase respiratory rate	Slowly rewarm if hypothermic
Decrease PaO$_2$	Add hyperosmolar treatment for edema
Abbreviation: CSF, cerebrospinal fluid.	

metabolism, fever, shivering, seizures, agitation, and pain. If left untreated, it could lead to ischemic injury. On the other side, high SjvO$_2$ can be caused by either an increase in O$_2$ supply, from severe hypercapnea, drug-induced vasodilation, hypertension, AVM, or increase in PaO2 or from a decrease in demand, from hypothermia, barbiturates, cerebral infarct, or brain death. If left untreated, it could cause cerebral edema or death. Understanding the etiology of the high or low SjvO$_2$ allows directed therapy (▶ Table 17.4).

Advantages

• Provides global assessment of brain oxygenation
• Use is supported by evidence-based professional guidelines

Limitations

• Fiberoptic catheter requires frequent calibration
• Accuracy may be compromised by clot formation on catheter or if catheter tip is directly apposed against vessel wall
• May not detect regional abnormalities in brain oxygenation
• Carries theoretical risk of aggravating intracranial hypertension. Thrombus formation within the dominant sinus may lead to decreased venous return from the brain.

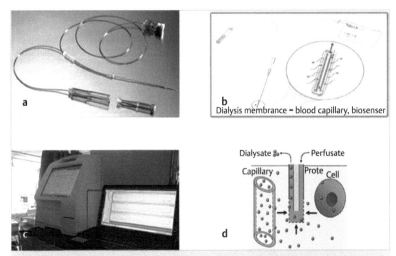

Fig. 17.6 (a) Cerebral microdialysis catheter and microvial used for cerebral microdialysis. (b) Microdialysis catheter as universal biosensor/blood capillary. (c) Bedside cerebral microdialysis analyzer used to monitor the values of dialysate. (d) Schematic picture showing principle of microdialysis with microdialysis in center collecting products of cellular metabolism from cell and interstitial fluid components from capillary by diffusion. Source: Gupta D, Mazzeo A. Cerebral microdialysis: Going deep into brain biochemistry for a better understanding of pathomechanisms of acute brain injury. Indian Journal of Neurosurgery. 2017.

Microdialysis Monitoring

Microdialysis (▶ Fig. 17.6) is a well-established laboratory method of assessing the metabolic state of tissues. The technique involves insertion of a double lumen catheter into the tissue of interest. A dialysate solution is pumped through the catheter. The dialysate is separated from the tissue by a semipermeable membrane which allows only particles < 20 kDa to pass from the tissue to the dialysate. The dialysate is returned and analyzed. The most common molecules studied include glucose, pyruvate and lactate, glycerol, and glutamate.[43]

Use

• SAH for early prediction of vasospasm
• Any indication having concern for delayed cerebral ischemia

Advantages

It provides metabolic profile of brain tissue with potential to measure numerous target molecules.

Limitations

- Technically demanding: Requires 24/7 personnel familiar with operation and maintenance
- Invasive: Requires insertion of intracranial probe
- Limited use in clinical practice
- Limited availability
- No evidence-based treatment protocols are based upon microdialysis measurements

17.2.3 Cerebral Blood Flow Monitors

QFlow 500 Perfusion Probe

Probe works in conjunction with the Bowman Perfusion Monitor to calculate regional blood flow via thermal diffusion.

Use

- SAH
- TBI
- Neurosurgical procedures requiring continuous blood flow monitoring (aneurysm clipping, EC/IC bypass)

Advantages

- Can be used for up to 10 days
- No calibration or zeroing required
- Computed tomography (CT) compatible

Disadvantages

- Small amount of tissue volume being measured ($27 \, mm^3$)
- Due to the small area being monitored, placement of catheter becomes critical

17.2.4 Intracranial Pressure Monitoring

Measurement of ICP and ICP-directed therapies are central to the care of patients with TBI as well as a variety of other neurologic conditions which result in intracranial hypertension. ICP can be measured using a ventriculostomy catheter (considered the gold standard) or a parenchymal monitor. Both of these devices are inserted into the brain via a twist-drill burr hole. In the case of a ventriculostomy, the catheter is positioned in the lateral ventricle, creating a continuous fluid column of cerebrospinal fluid (CSF). The height of the fluid column is a direct measurement of the ICP. The catheter can be connected to a pressure transducer to allow for continuous monitoring. There are several commercially available parenchymal ICP monitors. The Camino (Integra, Plainsboro, NJ, USA) and the Microsensor (Codman, Raynham, MA, USA) are two of the more widely used devices. The Camino probe contains a fiberoptic transducer,[44] whereas the Microsensor measures electrical conductance across a strain gauge mounted on the tip of the probe.[45] In patients who do not require CSF diversion, parenchymal monitors may be preferred over ventriculostomies, as they pose lower risk of infection. Subdural and epidural monitors are also available but are used less commonly in clinical practice.

The range of normal ICP values remains controversial. ICP > 22 mm Hg has been shown to be associated with poor neurologic outcome and increased mortality in TBI.[44] There is widespread expert consensus that control of intracranial hypertension, based upon monitoring of ICP, is crucial to mitigating secondary neurologic injury. Current professional guidelines recommend ICP monitoring in severe TBI[26] and this is considered standard of care in the United States and many other countries. Despite this general support, there is no Class 1 evidence of benefit of ICP monitoring.

ICP monitoring is commonly used in conjunction with cerebral perfusion pressure (CPP) monitoring. Under normal physiologic circumstances CPP is the difference between mean arterial pressure (MAP) and jugular venous pressure (JVP). In states of intracranial hypertension, ICP exceeds JVP. When this is the case CPP is calculated as follows:

$$CPP = MAP - ICP$$

Current professional guidelines recommend maintaining CPP between 60 and 70 mm Hg in patients with TBI.[26] This too is an area of controversy, with experts advocating both higher and lower target CPP ranges. Strong physiologic arguments can be made on both sides of the debate. Higher CPP can potentially lead to cerebral edema and increased ICP due to increased cerebral blood volume and increased trans-capillary hydrostatic pressure. On the other hand, cerebral autoregulation in the injured brain is not completely disrupted but rather is right-shifted. Consequently, at a higher CPP, the brain's afferent arterioles constrict, thus reducing cerebral blood volume and reduced ICP with stable cerebral blood flow.[45] In practice, each patient is different and the bedside physician must adjust his her approach accordingly.

Advantages: External Ventricular Drain

- Considered to be the "gold standard" method for measurement of ICP
- Allows for therapeutic drainage of CSF in addition to ICP measurement

Limitations: External Ventricular Drain

- Requires insertion of intracranial catheter
- Susceptible to infection of CSF space
- Measurement will not be accurate in the setting of ventricular collapse which is likely to occur in high ICP states
- Measurement may not be accurate in the setting of thick intraventricular hemorrhage or clot within the catheter tubing
- Insertion may be challenging in the setting of high ICP, midline shift, or ventricular effacement

Advantages: Parenchymal Monitor

- More accurate than ventricular catheter in the setting of high ICP and ventricular collapse
- Less susceptible to infection than ventricular catheter
- Can generally be placed easily and safely in almost any disease state

Limitations: Parenchymal Monitor

- Requires insertion of intracranial probe
- Measurements are subject to calibration error as well as "drift," becoming less reliable over time
- Fragile probe tip can be easily damaged with insertion, resulting in inaccurate measurement
- Most parenchymal monitors are not magnetic resonance imaging (MRI) compatible

References

[1] Gnaegi A, Feihl F, Perret C. Intensive care physicians' insufficient knowledge of right-heart catheterization at the bedside: time to act? Crit Care Med. 1997; 25(2):213–220
[2] Rajaram SS, Desai NK, Kalra A, et al. Pulmonary artery catheters for adult patients in intensive care. Cochrane Database Syst Rev. 2013(2):CD003408

[3]   Broch O, Renner J, Gruenewald M, et al. A comparison of third-generation semi-invasive arterial waveform analysis with thermodilution in patients undergoing coronary surgery. Scientific-WorldJournal. 2012; 2012:451081

[4]   Mutoh T, Ishikawa T, Kobayashi S, Suzuki A, Yasui N. Performance of third-generation FloTrac/Vigileo system during hyperdynamic therapy for delayed cerebral ischemia after subarachnoid hemorrhage. Surg Neurol Int. 2012; 3:99

[5]   Monnet X, Anguel N, Jozwiak M, Richard C, Teboul JL. Third-generation FloTrac/Vigileo does not reliably track changes in cardiac output induced by norepinephrine in critically ill patients. Br J Anaesth. 2012; 108(4):615–622

[6]   Ganter MT, Alhashemi JA, Al-Shabasy AM, et al. Continuous cardiac output measurement by uncalibrated pulse wave analysis and pulmonary artery catheter in patients with septic shock. J Clin Monit Comput. 2016; 30(1):13–22

[7]   Felbinger TW, Reuter DA, Eltzschig HK, Bayerlein J, Goetz AE. Cardiac index measurements during rapid preload changes: a comparison of pulmonary artery thermodilution with arterial pulse contour analysis. J Clin Anesth. 2005; 17(4):241–248

[8]   Friesecke S, Heinrich A, Abel P, Felix SB. Comparison of pulmonary artery and aortic transpulmonary thermodilution for monitoring of cardiac output in patients with severe heart failure: validation of a novel method. Crit Care Med. 2009; 37(1):119–123

[9]   Linton R, Band D, O'Brien T, Jonas M, Leach R. Lithium dilution cardiac output measurement: a comparison with thermodilution. Crit Care Med. 1997; 25(11):1796–1800

[10] Slagt C, Helmi M, Malagon I, Groeneveld AB. Calibrated versus uncalibrated arterial pressure waveform analysis in monitoring cardiac output with transpulmonary thermodilution in patients with severe sepsis and septic shock: an observational study. Eur J Anaesthesiol. 2015; 32(1):5–12

[11] Schmid B, Fink K, Olschewski M, et al. Accuracy and precision of transcardiopulmonary thermodilution in patients with cardiogenic shock. J Clin Monit Comput. 2016; 30(6):849–856

[12] Scully CG, Gomatam S, Forrest S, Strauss DG. Importance of re-calibration time on pulse contour analysis agreement with thermodilution measurements of cardiac output: a retrospective analysis of intensive care unit patients. J Clin Monit Comput. 2016; 30(5):577–586

[13] Broch O, Renner J, Gruenewald M, et al. A comparison of the Nexfin® and transcardiopulmonary thermodilution to estimate cardiac output during coronary artery surgery. Anaesthesia. 2012; 67 (4):377–383

[14] Fischer MO, Avram R, Cârjaliu I, et al. Non-invasive continuous arterial pressure and cardiac index monitoring with Nexfin after cardiac surgery. Br J Anaesth. 2012; 109(4):514–521

[15] Monnet X, Picard F, Lidzborski E, et al. The estimation of cardiac output by the Nexfin device is of poor reliability for tracking the effects of a fluid challenge. Crit Care. 2012; 16(5):R212

[16] Squara P, Denjean D, Estagnasie P, Brusset A, Dib JC, Dubois C. Noninvasive cardiac output monitoring (NICOM): a clinical validation. Intensive Care Med. 2007; 33(7):1191–1194

[17] Marqué S, Cariou A, Chiche JD, Squara P. Comparison between Flotrac-Vigileo and Bioreactance, a totally noninvasive method for cardiac output monitoring. Crit Care. 2009; 13(3):R73

[18] Fagnoul D, Vincent JL, Backer D. Cardiac output measurements using the bioreactance technique in critically ill patients. Crit Care. 2012; 16(6):460

[19] Kupersztych-Hagege E, Teboul JL, Artigas A, et al. Bioreactance is not reliable for estimating cardiac output and the effects of passive leg raising in critically ill patients. Br J Anaesth. 2013; 111 (6):961–966

[20] Miller C, Armonda R, Participants in the International Multi-disciplinary Consensus Conference on Multimodality Monitoring. Monitoring of cerebral blood flow and ischemia in the critically ill. Neurocrit Care. 2014; 21 Suppl 2:S121–S128

[21] Carrera E, Schmidt JM, Oddo M, et al. Transcranial Doppler for predicting delayed cerebral ischemia after subarachnoid hemorrhage. Neurosurgery. 2009; 65(2):316–323, discussion 323–324

[22] Foreman B, Claassen J. Quantitative EEG for the detection of brain ischemia. Crit Care. 2012; 16 (2):216

263

[23] Claassen J, Hirsch LJ, Kreiter KT, et al. Quantitative continuous EEG for detecting delayed cerebral ischemia in patients with poor-grade subarachnoid hemorrhage. Clin Neurophysiol. 2004; 115 (12):2699–2710

[24] Labar DR, Fisch BJ, Pedley TA, Fink ME, Solomon RA. Quantitative EEG monitoring for patients with subarachnoid hemorrhage. Electroencephalogr Clin Neurophysiol. 1991; 78(5):325–332

[25] Vespa PM, Nuwer MR, Juhász C, et al. Early detection of vasospasm after acute subarachnoid hemorrhage using continuous EEG ICU monitoring. Electroencephalogr Clin Neurophysiol. 1997; 103 (6):607–615

[26] Carney N, Totten AM, O'Reilly C, et al. Guidelines for the Management of Severe Traumatic Brain Injury, Fourth Edition. Neurosurgery. 2017;80(1):6–15.

[27] Bergsneider M, Hovda DA, Shalmon E, et al. Cerebral hyperglycolysis following severe traumatic brain injury in humans: a positron emission tomography study. J Neurosurg. 1997; 86(2):241–251

[28] Stewart C, Haitsma I, Zador Z, et al. The new Licox combined brain tissue oxygen and brain temperature monitor: assessment of in vitro accuracy and clinical experience in severe traumatic brain injury. Neurosurgery. 2008; 63(6):1159–1164, discussion 1164–1165

[29] Huschak G, Hoell T, Hohaus C, Kern C, Minkus Y, Meisel HJ. Clinical evaluation of a new multiparameter neuromonitoring device: measurement of brain tissue oxygen, brain temperature, and intracranial pressure. J Neurosurg Anesthesiol. 2009; 21(2):155–160

[30] Eriksson EA, Barletta JF, Figueroa BE, et al. The first 72 hours of brain tissue oxygenation predicts patient survival with traumatic brain injury. J Trauma Acute Care Surg. 2012; 72(5):1345–1349

[31] Chang JJ, Youn TS, Benson D, et al. Physiologic and functional outcome correlates of brain tissue hypoxia in traumatic brain injury. Crit Care Med. 2009; 37(1):283–290

[32] Stiefel MF, Udoetuk JD, Spiotta AM, et al. Conventional neurocritical care and cerebral oxygenation after traumatic brain injury. J Neurosurg. 2006; 105(4):568–575

[33] Bardt TF, Unterberg AW, Härtl R, Kiening KL, Schneider GH, Lanksch WR. Monitoring of brain tissue PO2 in traumatic brain injury: effect of cerebral hypoxia on outcome. Acta Neurochir Suppl (Wien). 1998; 71:153–156

[34] Valadka AB, Gopinath SP, Contant CF, Uzura M, Robertson CS. Relationship of brain tissue PO2 to outcome after severe head injury. Crit Care Med. 1998; 26(9):1576–1581

[35] van den Brink WA, van Santbrink H, Steyerberg EW, et al. Brain oxygen tension in severe head injury. Neurosurgery. 2000; 46(4):868–876, discussion 876–878

[36] Narotam PK, Morrison JF, Nathoo N. Brain tissue oxygen monitoring in traumatic brain injury and major trauma: outcome analysis of a brain tissue oxygen-directed therapy. J Neurosurg. 2009; 111(4):672–682

[37] Spiotta AM, Stiefel MF, Gracias VH, et al. Brain tissue oxygen-directed management and outcome in patients with severe traumatic brain injury. J Neurosurg. 2010; 113(3):571–580

[38] Martini RP, Deem S, Yanez ND, et al. Management guided by brain tissue oxygen monitoring and outcome following severe traumatic brain injury. J Neurosurg. 2009; 111(4):644–649

[39] Green JA, Pellegrini DC, Vanderkolk WE, Figueroa BE, Eriksson EA. Goal directed brain tissue oxygen monitoring versus conventional management in traumatic brain injury: an analysis of in hospital recovery. Neurocrit Care. 2013; 18(1):20–25

[40] McCarthy MC, Moncrief H, Sands JM, et al. Neurologic outcomes with cerebral oxygen monitoring in traumatic brain injury. Surgery. 2009; 146(4):585–590, discussion 590–591

[41] Shutter L. Brain Oxygen and Outcome in Severe TBI (BOOST) Phase 2 Presentation of Initial Results. Presentation to Neurocritical Care Society. September 2014

[42] Kett-White R, Hutchinson PJ, Al-Rawi PG, Gupta AK, Pickard JD, Kirkpatrick PJ. Adverse cerebral events detected after subarachnoid hemorrhage using brain oxygen and microdialysis probes. Neurosurgery. 2002; 50(6):1213–1221, discussion 1221–1222

[43] de Lima Oliveira M, Kairalla AC, Fonoff ET, Martinez RC, Teixeira MJ, Bor-Seng-Shu E. Cerebral microdialysis in traumatic brain injury and subarachnoid hemorrhage: state of the art. Neurocrit Care. 2014; 21(1):152–162

[44] Sorrentino E, Diedler J, Kasprowicz M, et al. Critical thresholds for cerebrovascular reactivity after traumatic brain injury. Neurocrit Care. 2012; 16(2):258–266

[45] Rosner MJ, Rosner SD, Johnson AH. Cerebral perfusion pressure: management protocol and clinical results. J Neurosurg. 1995; 83(6):949–962

[46] Schell RM, Cole DJ. Cerebral monitoring: jugular venous oximetry. Anesth Analg. 2000; 90 (3):559–566

18 Neuroimaging

Michael J. Lang

Abstract
This chapter is a brief introduction to neuroimaging, with attention to imaging modalities, indications, and limitations of use. Major modalities for brain and spine imaging will be discussed, with particular attention to types of imaging sequences commonly used in the neurocritical care patient population.

Keywords: neuroimaging, magnetic resonance imaging, computed tomography, angiography, ultrasound

18.1 Introduction

Neuroimaging plays an essential role in the diagnosis and management of critical neurological disease. Advances in the fields of neurology and neurosurgery have directly paralleled advances in neuroimaging, for which their inventors have won numerous Nobel Prizes since Röntgen developed X-rays.[1] An in-depth discussion of the physics of neuroimaging, interpretation of neuroradiography, and clinical application thereof are beyond the scope of this chapter. The following should serve as a brief introduction to commonly used imaging modalities in the neurocritical care patient.

18.2 Types of Imaging

18.2.1 Brain Imaging

In the modern era, computed tomography (CT) and magnetic resonance imaging (MRI) account for the vast majority of brain imaging studies. This is in large part due to their ease of acquisition, relatively noninvasive nature, multi-planar reconstruction (MPR) of multiple image sets from a single acquisition, and use of advanced imaging techniques. This chapter will also discuss cerebral angiography, which still plays a key role in diagnosis of cerebral vascular diseases, and is essential for neuroendovascular procedures.

18.2.2 Spine Imaging

As with brain imaging, CT and MRI form the core of modern neuroimaging for spinal disorders. They form a direct complement to one another, with CT most useful for imaging bony elements, and MRI most adept at demonstrating neural elements or soft-tissue pathology. The exception to this is CT myelography (CT-M), which uses lumbar puncture to inject iodinated contrast to image the intra-thecal contents. Unlike brain imaging, plain X-rays are used extensively in management of spine disease, particularly in order to demonstrate dynamic changes in spinal alignment to motion or weight-bearing.

18.3 Advantages and Limitations (▶ Table 18.1)

18.3.1 Brain Imaging

CT

A CT scan produces cross-sectional images (slices) from computer reconstruction of a series of X-rays taken from different angles. In general, findings on CT are described in terms of density: isodense, hypodense, and hyperdense.

- Isodense is grey and refers to brain tissue.
- Hypodense is dark grey or black and refers to cerebrospinal fluid (CSF) (dark grey) or air (black).
- Hyperdense is white and refers to bone, blood, or calcium.

The X-rays are absorbed by tissues depending on density, which is translated to different intensities on a grey scale. The scale of absorption is referred to in

Table 18.1 Imaging advantages and disadvantages

Image type	Advantages	Disadvantages	Cost	Risk
Computed tomography (CT)	• Fast acquisition of images • Best modality for trauma • Best modality to differentiate between ischemic stroke and hemorrhagic stroke • Best for acute screening for subarachnoid hemorrhage • Best for spinal bone anatomy • Allows for contrast imaging, venous imaging, perfusion imaging	• Poor tissue contrast (less sensitive than MRI) • Poor resolution of the brainstem and posterior fossa • Not compatible with functional imaging • Less sensitive for spinal cord injury/anatomy • Sensitive to bone artifact and beam hardening artifact • Exposure to ionizing radiation • Imaging processing time for perfusion studies	Low	Radiation exposure Iodinated contrast

(Continued)

Table 18.1 *(Continued)* Imaging advantages and disadvantages

Image type	Advantages	Disadvantages	Cost	Risk
Magnetic resonance imaging (MRI)	• Soft tissue contrast • Demyelination and cerebral edema clearly imaged • No radiation • Advanced (specialized) sequences (MRA, DTI, fMRI, MRS) • Best for spinal anatomy	• Long acquisition times • Susceptibility and motion artifact • Differentiation of age of blood • Magnetic safety regulations	High	RF heat deposition causing burn Gadolinium contrast low risk unless renal failure Device magnet compatibility Patients may require sedation to remain calm and not move
Functional MRI	• Provides anatomical and functional view of the brain • Metabolic studies track real-time brain activity which can be used preoperatively • Uses tissue oxygenation and use—records brain signals • High spatial resolution	• Same limitations with plain MRI • Skilled reader to interpret the imaging • Risk of false positive • Based on blood low as correlate of brain activity • "Noise" • Limited availability	Very high	Same as MRI
Digital subtraction angiography (DSA)	Gold standard for vascular imaging Supports cerebrovascular intervention	Invasive Poor surveillance imaging	Very high	Iatrogenic stroke or hemorrhage Large radiation dose Uses iodinated contrast
Ultrasound	• Fast • Ease of use • Available for bedside procedures • No radiation	• Operator dependent • Difficult in viewing retroperitoneal	Low	Procedural error (misinterpretation of image)
Transcranial Dopplers	• Fast • Noninvasive • Bedside testing can be performed • Screening of children with sickle cell disease for stroke risk	• Up to 20% of patients do not have insonable intracranial vessels • Technician dependent • Low sensitivity	Low	• No direct risk

Abbreviations: DTI, diffusion tensor imaging; fMRI, functional MRI; MRA, magnetic resonance angiography; MRS, magnetic resonance spectroscopy; RF, radiofrequency.

Table 18.2 Hounsfield units

Tissue/Substance	Hounsfield units
Air	−1,000
Fat	−30 to −70
Water	0
Muscle/Soft tissue	20 to 40
Brain white matter	25
Brain grey matter	35
Intracranial hemorrhage	60 to 100
Punctate calcification	30 to 500
Iodinated contrast	100 to 600
Bone or metal	+ 1,000

Note: Approximate values. May vary according to source.

terms of Hounsfield units (HU) and ranges from + 1,000 (bone) to −1,000 (air) (▶ Table 18.2). The higher the number the brighter it is on imaging and likewise the lower the number the darker it is.[17]

CT has significant advantages that often make it the initial study for patients with suspected intracranial pathology. The ease of acquisition makes it the ideal study for emergent or repeat brain imaging in the acute inpatient setting.[2] Routine head CT imaging (HCT) produces 5 mm thick axial sections, although multi-detector scanners can now generate submillimeter thickness images which accommodate MPR with minimal interpolation artifact. Routine HCT is full of clinically relevant information, such as the presence of brain edema or herniation, ventricular configuration, ischemia, and osseous imaging of the skull and sinuses (▶ Fig. 18.1). Generally speaking, it is the study of choice for intracranial hemorrhage for several reasons. First, the speed of acquisition allows interventional decisions to be made rapidly. Also, the evolution of blood products from the acute to subacute to chronic phase is much more straightforward than on MRI. Finally, the advent of portable CT scanners has meant that all but the most extremely unstable critical care patients can undergo HCT imaging as clinically indicated.[3]

However, CT does have several limitations. As with all X-ray-based imaging technologies, CT requires exposure to ionizing radiation, which is of particular concern with pediatric patients. HCT is also significantly limited in its ability to demonstrate parenchymal changes. Contrast-enhanced HCT can help improve tissue contrast for certain disease states, but does require iodinated contrast

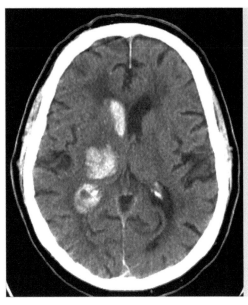

Fig. 18.1 Noncontrast head computed tomography (CT) demonstrating right thalamic intraparenchymal hemorrhage with intraventricular extension and nonspecific white matter changes. The mnemonic "Blood Can Be Very Bad" may aid in systematic review of intracranial structures for the novice (B: Blood, C: Cisterns, B: Brain, V: Ventricles, B: Bone) to avoid missing key findings.

administration, with its attendant renal and allergic risks. The major classes of image artifacts encountered in CT imaging include motion (though less so than MRI), streak artifact from metal in the image field, and beam hardening artifact (which limits the utility of HCT in imaging the posterior fossa).[4]

Since the time of its creation in the 1970s, CT imaging has continued to evolve and now detailed neurovascular imaging can be provided through angiography, perfusion, venography, and contrast enhancement.

CT Angiography

CT angiography (CTA) has become one of three core imaging techniques for imaging cervical and intracranial vascular disease (see below). High-resolution acquisition can be reconstructed in multiple planes, and can be rendered in three dimensions. In combination with CT perfusion (CTP), CTA is an essential component of neuroimaging in acute brain ischemia when considering endovascular thrombectomy.[5] Acute thrombus is identified as an abrupt cutoff in a vascular tree. CTA approaches the sensitivity and specificity of digital subtraction angiography (DSA) for detection of cerebral aneurysms and other intra-cranial vascular lesions, although without the benefit of dynamic imaging of cerebral blood flow. The presence of vascular intervention devices, such as aneurysm clips, coils, or stents, results in significant streak artifact that can limit the utility of CTA for long-term follow-up.[6] Poor bolus timing (as with cardiomyopathy) can result in poor arterial opacification or venous contamination.

CT Venography

CT venography (CTV) is a useful and rapid imaging technique used to diagnose cerebral venous thrombosis. The CTV is reported to have 95% sensitivity with multi-planar reformatting compared to traditional DSA.[19] It can provide detailed anatomy of intracranial venous system, both the deep and superficial veins. That being said, it is common to have normal variants of the venous system and should not be mistaken for pathologic event.[18] It carries the same limitation as any study that requires contrast and should be used with caution in pregnancy.

CT Perfusion

Described first by Axel in 1980,[22] perfusion imaging of the brain has taken on a core role in the acute management of ischemic stroke. At a basic level, perfusion imaging relies on dynamic imaging of a contrast bolus through a volume of tissue. Parenchymal blood flow parameters can be mapped on a voxel-by-voxel basis, and reconstruction of perfusion maps allows for identification of cerebral blood flow (CBF), mean transit time (MTT), and cerebral blood volume (CBV), which are related by the equation:

$$CBF = \frac{CBV}{MTT}$$

Clinical application of this imaging technique allows for delineation of ischemic/oligemic versus infarcted cerebral tissue. Regions of ischemia significant enough to produce cell death (less than 8–10 mL/100 cc tissue/minute) will have matched regions of decreased CBF and CBV (▶ Table 18.3). However, intermediate ranges of ischemia or oligemia can result in impaired neuronal function without cell death, resulting in potentially reversible clinical symptoms. This is seen as regions of decreased CBF but with preserved CBV, which receive enough collateral flow to preserve neuronal integrity for a period of time,

Table 18.3 Interpretation of CTP imaging

CTP	MTT	CBF	CBV	Significance
Penumbra	Prolonged	Moderately decreased	Normal or increased	Tissue at risk
Infarct	Prolonged	Decreased	Decreased	Completed infarct

Abbreviations: CBF, cerebral blood flow; CBV, cerebral blood volume; CTP, computed tomography perfusion; MTT, mean transit time.

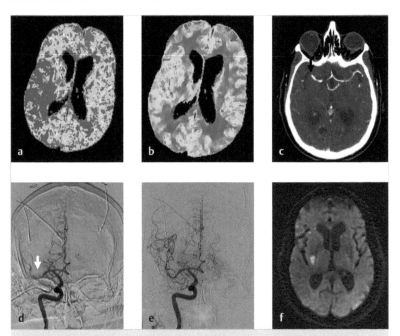

Fig. 18.2 Imaging studies in an acute stroke patient. Computed tomography (CT) perfusion imaging shows elevated mean transit time (**a**) in the territory of the right middle cerebral artery. Cerebral blood volume in the same region (**b**) was preserved, suggesting salvageable penumbra. CT angiography (CTA) demonstrated distal right M1 cutoff (**c**, *black arrow*). This finding correlated during emergent cerebral angiography (**d**, *white arrow*), with subsequent reperfusion following mechanical thrombectomy (**e**), and postoperative magnetic resonance imaging (MRI) demonstrating minimal ischemic changes on diffusion-weighted imaging (DWI) (**f**).

known as the ischemic penumbra, which can potentially be salvaged with thrombolytic or mechanical thrombectomy therapies (▶ Fig. 18.2).[7] CT-based perfusion imaging is, generally speaking, more reliable than MR perfusion (MRP) due to the fixed relationship between iodinated contrast concentration and density, unlike the nonlinear relationship between Gd-contrast and the $T2^*$ signal which forms the basis for MRP.

Contrast

While brain MRI is the imaging modality of choice for evaluation of intracranial pathology, contrast-enhanced head CT still has some utility. Most commonly, it is utilized for patients with non-MRI compatible metallic or implantable hardware. Additionally, in some cases, contrast imaging is preferred or required. Patients with renal failure are unable to receive gadolinium (Gd)-based contrast due to the risk of development of nephrogenic systemic fibrosis (NSF) and CT contrast is iodinated which can be dialyzed.

MRI

MRI is based on the principle in physics of nuclear magnetic resonance.[8] It uses interactions of hydrogen nuclei, radiofrequency energy, and a magnetic field. The majority of images are created from the magnetic properties of the hydrogen nuclei contained with water molecules within tissue, of which the human body is abundant. The exact physics behind the individual sequences are beyond the scope of this chapter.

MRI has far greater brain tissue contrast compared to CT. This is particularly true for new higher field strength magnets (3 Tesla or greater), although with notable limitations for certain types of artifacts.[9] MR-based imaging is also capable of a wide array of advanced imaging techniques such as diffusion imaging or spectroscopy, and does not use ionizing radiation. Conversely, MRI is significantly more susceptible to motion artifact than CT, requires longer image acquisition times, is significantly more expensive to install and maintain, and requires safety protocols for patients and equipment in the magnetic environment. In comparison to CT, findings are referred to in terms of intensity: hypointense, hyperintense, and isointense. There are various sequences that are completed with routine MRI which are noted within ▶ Table 18.4.

Diffusion

Diffusion-weighted imaging (DWI) is currently the imaging modality of choice for the evaluation of cerebral infarction. DWI utilizes motion of water molecules for tissue contrast. Normal brain tissue has relatively low diffusion restriction, as the majority of water is contained in the interstitial space. However, in the setting of stroke, Na^{2+}/K^+ pump failure results in loss of cellular homeostasis, sodium influx, and net inflow of water into the intracellular space. This results in an extremely conspicuous hyperintense signal in the region of infarction referred to as *diffusion restriction*. A similar effect is seen with cerebral abscesses and epidermoid cysts, both of which show diffusion restriction on MRI. Due to short acquisition times, DWI can be performed quickly and is relatively resistant to motion artifact. However, DWI can be significantly limited by susceptibility artifact, particularly near the skull base due to air–tissue interface, in the region of blood/blood products or from metal-containing hardware. Diffusion imaging can also be complicated by the presence of underlying edema, which independently shows up hyperintense on DWI with the absence of true diffusion restriction. This is called T2 shine-

Table 18.4 MRI sequences

MRI sequence	Property	Practicality or usefulness
DWI/ADC	DWI—maps the diffusion of water molecules ADC—measure of diffusion	• Rapid changes with ischemia • Acute ischemia • Cytotoxic edema • Cerebral abscess or encephalitis • Highly proteinaceous tumor • Diffuse axonal injury • Anoxic injury/HIE • Acute demyelination • Tumors with necrosis or high nuclear to cytoplasmic ratio ADC—useful for estimating and distinguishing acute from subacute stroke and age of lesion. Hypointensity in ADC: • Abscess • Lymphoma • MS • Seizures • Metabolic d/o (Canavan)
T1-weighted	Image is created based on relaxation times between fat and water High fat signal (white) Low water signal (black)	Anatomical identification: White on T1: Fat, subacute blood, melanin, proteinaceous fluid, paramagnetic substances (gadolinium contrast) Dark on T1: Edema (water), tumor, infection, inflammation, blood (hyperacute and chronic)
T2-weighted	Images is created based on relaxation times between water and fat High water signal (white) Low fat signal (black)	Evaluation of pathology: Bright on T2: Vasogenic edema, tumor, infection, inflammation, subdural blood, late subacute blood
FLAIR	T2-weighted with suppression of the CSF signal (CSF is dark)	Detects white matter abnormalities (diseases affecting paraventricular tissue) Mesial temporal sclerosis hamartomas Is sensitive but not specific
GRE	Single radiofrequency pulse + gradient reversal	Detection of blood products

Abbreviations: ADC, apparent diffusion coefficient; CSF, cerebrospinal fluid; DWI, diffusion-weighted imaging; GRE, gradient recalled echo; HIE, hypoxic-ischemic encephalopathy; MRI, magnetic resonance imaging; MS, multiple sclerosis.

through which refers to a hyperintense signal on DWI image without restricted diffusion but due to a high T2 signal which "shines through."[10] Use of apparent diffusion coefficient (ADC) maps can help delineate the difference between true diffusion restriction and T2 shine-through, with dark regions on ADC correlating with diffusion restriction. ADC changes also are the earliest identifiable features on MRI in the setting of acute stroke.

Perfusion

MRP imaging is used to demonstrate similar measures of cerebral blood flow and perfusion as CTP. As noted above, computational challenges exist for contrast-based MRP methods due to the nonlinear dose-dependent enhancement. However, acquisition time can limit its utility for acute stroke by delaying intervention relative to CTP.[11] At our institution, MRP is most commonly used as an adjunct to anatomic MRI and MR spectroscopy in the determination of recurrent tumor versus radiation necrosis in the glioma patient population.

T1-weighted

The sequence is good in identification of anatomy. It is best for viewing post-contrast images. Hyperintense signal can be caused by fat, methemoglobin, Gd contrast, or other paramagnetic contrast, melanin.

T2-weighted FLAIR and GRE

T2-weighted fluid-attenuated inversion recovery (FLAIR) imaging is a particularly useful sequence in the evaluation of cerebral pathology. Due to magnetic differences in the local environment, CSF signal can be nulled while accentuating intraparenchymal edema (▶ Fig. 18.3). As a result, FLAIR imaging is particularly useful for identifying regions of periventricular edema (such as trans-ependymal flow in hydrocephalus or periventricular white matter lesions in multiple sclerosis). Furthermore, FLAIR imaging (along with T_2*-gradient recalled echo [GRE] imaging) is considered the single most sensitive test for the identification of subarachnoid hemorrhage (SAH), and calls into question the utility of lumbar puncture in the evaluation of thunderclap headache.

Structures have different appearance when looking at T1 and T2 images (▶ Table 18.5). Blood and blood products in particular have varying signal characteristics which make it useful in determining the age of a hemorrhage at the time of MRI (▶ Table 18.6).

Role of Contrast

Gd-based contrast agents are utilized for intravenous contrast enhancement due to their paramagnetic properties at room temperature. A full accounting of

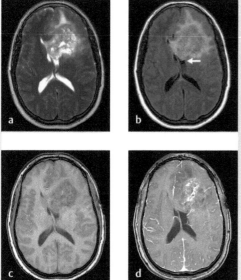

Fig. 18.3 Brain magnetic resonance imaging (MRI) study for a patient with suspected glial neoplasm. T_2 (**a**) and fluid-attenuated inversion recovery (FLAIR) (**b**) images demonstrate a left frontal glial tumor with significant mass effect on the left frontal horn, which is more sharply demarcated on the FLAIR images (*arrow*). T_1-weighted images, before and after contrast administration (**c** and **d**, respectively), show evidence of enhancement in a tumor which was found to be anaplastic astrocytoma.

Table 18.5 Appearance of structures on T1- and T2-weighted images on MRI

Structure	T1-weighted	T2-weighted
Fat	White	Dark
Cerebrospinal fluid	Dark	White
Air	Dark	Dark
Edema	Dark	Bright
Calcification	Dark	Dark
Gadolinium contrast	White	White

Abbreviation: MRI, magnetic resonance imaging.

contrast-enhancing lesions is beyond the scope of this text, but contrast should be administered during MRI evaluation of any nonischemic focal lesion of the parenchyma. Compared to iodinated contrast, Gd agents have a significantly improved safety profile. Although Gd can cause mild renal injury, causation of overt renal failure is very rare, and allergy is extremely rare. The feared complication of Gd-contrast administration is NSF, in which large fibrosing plaques developing on the skin and internal organs, resulting in severe flexion

Table 18.6 Appearance of blood products

Hemorrhage	Time	Hemoglobin	T1-weighted	T2-weighted
Hyperacute	<24	Oxyhemoglobin (intracellular)	Isointense	Hyperintense
Acute	1–3 days	Deoxyhemoglobin (intracellular)	Isointense	Hypointense
Early subacute	3–7 days	Methemoglobin (intracellular)	Hyperintense	Hypointense
Late subacute	7–14 days	Methemoglobin (extracellular)	Hyperintense	Hyperintense
Chronic	>14 days	Hemosiderin	Hypointense	Hypointense

Adapted from Greenberg MS. Handbook of Neurosurgery. 6th ed. New York, NY: Thieme; 2006.

contractures and pain. NSF is an extremely rarely reported disease, which has been nearly uniformly identified in patients on chronic hemodialysis (though a few cases in patients with a history of peritoneal or pre-dialysis patients have been reported in the literature).[12]

Angiography and Venography

Magnetic resonance arteriography (MRA) and magnetic resonance venography (MRV) are commonly utilized in clinical practice. Time of flight (TOF) imaging can be used to image either arteries or veins without contrast, although contrast-enhanced methods are also used. Venography is most commonly used in the evaluation of venous sinus thrombosis or to evaluate sinus patency in the region of dural-based lesions. MR-based vascular imaging is an important screening tool in the evaluation of vascular disease, given the benefits of MRI in general. However, certain important artifacts are associated with MRA/MRV. As with any MR technique, susceptibility artifact in the region of vascular devices can limit evaluation of nearby structures, although often less significant than CT streak artifact. Regions of turbulent flow result in spin dephasing which can result in overestimation of vascular stenosis or underestimation of vessel diameter due to nonlaminar flow at the vessel–blood interface. Furthermore, MRA/MRV may have difficulty differentiating between severe stenosis and complete occlusion.[13]

Angiography

Cerebral angiography remains the gold standard for diagnostic evaluation of cerebrovascular disease, and the sensitivity and specificity of catheter-based angiography for identification of cerebrovascular lesions remains unsurpassed (▶ Fig. 18.4). However, angiography has several inherent limitations. Diagnostic cerebral angiography is associated with a complication rate on the order of 0.5 to 1%, which can include iatrogenic injury to any of the vessels crossed with a

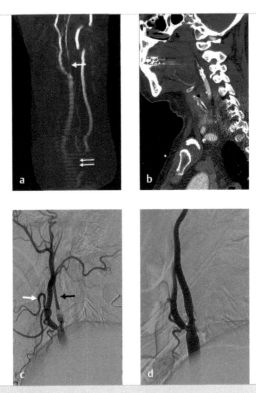

Fig. 18.4 Three modalities of vascular imaging are shown. Time of flight magnetic resonance arteriography (MRA) (**a**) shows a right carotid bifurcation with high-grade stenosis (*arrow*), but cannot clearly demonstrate flow through the stenotic lesion. "Venetian blind" artifact is evident throughout due to stacking of adjacent slab acquisition for three-dimensional reconstruction (*double arrow*). Computed tomography angiography (CTA) (**b**) shows evidence of extensive calcification in the plaque and the anatomic position of the carotid bifurcation. Given the plaque extended to the C2–C3 level, a carotid artery stent was selected instead of carotid endarterectomy. Cervical carotid artery angiogram demonstrates the complex plaque with high-grade stenosis (**c**) and resulting delayed opacification of the internal carotid artery (*black arrow*) relative to the external carotid artery (*white arrow*). Post-stent angiography (**d**) shows significantly improved intracranial flow.

catheter.[14] These risks are increased in patients with atherosclerotic vessel disease or connective tissue disorders. The use of iodinated contrast agents, often at significantly higher doses than those required for CTA, is also a limitation.

18.3.2 Spine Imaging

CT

CT spine imaging is essential to the management of spinal disease, and is unrivaled in its ability to delineate static body anatomy of the vertebral column. Subtle differences in fracture pathology can dictate significantly different management. Likewise, CT imaging is extremely useful in planning for instrumented fusion procedures, especially for osteoreductive corrections. Spinal CT also helps to demonstrate changes in bone quality from endocrinologic or oncologic pathology. In general, spinal CT has poor resolution of the underlying neural elements, but is complementary to MRI, which images bony anatomy poorly. Contrast-enhanced spinal CT can be of use in patients unable to undergo MRI. When lesions of the thoracic spine are being evaluated, we recommend contiguous imaging of the adjacent cervical and/or lumbar spine so that accurate counting of vertebral levels can be performed, and serve as a reference for intraoperative X-ray localization. Finally, it is essential to remember that the spinal column is a dynamic structure, and CT acquired in the supine position may poorly reflect the alignment of the spine in weight-bearing conditions. At our institution, full-length weight-bearing scoliosis X-rays are routinely acquired to assess segmental and global measures of stability and alignment.

MRI

MRI of the spine is the current gold standard for evaluation of the neural elements. In particular, spinal MRI should be pursued, if feasible, in all patients being considered for surgical intervention of degenerative spinal disease, with osteoarthritis, disk herniation, and vertebral endplate Modic changes all well-visualized.[15] Most importantly, however, MRI provides an important means to evaluate concordance of clinical presentation with imaging changes. Patients are frequently seen with pain syndromes which mimic spinal pathology without radiographic correlate, and asymptomatic imaging changes become increasingly frequent with age. It should also be considered the modality of choice for evaluating oncologic pathology of the spinal cord or vertebral column (including intramedullary, intradural-extramedullary, and extradural lesions), with the use of Gd contrast (▶ Fig. 18.5). T_2-weighted imaging is of particular use in spinal MRI; impingement of the spinal cord and nerve roots (including in the lateral recess and neural foramen) is identified clearly as a loss

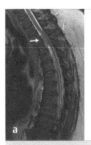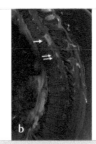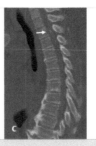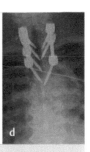

Fig. 18.5 Imaging evaluation of a patient presenting with paraparesis demonstrates the presence of an intradural-extramedullary mass on thoracic T_2-weighted magnetic resonance imaging (MRI), T_1-weighted MRI with contrast, and computed tomography (CT) (**a–c**, *arrow*), consistent with meningioma. A small syrinx and cord edema are seen on T_2-weighted images, and a secondary intramedullary mass can be seen on post-contrast images (**c**, *double arrows*). A trans-pedicular approach was chosen for resection of the extramedullary tumor and biopsy of the intramedullary lesion, necessitating instrumented fusion, which can be seen on intraoperative X-rays (**d**).

of normal spinal fluid cushion. Advanced spinal MRI techniques, such as time-resolved MRA, has been utilized extensively in our institution to aid localization of spinal dural arteriovenous fistulas (dAVFs), thereby reducing operative times, radiation exposure, and contrast dosage during catheter angiography of the segmental arteries.[16] Finally, emergent MRI is frequently indicated to assess pathologies associated with impending severe or permanent neurologic injury, such as epidural abscess, cauda equine syndrome, and metastatic tumors invading the epidural space.

Myelography

Despite the widespread use of MRI, CT-M still plays an important role in the evaluation of spinal disease. It is the imaging study of choice when visualization of spinal neural elements is necessary in patients unable to undergo MRI, such as those with non-MRI compatible pacemaker or spinal cord stimulator devices. Finally, the combined visualization of the vertebral column and underlying CSF space in a single image-space provides a particularly useful tool in preoperative planning. These benefits, however, must be weighed against the invasive nature of the procedure, as well as the inability to visualize beyond a complete CSF block in the setting of severe spinal stenosis.

18.3.3 Systemic

Ultrasonography

Ultrasound has become an essential tool for clinicians of nearly every specialty. Its diagnostic uses in routine critical care settings include echocardiography, deep venous thrombosis screening, acute arterial occlusion, carotid artery stenosis, and intra-abdominal imaging (such as the focused assessment with sonography in trauma [FAST]). Likewise, bedside ultrasound performed by the intensivist is common for procedures such as arterial line/central venous line placement, bedside volume assessment as well as thoracentesis and paracentesis. It is important for critical care clinicians to become comfortable with use of the ultrasound probe (including radiographic conventions such as the orientation of the probe's leading edge), and understand the sonographic qualities of fluid versus solid tissue and artifacts related to interference from hyperechoic bone and hypoechoic air signals.

Ultrasound-based transcranial Doppler (TCD) is a type of noninvasive ultrasound which measure blood flow velocity and direction from intracranial and extracranial arteries. It plays an important role as a tool in evaluating cerebrovascular disease. It can be used to identify and follow intracranial stenosis, intra-arterial emboli, or recanalization of vessel after thrombolytic therapy as well as early detection of cerebral vasospasm following SAH. ▶ Fig. 18.6 and ▶ Fig. 18.7 are examples of waveforms seen during the evaluation for vasospasm with SAH. ▶ Fig. 18.6 is a patient who has no evidence of vasospasm while ▶ Fig. 18.7 has moderate vasospasm based on the Lindegaard ratio noted in ▶ Table 18.7. TCDs are a recommended ancillary test for the diagnosis of brain death.[20] However, poor acoustic windows or insonable windows are found in approximately 5 to 20% patients.[21] In SAH, elevation in transcranial velocities may occur 1 to 2 days before clinical findings. TCDs are reported as the mean flow velocity (MFV) of both anterior and posterior intracranial vessels (cm/s). A MFV of the MCA vessel of > 200 cm/s has a positive predictive value of 86%.[21] The Lindegaard ratio which the mean flow velocity in the MCA/mean velocity in the ipsilateral extracranial internal carotid artery. It adjusts for other causes of increased cerebral blood flow (anemia, fever, vasopressor use, etc). The ratio has been correlated to angiographic vasospasm with or without clinical symptoms or delayed cerebral ischemia (▶ Table 18.7). Our institutional practice is to check TCDs twice a day on all SAH patients. We follow the values listed in ▶ Table 18.6 when screening for vasospasm.

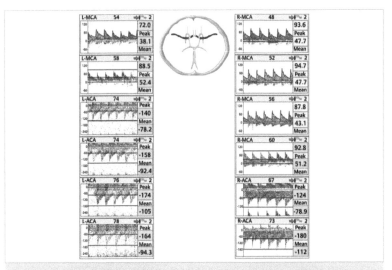

Fig. 18.6 B-Mode data from transcranial Doppler examination of a patient 7 days after rupture of an anterior communicating artery aneurysm. The patient was found to have elevated mean and peak velocities in bilateral anterior cerebral arteries.

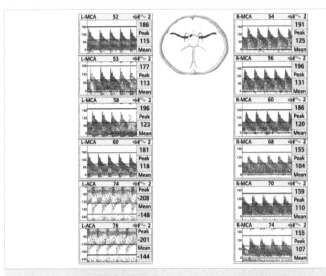

Fig. 18.7 Trans-cranial Dopplers (TCDs) for patient with subarachnoid hemorrhage. Elevated Lindegaard ratios: Right 4.74 and Left 4.44 indicating moderate vasospasm.

Table 18.7 MFV, LR, and Vasospasm

MCA mean flow velocity (cm/s)	Lindegaard ratio	Significance
<90	<3	Normal
90–120	<3	Hyperemia
120–150	3–4.5	Mild vasospasm
150–200	4.5–6	Moderate vasospasm
>200	>6	Severe vasospasm

Abbreviations: MCA, middle cerebral artery; MFV, mean flow velocity; LR, Lindegaard ratio.

References

[1] Kirkman MA. The role of imaging in the development of neurosurgery. J Clin Neurosci. 2015; 22 (1):55–61

[2] Mirvis SE, Shanmuganathan K. Trauma radiology: Part IV. Imaging of acute craniocerebral trauma. J Intensive Care Med. 1994; 9(6):305–315

[3] Carlson AP, Yonas H. Portable head computed tomography scanner—technology and applications: experience with 3421 scans. J Neuroimaging. 2012; 22(4):408–415

[4] Imhof H, Czerny C, Dirisamer A. Head and neck imaging with MDCT. Eur J Radiol. 2003; 45 Suppl 1:S23–S31

[5] Menon BK, Campbell BCV, Levi C, Goyal M. Role of imaging in current acute ischemic stroke workflow for endovascular therapy. Stroke. 2015; 46(6):1453–1461

[6] Kovács A, Möhlenbruch M, Hadizadeh DR, et al. Noninvasive imaging after stent-assisted coiling of intracranial aneurysms: comparison of 3-T magnetic resonance imaging and 64-row multidetector computed tomography—a pilot study. J Comput Assist Tomogr. 2011; 35(5):573–582

[7] Mangla R, Ekhom S, Jahromi BS, Almast J, Mangla M, Westesson P-L. CT perfusion in acute stroke: know the mimics, potential pitfalls, artifacts, and technical errors. Emerg Radiol. 2014; 21(1):49–65

[8] Plewes DB, Kucharczyk W. Physics of MRI: a primer. J Magn Reson Imaging. 2012; 35(5):1038–1054

[9] Springer E, Dymerska B, Cardoso PL, et al. Comparison of routine brain imaging at 3 T and 7 T. Invest Radiol. 2016; 51(8):469–482

[10] Oshio K, Okuda S, Shinmoto H. Removing ambiguity caused by T2 shine-through using weighted diffusion subtraction (WDS). Magn Reson Med Sci. 2016; 15(1):146–148

[11] Menjot de Champfleur N, Saver JL, Goyal M, et al. Efficacy of stent-retriever thrombectomy in magnetic resonance imaging versus computed tomographic perfusion-selected patients in SWIFT PRIME trial (solitaire FR with the intention for thrombectomy as primary endovascular treatment for acute ischemic stroke). Stroke. 2017; 48(6):1560–1566

[12] Fraum TJ, Ludwig DR, Bashir MR, Fowler KJ. Gadolinium-based contrast agents: a comprehensive risk assessment. J Magn Reson Imaging. 2017; 46(2):338–353

[13] Huang BY, Castillo M. Neurovascular imaging at 1.5 Tesla versus 3.0 Tesla. Magn Reson Imaging Clin N Am. 2009; 17(1):29–46

[14] Chalouhi N, Theofanis T, Jabbour P, et al. Safety and efficacy of intraoperative angiography in craniotomies for cerebral aneurysms and arteriovenous malformations: a review of 1093 consecutive cases. Neurosurgery. 2012; 71(6):1162–1169

[15] Modic MT, Steinberg PM, Ross JS, Masaryk TJ, Carter JR. Degenerative disk disease: assessment of changes in vertebral body marrow with MR imaging. Radiology. 1988; 166(1 Pt 1):193–199

[16] Koizumi S, Takai K, Shojima M, et al. Spinal extradural arteriovenous fistulas with retrograde intradural venous drainage: diagnostic features in digital subtraction angiography and time-resolved magnetic resonance angiography. J Clin Neurosci. 2017; 45(August):276–281

[17] Lev MH, Gonzalez RG. CT angiography and CT perfusion imaging. In: Toga A, Mazziotta JC, eds. Brain Mapping: The Methods. San Diego, CA: Academic Press; 2002:427–484 . DOI:

[18] Rodallec MH, Krainik A, Feydy A, et al. Cerebral venous thrombosis and multidetector CT angiography: tips and tricks. Radiographics. 2006; 26 Suppl 1:S5–S18, discussion S42–S43

[19] Wetzel SG, Kirsch E, Stock KW, Kolbe M, Kaim A, Radue EW. Cerebral veins: comparative study of CT venography with intraarterial digital subtraction angiography. AJNR Am J Neuroradiol. 1999; 20(2):249–255

[20] Wijdicks EF, Varelas PN, Gronseth GS, Greer DM, American Academy of Neurology. Evidence-based guideline update: determining brain death in adults: report of the Quality Standards Subcommittee of the American Academy of Neurology. Neurology. 2010; 74(23):1911–1918

[21] Sarkar S, Ghosh S, Ghosh SK, Collier A. Role of transcranial Doppler ultrasonography in stroke. Postgrad Med J. 2007; 83(985):683–689

[22] Axel L. Cerebral blood flow determination by rapid-sequence computed tomography: theoretical analysis. Radiology 1980;137:679–86

19 Ventilation Strategies in Neuro-ICU

Amandeep S. Dolla and M. Kamran Athar

19.1 Introduction

Mechanical ventilation has become the cornerstone of modern intensive care unit (ICU) care. The term "ventilate" is derived from Latin word "ventus" meaning wind. Its history dates back to biblical times.[1,2] This chapter describes the basic concept of positive pressure ventilation (PPV), the initial settings on a ventilator, and various indications for initiating mechanical ventilation. We will learn how to troubleshoot commonly encountered errors during mechanical ventilation. Lastly, we will discuss the liberation strategies from mechanical ventilation and various factors which can hamper vent liberation.

19.2 Respiratory Failure

It is not uncommon to find patients intubated in the neuro-intensive care unit (neuro-ICU). There are multiple causes of respiratory failure usually broken up into categories based on the system affected (▶ Table 19.1). The causes can be broken up to categories (▶ Fig. 19.1):

There are two main types of respiratory failure:

- **Type I:** Hypoxic respiratory failure defined as PaO2 < 60 mm Hg without hypercapnia
- **Type II:** Hypercapnic respiratory failure defined as PaCO2 > 50 mm Hg

Some of the main causes of respiratory failure are listed in ▶ Table 19.2.

19.2.1 Noninvasive Oxygenation and Ventilation

Not all patients with respiratory failure require mechanical ventilation. Many patients can be successfully managed using supplemental oxygen. Nasal cannula, non-rebreathers, and Venturi masks are considered low-flow devices with a limit of 15 lpm. However, supplemental oxygen via nasal cannula or face mask is limited by its flow rate, inability to provide humidity/heat, and delivery of O_2 will be lowered when mixed with inspired room air.[3] The patient's tolerance will be impacted by these limitations and also by the method of delivery, nasal cannula, or face mask. ▶ Table 19.3 lists different methods of oxygen delivery that can be utilized in the neuro-ICU.

Noninvasive systems to provide humidified high-flow oxygen or positive airway pressure ventilation are additional methods which can be utilized as a bridge to intubation or post-extubation in the appropriate patient. Humidified

Table 19.1 Causes of respiratory failure

Location	Cause
CNS	Brainstem stroke Central hypoventilation Drug overdose Anoxic brain injury Subarachnoid hemorrhage Intracranial hemorrhage Bulbar poliomyelitis Meningitis Encephalitis Status epilepticus
Spinal cord anterior horn cell	Acute spinal cord injury Multiple sclerosis/transverse myelitis Amyotrophic lateral sclerosis (ALS) Poliomyelitis
Neuromuscular system motor nerves muscle	Myasthenia gravis Guillain-Barré syndrome Neuromuscular blockade Muscular dystrophy Critical illness myopathy Tetanus/botulism/toxins Hypokalemia period paralysis
Thoracic cage and pleura	Pneumothorax Large pleural effusion Pulmonary fibrosis Flail chest Morbid obesity Kyphoscoliosis
Upper airway	Vocal cord paralysis Epiglottitis Laryngotracheitis Post-extubation airway edema Tracheal obstruction Obstructive sleep apnea
Lower airway	Pneumonia Asthma Aspiration ARDS COPD Atelectasis Interstitial lung disease Traumatic pulmonary contusion

Table 19.1 (*Continued*) Causes of respiratory failure

Location	Cause
Cardiovascular system	Left ventricular failure Biventricular failure Valvular failure Pulmonary embolism

Abbreviations: ARDS, acute respiratory distress syndrome; CNS, central nervous system; COPD, chronic obstructive pulmonary disease.

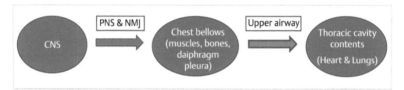

Fig. 19.1 Etiological categories of respiratory failure.

Table 19.2 Causes of type 1 and type 2 respiratory failure

Type 1	Causes	Type 2	Causes
Hypoxic respiratory failure	• Inadequate oxygenation without hypercapnia • Parenchymal diseases causing shunt physiology (pain, edema, ARDS, ILD) • Ventilation/perfusion mismatch • Diffusion defects • Alveolar hypoventilation • Decreased inspired oxygen • Acute tissue hypoxia	Hypercapnic respiratory failure	• Failure of the lungs to adequately remove CO_2 • Reduced respiratory drive due to CNS depressants, brain or brainstem lesions (stroke, trauma, tumors), hypothyroidism • Increased drive to breathe due to increased metabolic rate (increased CO_2 production), metabolic acidosis, anxiety associated with dyspnea • Paralytic disorders (myasthenia gravis, Guillain-Barré syndrome, poliomyelitis, etc.) • Paralytic drugs (curare, sarin/nerve gas, succinylcholine, insecticides) • Drugs that affect neuromuscular transmission (calcium channel blockers, long-term adrenocorticosteroids, etc.)

Abbreviations: ARDS, acute respiratory distress syndrome; ILD, interstitial lung disease; PNA.

Table 19.3 Methods of oxygen delivery, flow rate, and percentage of oxygen delivered

Device	Flow rate (in lpm)	Delivered O_2 (%)
Nasal cannula	1	21–24
	2	25–28
	3	29–32
	4	33–36
	5	37–40
	6	41–44
Simple face mask	6–10	35–60
Face mask with O_2 reservoir (non-rebreather)	6	60
	7	70
	8	80
	9	90
	10–15	100
Venturi mask Flow rate depends on color-coded jet adapter	Blue 2	24
	White 4	28
	Orange 6	31
	Yellow 8	35
	Red 10	40
	Green 15	60

high-flow devices provide a mechanism to deliver O_2 flow up to 60 lpm depending on the device, thereby increasing the FiO_2 to nearly 100%. The flow rate can be set to match the severity of the patient's respiratory distress/inspiratory demand.[4]

Benefits from humidified high-flow nasal cannula:
• Improve oxygenation
• Improve ventilation
• Decrease work of breathing
• Improve tachypnea
• Can provide positive airway pressure in the pharynx of up to 8 cm H_2O.[4]

CPAP—continuous positive airway pressure
BiPAP—provides inspiratory and expiratory pressure
Venturi mask—constant flow of oxygen through various port size
HHFNC—Humidified High-Flow Nasal Cannula: Allows for high-flow oxygen of up to 60 L/minute to be given via nasal cannula.
Problems:
• Air leak from poor seal
• Pressure sores
• Mucosal dryness

- Sensitivity of front teeth
- Claustrophobia

Not all patients are suitable for noninvasive ventilation (NIV). Patients who have a poor mental status, bulbar weakness, and hemiplegia/paresis are unable to clear secretions or have copious secretions, and facial fracture/deformity have a higher risk of aspiration and NIV may be contraindicated.

19.2.2 Invasive Mechanical Ventilation

Indications for Initiating Mechanical Ventilation

Roughly 5% of oxygen (VO_2) is utilized for work of breathing.[5] In a critically ill patient this may rise to more than 20%.[5] Invasive mechanical ventilation eliminates the metabolic cost of breathing.

- Type I respiratory failure with PaO2 < 60 mm Hg with FiO_2 > 50%
- Type II respiratory failure with PaCO2 > 55 mm Hg with progressive acidosis
- Progressive acidosis, pH < 7.3
- Hyperventilation for a central nervous system (CNS) event (to rapidly reduce intracranial pressure)
- Tachypnea, paradoxical breathing, and use of accessory muscles
- Upper airway obstruction
- Glasgow coma score < 8
- Bulbar weakness or inability to clear oral secretions
- Weakness of neck flexor/extensors
- Failure of noninvasive methods of oxygenation and ventilation
- Ventilatory mechanics:
  - Vital capacity: < 15 mL/kg
  - Negative inspiratory force < −20 cm H_2O
  - Respiratory rate > 35 bpm

Basic Ventilator Parameters

- Fractional concentration of inspired oxygen delivered (FiO_2): Expressed as a percentage (%) (21–100). The goal is to keep the FiO_2 below 50% as much as possible
  - Desired FiO_2 = PaO_2 (desired) × FiO_2 (known)/PaO_2 (known)[6,7]
- **Respiratory rate (f):** The number of times inspiration is initiated in 1 minute (breaths per minute or bpm).
- **Tidal volume (V_T):** The amount of gas that is delivered during inspiration expressed in milliliters (mL) or liters (L). Inspired or exhaled.
- **Flow:** The velocity of gas flow or volume of gas per minute. Typical flow rate is 60 L/minute (40–80 L/minute). Minimum flow of at least two times the

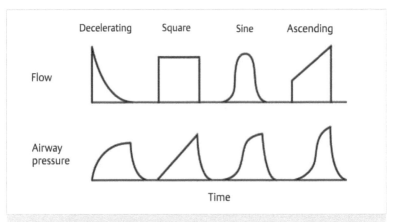

Fig. 19.2 Flow patterns. Modified from Pontoppidan H, Geffin B, Lowenstein E. Acute respiratory failure in the adult. 3. N Engl J Med. 1972;287.

minute ventilation volume is required. High-flow rate may increase the risk of alveolar rupture.

- **Flow pattern:** Selection of flow pattern (▶ Fig. 19.2) and rate may depend on the patient's lung condition. Most common flow pattern is **descending ramp**. Studies have shown that it improves the distribution of gas in the lungs, reduces dead space, and increases oxygenation by increasing mean and plateau airway pressures.
- **Sensitivity setting:** Sensitivity is normally set so that patients can easily flow or pressure-trigger a breath.
  - Flow triggering is set in a range of 1 to 10 L/minute below the base flow, depending on the ventilator.
  - Pressure sensitivity is commonly set between −1 and −2 cm H_2O.

Flow triggering is now the preferred method of triggering, because it has a faster response time compared with pressure triggering.

- **Extrinsic positive end-expiratory pressure (PEEP):** It is the application of positive pressure at end exhalation. This prevents pressure from returning to zero, or atmospheric, at the end of the breath. When positive pressure is applied at the end of a mechanical breath, it is referred to as extrinsic PEEP. When positive pressure is applied throughout the *spontaneous* breathing cycle, it is referred to as CPAP, or continuous positive airway pressure. It increases functional residual capacity (FRC) and improves oxygenation. It recruits collapsed alveoli, splints and distends patent alveoli, and redistributes lung fluid from alveoli to perivascular space.

- **Intrinsic PEEP or Auto-PEEP**: It is a complication of positive pressure ventilation in which air is accidentally trapped in the lung. This occurs in three situations:[8]
  - Strong active expiration, often with normal or even with low lung volumes; e.g., Valsalva maneuver.
  - High minute ventilation (> 20 L/minute) where expiration time is too short to allow full exhalation or when expiration is inhibited by resistance external to the patient such as a partially obstructed expiratory filter.
  - Expiratory air flow limitation due to increased airway resistance, as may occur in patients with chronic obstructive pulmonary disease (COPD) on mechanical ventilation or with small endotracheal (ET) tubes.
    - It is *measured* by doing inspiratory pause and then subtracting extrinsic PEEP from total PEEP.

19.2.3 Basic Principles of Mechanical Ventilation

- Gas is pumped in during inspiration (Ti) and the patient passively exhales during expiration (Te). The sum of Ti and Te is the respiratory cycle or "breath."

(PIP = peak inspiratory pressure, PEEP = positive end-expiratory pressure, Ti = time for inspiration, Te = time for expiration)
- Each ventilatory cycle can be divided into two phases: Inspiration is the point at which exhalation valve closes and fresh gas enters the chest. The amount of gas delivered during inspiration is limited by three **parameters** that can be set in the ventilator[9]:
  - Volume
  - Pressure and/or
  - Flow
- **Cycling**[9]: Changeover from the end of inspiration to the second phase → expiration. Cycling can occur in response to elapsed time, delivered volume, or a decrease in flow rates. Expiration begins when the gas flow from the ventilator is stopped and exhalation circuit is opened to allow gas to escape from the lungs.
- **Triggering**[9]: Changeover from expiration to inspiration. All ventilators require some signal from the patient to determine when inspiration should begin. Triggering signal results when patient's inspiratory effort produces a drop in airway pressure or diversion of a constant gas flow in ventilator circuitry.

In the absence of patient's interaction with the ventilator, *breaths are delivered based on elapsed time (time triggering)*.

19.2.4 Modes of Ventilation[10,11,12,13]

The breath type and pattern of breath delivery during mechanical ventilation constitute the mode of ventilation. The mode is determined by the following factors
- Type of breath (mandatory, spontaneous, assisted)
- Targeted control variable (volume/flow or pressure)
- Timing of breath delivery (continuous mandatory ventilation [CMV], synchronized intermittent mandatory ventilation [SIMV], or spontaneous)

Type of Breath

- Mandatory breaths are breaths for which the ventilator controls the timing or tidal volume (or both).
- Spontaneous breaths are controlled by patient in terms of timing and the tidal volume. The volume or pressure (or both) delivered is based on patient's demand, and the patient's lung compliance and not on a set value.
- Assisted breaths have characteristics of both mandatory and spontaneous breaths. In an assisted breath, all or part of the breath is generated by the ventilator, which does a part of the work of breathing for the patient. If the airway pressure rises above baseline during inspiration, the breath is assisted.

Targeted Control Variable
Volume/Flow-Targeted Ventilation

In volume-targeted ventilation, the volume provided is constant and independent of what happens to pressure when the patient's lung compliance changes or when the patient's effort changes.
- The main advantage of volume-targeted ventilation is that it guarantees a specific volume delivery regardless of changes in lung compliance and resistance or patient's effort.
- Volume-targeted ventilation is used when the goal is to maintain a certain level of PaCO2.
- The main disadvantage becomes evident when the lung compliance worsens. This can cause the peak and alveolar pressures to rise, leading to alveolar over distention.
- The controls for setting volume-targeted ventilation usually are tidal volume, respiratory rate, inspiratory flow, and a flow pattern.

Pressure-Targeted Ventilation

It allows the clinician to set pressure as an independent variable, that is, the pressure remains constant whereas volume delivery (the dependent variable) changes as lung compliance changes.

- Pressure-targeted ventilation has several advantages.
  - First, it allows the clinician to set a maximum pressure, which reduces the risk of overdistention of the lungs by limiting the pressure put on the lung.
  - Second, the ventilator delivers a descending flow which spares more normal areas of the lungs from overinflation.
  - It also may be more comfortable for patients who can breathe spontaneously.
- Disadvantages of pressure-ventilation include: Volume delivery varies, so VT and VE can decrease when lung compliance deteriorates.

▶ Fig. 19.3 compares volume/flow-versus pressure-targeted wave forms.

Timing of Breath Delivery

- **Continuous mandatory ventilation** (**CMV**): All breaths are mandatory and can be volume or pressure targeted. Breaths also can be patient triggered or time triggered. When they are patient triggered, the CMV mode sometimes is called *assist/control (A/C)*. When they are time triggered, the CMV mode is called controlled ventilation or the control mode.

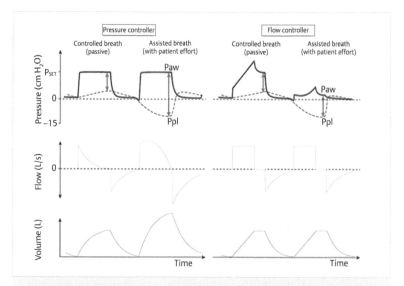

Fig. 19.3 Flow and volume tracings during pressure-controlled ventilation (PCV, left panel of curves) and during flow/Volume-controlled ventilation (VCV, right panel of curves). Reproduced with permission from Pressure-Controlled and Inverse-Ratio Ventilation, Tobin MJ. Chapter 9. *Principles and Practice of Mechanical Ventilation, 3e;* The McGraw-Hill Companies, 2013.

- In the control mode, the patient usually makes no spontaneous effort. *The only difference between control and assist/control is the trigger; the control mode is time triggered, whereas the A/C mode can be either patient triggered, or time triggered.*
- **Intermittent mandatory ventilation** (IMV) **and SIMV**: In IMV, periodic volume or pressure-targeted breaths occur at set intervals (time triggering). Between mandatory breaths, the patient breathes spontaneously at any desired baseline pressure without receiving a mandatory breath.

Spontaneous Modes

The two basic means of providing support for continuous spontaneous breathing (CSV) during mechanical ventilation are:

- **Spontaneous breathing**: Patients can breathe spontaneously through a ventilator circuit; this is sometimes called a T-piece method.
- **Pressure support ventilation** (PSV): It is a special form of assisted ventilation. For PSV, the patient must have a consistent and reliable spontaneous respiratory pattern. The ventilator provides a constant pressure during inspiration once it senses that the patient has inspiratory effort.
  - The operator sets the inspiratory pressure, PEEP, and sensitivity level. The patient establishes the rate, inspiratory flow, and T_i (time for inspiration). PSV is always in assist mode (patient triggered). The flow curve resembles a descending ramp, and the patient can vary the inspiratory flow on demand.
  - PS breath is patient triggered, pressure limited, and flow cycled. The machine senses a decrease in flow and determines that inspiration is ending. The decrease in flow corresponds to the decrease in the pressure gradient between the mouth and lungs as the lungs fill.

19.2.5 Initial Ventilator Settings

Determining pressure, tidal volume, respiratory frequency, and minute ventilation for volume and pressure ventilation.

For Volume-Targeted Ventilation

Minute Ventilation (V_E)

V_E for a male = $4 \times$ BSA
  V_E for a female = $3.5 \times$ BSA
  Estimate Free Water deficit: = Current TBW × ([Serum Na /140] -1)

Tidal Volume (V_T)[15]

Minimum of 4 mL/kg of IBW

Maximum of 12 mL/kg of IBW. IBW, where IBW = ideal body weight. For calculating IBW:[16,17]

Men: 50 kg + 2.3 kg/each inch over 5 feet
Women: 45.5 kg + 2.3 kg/each inch over 5 feet
(To convert to lbs, multiply by 2.2).

Keep alveolar pressure < 30 cm H_2O (assumes thoracic compliance is normal)

Respiratory Frequency (f)

$f = V_E/V$

19.2.6 For Pressure Ventilation

Pressure Support Ventilation (PSV)

To overcome system resistance in the spontaneous or IMV/SIMV mode, set pressure at peak inspiratory pressure (PIP)—plateau achieved in a volume breath or at 5 to 10 cm H_2O.[10] To provide ventilatory support, set pressure to achieve a target V_T as described for volume-targeted ventilation.

Pressure-Targeted Ventilation

Set pressure to achieve VT as described for VV. Set frequency to achieve same VE.

$f = V_E /V_T$

Set inspiratory percentage to achieve an I/E ratio of greater than or equal to 1:1.5

19.2.7 Common Ventilator Problems

See ▶ Table 19.4.

19.2.8 Weaning from Ventilator

See ▶ Table 19.5 for parameters that predict successful weaning from mechanical ventilation.

19.2.9 WHEANS NOT Mnemonic[18]

For assessing various issue which can making weaning difficult:
- **W**—wheeze (especially COPD and asthma)
- **H**—heart disease and fluid overload

Table 19.4 Common ventilator problems and their possible causes

Problem	Possible causes
High peak and plateau pressures	Pulmonary edema, consolidation, atelectasis, mainstem intubation, tension pneumothorax, chest wall constriction
Increased difference in peak and plateau pressure	Bronchospasm, secretions, inspiratory circuit obstruction
Auto-PEEP	Insufficient flow rate or expiratory time, expiratory circuit obstruction, AC circuit with agitated patient
Low exhaled volume	Circuit or cuff leak, insufficient flow rate, bronchopleural fistula
Increased respiratory rate	Change in clinical status, low tidal volume, insufficient flow rate or set ventilator rate
High exhaled volume	In-line nebulizer therapy
High minute ventilation	Hyperventilation (central, agitation, wrong ventilator settings), hypermetabolism (increased CO_2 production, excess caloric intake, sepsis, fever, seizures), inefficient ventilation (increased dead space due to COPD, PE, ARDS, or auto-PEEP)

Abbreviations: ARDS, acute respiratory distress syndrome; auto-PEEP, auto-positive end-expiratory pressure; COPD, chronic obstructive pulmonary disease; PE, pulmonary embolism.

Table 19.5 Predictors of successful weaning from mechanical ventilation

Parameters	Assessment
Resolution of primary process	
Oxygenation	pO2 > 80 on FiO_2 < 0.40
Ventilation	V_E < 10–15 L/min for PCO2 = 40 mm Hg
Ventilatory drive	Spontaneous respiratory rate > 10 bpm and < 20 bpm
Ventilatory muscle strength	V_C > 10 mL/kg (V_C = Vital Capacity) NIF > neg 20–25 cm H_2O V_T > 5 mL/kg
Breathing pattern	RR/V_T < 100 (during spontaneous breathing)
Clear respiratory tract secretions	Adequate cough reflex, frequency, and amount of suctioning required
Patency of airway	Air leak around cuff when deflated
Electrolytes	K, Ca, Mg, and Phos are within normal values

- **E**—electrolytes and metabolic derangement
- **A**—anxiety and delirium
- **N**—neuromuscular disease and weakness
- **S**—sepsis
- **N**—nutrition insufficiency
- **O**—opiates and other sedatives
- **T**—thyroid disease

19.2.10 Extubation Procedure

- Explain procedure to the patient.
- **Prepare equipment**: laryngoscope, ET tube, bag-mask-valve system with O_2 hook-up, wall suction with Yankauer extension, and 10 mL syringe.
- Suction ET tube inside and around top of cuff.
- Instruct patient to take deep breath.
- Deflate cuff.
- Withdraw ET tube as patient exhales.
- Support patient with aerosol mask (FiO_2 of 10% over previous settings).
- Monitor respiratory rate and SaO2. Encourage incentive spirometry and coughing.

References

[1] Kacmarek RM. Respir Care. 2011; 56(8):1170–1180

[2] Kotur P. Mechanical ventilation—past, present, and future. Indian J Anaesth. 2004; 48(6):430–432

[3] Spoletini G, Alotaibi M, Blasi F, Hill N. Heated humidified high-flow nasal oxygen in adults: mechanisms of action and clinical implications. Chest. 2015; 148(1):253–261

[4] Papazian L, Corley A, Hess D, et al. Use of high-flow nasal cannula oxygenation in ICU adults: a narrative review. Intensive Care Med. 2016; 42(9):1336–1349

[5] Roussos C, Macklem PT. The respiratory muscles. N Engl J Med. 1982; 307(13):786–797

[6] Manthous CA, Hall JB, Kushner R, Schmidt GA, Russo G, Wood LD. The effect of mechanical ventilation on oxygen consumption in critically ill patients. Am J Respir Crit Care Med. 1995; 151(1):210–214

[7] Mithoefer JC, Karetzky MS, Mead GD. Oxygen therapy in respiratory failure. N Engl J Med. 1967; 277(18):947–949

[8] Karetzky MS, Keighley JF, Mithoefer JC. The effect of oxygen administration on gas exchange and cardiopulmonary function in normal subjects. Respir Physiol. 1971; 12(3):361–370

[9] Cairo JM. Chapter 7/Final considerations in ventilator setup. In: Pilbeam's Mechanical Ventilation: Physiological and Clinical Applications. 6th ed. St. Louis, MO: Elsevier; 2016:99–101

[10] Fuller BM, Cinel I, Phillip Dellinger R. Chapter 9/General principles of mechanical ventilation. In: Parrillo JE, Dellinger RP, eds. Critical Care Medicine: Principles of Diagnosis and Management in the Adult. Philadelphia: Elsevier/Saunders; 2014:138–44

[11] Cairo JM. Chapter 5/Selecting the ventilator and the mode. In: Pilbeam's Mechanical Ventilation: Physiological and Clinical Applications. 6th ed. St. Louis, MO: Elsevier; 2016

[12] Beier M, Weismann D, Roelleke Th. Classification of ventilation modes. White paper for discussion at the ISO TC121/SC3 meeting, Helsinki, June 5–9, 2006

[13] Chatburn RL. Classification of mechanical ventilators. Respir Care. 1992; 37(9):1009–1025

[14] Chatburn RL, Primiano FP, Jr. A new system for understanding modes of mechanical ventilation. Respir Care. 2001; 46(6):604–621

[15] Du Bois D, Du Bois EF. A formula to estimate the approximate surface area if height and weight be known. Arch Intern Med. 1916; 17:863–871

[16] Brower RG, Matthay MA, Morris A, Schoenfeld D, Thompson BT, Wheeler A, Acute Respiratory Distress Syndrome Network. Ventilation with lower tidal volumes as compared with traditional tidal volumes for acute lung injury and the acute respiratory distress syndrome. N Engl J Med. 2000; 342(18):1301–1308

[17] Devine BJ. Gentamicin therapy. Drug Intell Clin Pharm. 1974; 8:650–655

[18] Ely EW. The utility of weaning protocols to expedite liberation from mechanical ventilation. Respir Care Clin N Am. 2000; 6(2):303–319, vi

Index

1

1-desamino-8D-arginine vaso-pressin (DDAVP)   163

A

ABCDEF bundle   222
Absence of Respiratory Drive   **171**
Academy of Nutrition and Dietetics Malnutrition   196
Acetaminophen   52, 225
Acetylcholinesterase (ache)   141
Acinetobacter   100
Acute Asymptomatic Moderate Hyponatremia   **185**
Acute Bacterial Meningitis   **92**
Acute encephalopathy   3
Acute hydrocephalus   50
Acute infectious myelitis (West Nile virus, coxsackie, echovirus)   133
Acute Inflammatory Demyelinating Polyradiculoneuropathy (AIDP)   **132**
Acute inflammatory or metabolic myopathies   133
Acute ischemic stroke   194
Acute motor and sensory axonal neuropathy (AMSAN)   133
Acute motor axonal neuropathy (AMAN)   133
Acute poisoning   141
Acute postoperative period   157
Acute respiratory distress syndrome (ARDS)   242
Acute SCI, medical treatment of   **119**
Acute spinal cord injury   **119**
Acute stroke
– management   **11**
– therapy   23
Acute stroke   30, *272*

Acute Symptomatic Moderate to Severe Hyponatremia   **184**
Acute viral myositis   133
Adequate oral intake   200
ADH receptor antagonists   186
Adjuvant anesthetic agent   220
Adrenal insufficiency   56
Adrenocorticotropic hormone (ACTH)-secreting tumors   162
Adult weight categories/BMI   200
Advanced Trauma Life Support (ATLS) protocols   119
Air bubble sign   161, *162*
Airway management   **152**, 153
Alberta Stroke Program Early CT Score (ASPECTS)   22
Albuminocytologic dissociation   134
Alcoholism   231
Alpha-2 agonists   127
Alteplase (tpa)   39
Amantadine   146
American Epilepsy Society Guidelines for Convulsive Status Epilepticus   *113*
American Heart Association (AHA)   62
American Heart Association/American Stroke Association   18
American Society for Parenteral and Enteral Nutrition (ASPEN)   196
American Spinal Injury Association (ASIA) scale   120
American Spinal Injury Association impairment scale   121
American Stroke Association (ASA)   62
Amiodarone   182
Amitriptyline   182
Amoxapine   146
Amyloid bleed   34
ancillary test
– indications for   174
– list   175

Ancillary test   **134**, **171**
Ancillary tests   137, 169
Anemia, in ICU   **58**
Anemia   **55**
Aneurysm   33
Aneurysm formation   46
Aneurysm treatment   **50**
Aneurysmal SAH   72
Aneurysmal subarachnoid hemorrhage   **45**
Angioedema   24
Angiography   **277**
Angiotensin-converting enzyme (ACE)   189
Anterior cerebral artery   13
Anterior horn cell   286
Anterior spinal artery syndrome   133
Anti-emetics   146
Anti-fibrinolytics   48
Anti-shivering protocol   88
Antibiotic prophylaxis   153, **158**
Antibiotic therapy, for meningitis   95
Antibiotic therapy   106
Anticoagulants   **64**
Anticoagulation   **58**
Antidiuretic hormone (ADH)   163, 181
Antidopaminergic agents   146
Antiepileptic drugs (aeds)   156
Antihypertensive Treatment of Acute Cerebral Hemorrhage (ATACH)   37
Antimicrobial agent   100
Antimicrobial selection   100
Antiplatelet agent   38, 64
Antiplatelet Reversal   **62**
Antiplatelets   *41*
Antipsychotics   182
Antiretroviral therapy (ART) initiation   101
Antiseizure meds   182
Antiviral treatment   96
Aortic waveform   248
Apixaban   39, **66**
Apixiban   66
Arachnoid cyst   151

299

Argatroban 39, **69**

Aromatization 69

Arousability Assessment Tools 5

Arrhythmias 30

Arterial and venous thromboses 64

Arterial line 239

Arteriovenous oxygen content difference (AVDO2) 254, **257**

Aseptic (chemical) meningitis 158

Aseptic Meningitis **96**

Aspergillosis 97

Aspergillus 100

Assisted breaths 292

Astrocytoma 151

Atypical antipsychotics 9

Auto-PEEP 291

Azotemia 183

B

Baclofen 127

Bacterial meningitis 96, 158

Barbiturate coma 204

Basal ganglia hemorrhage 34

Basilar artery 13

Bedside cerebral microdialysis analyzer 259

Bedside shivering assessment score 88

Benzodiazepines 9, 114, 116, 127, 145, 212

Beta-blockers 30, 127

Bickerstaff encephalitis 134

Bilateral strokes 133

Bipap—provides 288

Bivalirudin 39

Blastomyces 97

Bleeding, treatment of **62**

Blood pressure control **156**

Blood pressure monitoring 238

blood products, appearance of 277

Blood—brain barrier (BBB) 159

Body movements 235

BOOST Trial 256

Botulism 133, **139**

Botulism Immune Globulin Intravenous (Human) 140

Brain **91**

Brain death, in adults **169**

Brain death **169**

Brain herniation, subtypes *82*

Brain herniation 80

Brain imaging **266–267**

Brain injuries alter metabolism 194

Brain retraction 159

Brain tissue oxygen monitor *255*

Brain tissue oxygen tension monitor (pbto2) 250

Brain tumor 73, 81

Brain Tumor Postoperative Management **149**

Brain-dead patient for organ donation **172**

Brainstem parenchyma or edema 152

Breath, types of **292**

Broad-spectrum antibiotics 126, 158

Bromocriptine 145

Brudzinski's sign 91

C

Calcium channel blockers 30

Calculation 178

Calorie Needs **198**

Candida 97

Carbamazepine 202

Cardiac disease 231

Cardiac function index (CFI) 242

Cardiac index (CI) 241

Cardiac output (CO) 241

Cardiopulmonary Complications **50**

Cardiovascular system 286

Carotid endarterectomy 31

Catheter-based angiography 277

Caudal excitatory pathways 127

Causative occlusion 21

Cefepime 106

ceftazidime 106

Centers for Disease Control and Prevention (CDC) 92

Central (Neurogenic) Diabetes Insipidus **187**

Central (Transtentorial) herniation 81

Central alpha receptors 88

Central fever **108**

Central nervous system (CNS) 99

Central neurocytoma 151

Central pontine myelinolysis 184

Central poststroke pain **234**

Central venous catheter 239

Central venous O2 saturation (SCVO2) 241

Central venous pressure (CVP) 173, 241

Cerebellar (Tonsillar) downward herniation 81

Cerebellar strokes 28

Cerebellum 34

Cerebral amyloid angiopathy 33

Cerebral angiography 175, 277

Cerebral autoregulation curve 77

Cerebral blood flow monitors **260**

Cerebral blood volume (CBV) 224

Cerebral contusion 81

Cerebral edema 28, **75**, 81, **152, 159**

Cerebral infarction 159

Cerebral metabolic rate (CMRO2) 257

Cerebral microdialysis catheter *259*

Cerebral oximetry **254**

Cerebral oxygen delivery (DO2) 257

Cerebral perfusion pressure (CPP) 75, 249, 261

Cerebral salt wasting (CSW) 178

Cerebral saltwasting (CSW) **181**

Cerebral scintigraphy 175

cerebral toxoplasmosis, treatment for 101
Cerebral toxoplasmosis **99**
Cerebrospinal fluid (CSF) 124, 249
Cerebrovascular **45**
Cerebrovascular emergency **11, 33**
Cervical SCI 119
Cetaminophen 231
Cheetah NICOM **248**
Chemical thromboprophylaxis 157
Chemoprophylaxis 53
Chemoprophylaxis initiation 72
Chemotherapeutics 182
Cholinergic Crisis **137**
Chordoma 151
Choroid plexus papilloma 151
Chronic encephalopathy 3
Chronic hypernatremia 191
Chronic liver disease 231
Chronic renal failure 87
Clearsight system **247**
Clonidine 127
Clostridium botulinum 139
Coagulase-negative staphylococci 100
Coagulation Cascade **64**
Coagulopathies **38**
Coagulopathy 33
Coccidioides 97
Cognitive dysfunction (dementia) 211
Compliance with ventilation 235
Compressive myelopathy 133
Computed tomography (CT) 35, 266–267
Confusion Assessment Method for the ICU (CAM-ICU) 6
Confusion assessment method for the intensive care unit (CAM-ICU) 7
Congenital disorders 190
Conivaptan 186
Continuous Electroencephalogram (ceeg) **249**
Continuous electroencephalography (ceeg) 114
Continuous infusions 127

Continuous mandatory ventilation (CMV) 293
Convenient noninvasive test 249
Convulsive SE (CSE) 111
Convulsive Status Epilepticus Management **112**
Cortical inhibitory circuits 127
Corticosteroids 159
CPAP—continuous positive airway pressure 288
cranial nerve reflexes, absence of **171**
Craniectomy **38**, 124
Craniopharyngioma 151, 187
craniopharyngiomas 158
Craniotomy **38**, 231
Critical Care Medicine (CCM) 222
Critical care pain observation tool 235
Crohn's disease 205
Cryptococcal meningitis 102
Cryptococcus 97
Cryptococcus neoformans 101
CT angiography (CTA) 35, 270
CT perfusion (CTP) 270, **271**
CT spine imaging 279
CT venography (CTV) 271
Cushing's disease 162
Cyproheptadine 145
Cytotoxic edema 82, 159

D

Dabigatran 39, **67**
Dantrolene 145
Decompression of neural elements 121
Deep sedation 86
Deep vein thrombosis (DVT) **72**
Deep venous thrombosis prophylaxis **52**
Degenerative spinal disease 279
Delayed Cerebral Ischemia (DCI) **53**
Delayed Neurological Deterioration (DND) **53**
Delirium

– medications used to treat 9
– risk factors for 5
– types of 4
Delirium **3**
Delirium Assessment **6**
Dementia 231
Demyelinating/Neuroinflammatory disorders 182
Detection and Management of Vasospasm and DCI **54**
Dexamethasone 95, 162
Dexmedetomidine 212, 225, **233**
Dexmedetomidine (Precedex) **218**
Diabetes insipidus (DI) 153, 163, 187
Diagnostic and Statistical Manual of Mental Disorders (DSM) 3
Diagnostic criteria for GBS/ AIDP 134
Diaphoresis 127
Diffusion-weighted imaging (DWI) 273
Digital subtraction angiography (DSA) 267, 270
Dilution Cardiac Output (lidco) **244**
Direct brain tissue oxygen (pbto2) monitoring 254, **255**
Direct parenchymal monitors 125
Direct tissue injury 123
Disk Herniation **233**, 279
Distal renal tubular necrosis 190
Dosage Forms **219**
Dose adjustment **71**
Drug-induced meningitis 96
Drugs—cocaine and appetite suppressants 33
Drug–nutrient interactions 202
Dysembryoplastic neuroepithelial tumors (DNET) 156
Dysfunctional vascular autoregulation 120
Dystonic posturing 127

E

Edoxaban **66**, 67
EEG 250
Electroencephalogram (EEG) 249
Elevated ICP, management of **125**
Elevated Intracranial Pressure 75, 77
Elevated troponin 30
Emotional experience 222
Empyema **103**
Encephalitis/Meningitis 182
Encephalopathy
– causes of 2
– diagnosis of 1
Encephalopathy 1
End stage renal disease 231
Endemic pathogens 106
Endocrine Dysfunction **56**
Endogenous corticosteroid function 162
Endoscopic transsphenoidal surgery 161
Endovascular intra-arterial vasodilation 55
Endovascular Therapy **18**
Enoxaparin 157
Enteral Nutrition **200**
Enteroviruses 96
Eosinophilic granuloma 187
Ependymoma 151
Epidermoid 151
Epidermoid cysts 158
Epidural Abscess **104**
Epidural and subdural monitors 125
Epidural empyema 103
Epidural hematoma 124
Epilepticus in Adults **111**
Equate dural closure 160
Euvolemia 51
Exserohilum 100
External or transcalvarial herniation 81
External ventricular drain (EVD) 250, **262**
External ventricular drainage (EVD) 50
Extra-axial tumors 151

Extracorporeal membrane oxygenation (ECMO) 253
Extravascular lung water (EVLW) 242
Extravascular lung water index (ELWI) 241
Extravascular lung water index (EVLWI) 242
Extrinsic positive end-expiratory pressure (PEEP) 290
Extubation Procedure **297**

F

Faces Pain Scale *235*
Facial expression 235
Fanconi syndrome 190
Febrile nonhemolytic transfusion reaction 59
Femoral artery site 25
Fentanyl (Sublimaze) **219**
Fever, defined 52
Fevers and Infections in the Neuro-ICU **91**
Flotrac. 244
Flotrac./Vigileo **245**
Flow patterns *290*
Flow targeted ventilation **292**
Fluid restriction 186
Fluid resuscitation 153
Fluoroquinolones 202
Focal neurologic deficits 159
Focused assessment with sonography in trauma [FAST]) 281
Fondaparinux **71**
Foreign-body-associated infection 106
Fresh frozen plasma (FFP) 66
Functional MRI 267
Fungal Meningitis **97**

G

Gabapentin 127, 225
Gabapentin and Pregabalin **232**
Ganglioglioma 151
Gangliogliomas 156
Gastric residual volumes (GRVs) 202

Gastrointestinal complications of enternal nutrition 203
Gastrointestinal fistula 205
Gd-based contrast agents 275
Glasgow Coma Scale (GCS) 123
Glasgow Coma Scale (GCS) score 122
Glioblastomas (GBM) 156
Global ejection fraction (GEF) 242
Global end diastolic volume (GEDV) 242
Global end diastolic volume index (GEDI) 241–242
Glucose management **52**, 194
Glucose Utilization **194**
Godendrogliomas 156
Grading System **46**
Guillain-Barri Syndrome (GBS) **132**

H

Head CT imaging (HCT) 269
Hemangioblastoma 151
Hemodynamic and Neurological Monitoring in the Neuro-ICU **238**
Hemodynamic instability 238
Hemodynamic monitoring **238**
Hemodynamic monitors 239
Hemodynamic stability 165
Hemoglobin "Triggers" **60**
Hemorrhagic classification 24
Hemorrhagic shock classification 60
Hemorrhagic stroke algorithm 63
Hemorrhagic transformation of infarction 33
Hemorrhagic transformation of ischemic stroke 24
Heparin 157
Heparin-induced thrombocytopenia (HIT), 61
Heparins **70**
Hepatic hydroxylation 69
Herbal products 146
Herniation syndromes 80–81

HHFNC–Humidified High Flow Nasal Cannula 288
Histoplasma 97
HIV related infections **99**
Hormonal dysregulation **162**
Hormonal replacement 162
Hormone replacement therapy 165
Hounsfield units 269
Humidified high flow oxygen 285
Hunt and Hess Grade6 **46**
Hunter criteria for serotonin syndrome–serotonergic agent 144
Hydrocephalus **50**, 160, 182
Hydromorphone 225
Hydronephrosis 190
hyperactive level of psychomotor activity 4
Hyperacute hyponatremia 184
Hypercatabolism. 199
Hyperglycemia 52, 194
hypernatremia, causes of 188
Hypernatremia 178, **187**, **189**
Hypertension 33, 127
Hypertensive hemorrhage 34
Hyperthermia 127
Hypertonic saline (HTS) for cerebral edema 28
Hypervolemia 55
Hypoactive level of psychomotor activity 4
Hypocortisolemia 153, 162, 165
hyponatremia
– based on classification 180
– causes of **179**
– classification **178**
– diagnostic approach to *179*, **183**
Hyponatremia **56**, 153, 178, 181, **186–187**
Hyponatremia treatment **184**
Hypotension 120, 217
Hypothalamic-pituitary axis (HPA) 162
Hypothyroid 180
Hypovolemic hyponatremia 181

Hypoxic respiratory failure 287

I

Ibuprofen 52, 225
ICH score 42–43
ICP monitoring 261
Immunocompromised state (T-cell deficiency) 101
Impaired thirst 188
Inadequate nutrition 194
Incomplete cervical SCI 121
Indications for Sedation **210**
Indirect calorimetry (IC) 198
Indirect calorimetry measurement 199
Individualizing Therapy in NICU **224**
Infectious Diseases Society of America (IDSA) 98
Inflammatory cytokine release 201
Inflammatory cytokines 159
Infra-axial tumors 151
Infratentorial Tumors **152**
Initial medical therapy 114
Initial Ventilator Settings **294**
Initiating aggressive nutrition 198
Inotropic agents 55
Inspiratory and expiratory pressure 288
Insufficient intraoperative hemostasis 156
Intensive Blood Pressure Reduction in Acute Cerebral Hemorrhage (INTERACT) 37
Intensive insulin therapy (IIT) 194–195
intermittent mandatory ventilation (IMV) 294
International normalized ratio (INR) 64
International Surgical Trial 38
Intra-axial tumor 151
Intra-venous contrast 275
Intracerebral hemorrhage (ICH) 33, 38, 62, 182
Intracranial compliance 76

Intracranial compliance curve *78*
Intracranial hemorrhage **62**, 124, 269
Intracranial hypertension 75
Intracranial monitors *255*
Intracranial pressure (ICP) 220, 249
Intracranial pressure monitor (microsensors) 250
Intracranial pressure monitoring **261**
Intraoperative X-ray localization 279
Intrathecal fluorescein administration 160
Intravenous **69**
Intraventricular monitor 125
Intraventricular rtpa 38
Intraventricular tumor 151
Intraventricular tumors 151
Intrinsic PEEP 291
Invasive Mechanical Ventilation **289**
Invasive monitors 240, **254**
Irreversible cessation of cerebral function 169
Irreversible inhibitors 146
Ischemic penumbra 271
Ischemic stroke 72
Ischemic Stroke and Assessment for intravenous Tpa *21*
Isotonic fluids 51

J

Jugular Bulb Monitoring **257**
Jugular venous oximetry 250
Jugular venous pressure (JVP) 261
Jugular venous saturation *257*

K

Kernig's sign 91
Ketamine 225, **233**
Ketamine (Ketalar) **220**
Ketorolac 225

L

Labetalol 127
Lacosamide 156
Lambert-Eaton myasthenic syndrome 136
Left hemispheric hemorrhage 34
Leptomeninges 91
Less Invasive 241
Lethal syndrome 216
Leukocyte Reduction Indications 59
Leukotrienes 159
Levenson's clinical criteria 143
Levetiracetam 156
Lidco 239
Lidocaine 225
Long-term glucocorticoid replacement 162
Low and high jugular venous oxygen saturation 258
Low molecular weight heparin 39
Low Molecular Weight Heparin (LMWH) 70
Low-density lipoprotein receptor-related protein 4 (LRP4) antibodies 137
Low-dose prophylactic anticoagulation 157
Lower airway 286
Lumbar drain 102
Lundberg Waves 80
Lyme disease 133
Lymphoma/Leukemia 182

M

Magnesium 53
Magnetic resonance imaging (MRI) 266–267
Magnetic resonance venography (MRV) 277
Malignant edema 28
Malnutrition 194, 196
Mandatory breaths 292
Matrix metalloproteinases (mmps) 159
Mean arterial blood pressure (MAP) 241

Mean arterial pressure (MAP) 120, 261
Mechanical ventilation 285, 291
Mediastinal tumors 182
Medulloblastoma 151
Membrane channel stabilizers 225
Membrane Stabilizing Agents 232
Meningioma 151
Meningitis 91
Mesenteric ischemia 205
Metasatases 151
Metastatic brain tumors 151
Methicillin-resistant S. Aureus 100
Methicillin-susceptible S. Aureus 100
Methylprednisolone 120
Metoprolol 127
Microdialysis 250
Microdialysis catheter 259
Microdialysis Monitoring 259
Microdialysis monitoring of extracellular glutamate 254
Midazolam 217
Middle cerebral artery 13
Miller-Fisher syndrome (MFS) 133
Minimally invasive aspiration of hemorrhage 40
Minimally Invasive Monitoring 245
Minimally Invasive Surgery Plus Recombinant Tissue-Type Plasminogen Activator for ICH Evacuation Trial II (MISTIE II) 40
Minimally Invasive Surgical Evacuation 40
Minute Ventilation (VE) 294
Mixed venous O2 saturation (SVO2) 241
Moderate hyponatremia 181
Modes of Ventilation 292
Modified Fischer Scores 47
Monophasic course 132
Monro-Kellie doctrine 75, 76
Morphine 127, 225
Mount Fuji sign 162
Movement Disorders 234

MRI sequences 274
Multi-planar reconstruction (MPR) 266
muscarinic receptors, activation of 141
Muscle tension 235
Muscle-specific kinase (musk) antibodies 137
Myasthenia Gravis (MG) 133, 136
Myasthenic crisis 137
myasthenic crisis, management of 137
Myelography 280

N

Naproxen Sodium 225
National Institute of Neurological Disorders and Stroke (NINDS) 1
National Institutes of Health Stroke Scale (NIHSS) 12
Near-infrared spectroscopy (NIRS) 249, 253, 254
Near-infrared Spectroscopy Measurement 253
Neonatal intensive care unit (NICU) 187
Neoplasm 33
Nephrogenic DI 189
Nephrogenic DI Treatment 192
Nephrogenic Diabetes Insipidus 189
Nephrogenic systemic fibrosis (NSF) 272
Nerve-conduction studies (NCS) 134
Neuro-specific Diseases 233
Neurocognitive Disorders7 3
Neurocritical Care Management of Ischemic Stroke 23
Neurocritical Care Society guidelines 64
Neurogenic Stress Cardiomyopathy 51
Neuroimaging 35, 266
Neuroleptic Malignant Syndrome (NMS) 142, 145
Neurologic injury 210
Neurological Monitoring 249

Neuromonitors 250
Neuromuscular and Other Neurologic Emergencies **132**
Neuromuscular blockade (NMB) 87
Neuromuscular blocking agents 133
Neuromuscular junction (NMJ) 136
Neuromuscular system 286
Neuroparalytic syndrome 139
Neuroscience ICU 210
Neuroscience intensive care unit **210**
Neurovent probe contains luminescent ruthenium 255
nicotinic receptors, activation of 141
NIH Stroke Scale 15
NIRS 250
Non-nociceptive external stimuli 127
Non-ST elevation myocardial infarction 70
Noncompetitive calcium antagonist 53
Nonconvulsive SE (NCSE) 111
Nonconvulsive Status Epilepticus (NCSE) **115**
Noninvasive Hemodynamic Monitoring **247**
Noninvasive monitoring system 248
Noninvasive Monitors **249**
Noninvasive Oxygenation **285**
Noninvasive systems 285
Noninvasive ventilation (NIV) 289
Nonopioid Analgesics 231
Nonpharmacologic Treatments for Delirium **8**
Nonpharmacological Approach **233**
Nonpsychotropic drugs 146
Nonsteroidal anti-inflammatory drug 225
Nonsteroidal anti-inflammatory drug (NSAID) 192
Nonsteroidal anti-inflammatory drugs (nsaids) 224

Nonvalvular atrial fibrillation stroke prevention 66–67
Norepinephrine 55
Normal hemodynamic values 241
Normal intracranial pressure waveforms 79
Normothermia 87
Nuclear Medicine 175
Numerical rating scale 235
Nutrition **194**
Nutrition Assessment **198**
Nutrition in Critical Care **194**
Nutrition regimen 196
Nutrition status **196**
Nutrition support **200**
Nutrition with combination therapy 207
Nutrition with therapeutic hypothermia or paralytics 206
Nutrition-related Laboratory Tests **198**

O

Obstructive hydrocephalus 76
Oculocephalic reflex (doll's eyes) 172
Oligodendroglioma 151
One-way valve mechanism 161
Ongoing Continuous Pain Monitoring in NICU **234**
Opioid analgesics 146, **224**
Opioid therapy 223
Opioid tolerant 231
Opioids 225
Oral 67
Oral Factor Xa Inhibitors **66**
Oral nimodipine 54
organophosphate overdose, treatment of 142
Organophosphate Toxicity **141**
Organophosphates 141
Orthostatic hypotension 187
Osmolality 178
Osmolarity 178
Osmotic demyelination 184
Osmotic myelinolysis 86
Osteoarthritis 279

Osteomyelitis **106**
Osteosarcoma 182
Oversedation 217
Oxycodone 225
Oxygen consumption (VO2) 241
Oxygen delivery (DO2) 241
oxygen delivery methods 288

P

Packed red blood cell (PRBC) 59
Pain from agitation and delirium (PAD) 222
Pain management 153
Pain Management in ICU Liberation **223**
Pain Management in NICU **224**
Pain Scales **234**
Parasellar Tumors **162**
Parenchymal Hematomas 124
Parenchymal monitor **262**
Parenteral Nutrition **204**
parenteral nutrition use 205
Parkinson's disease 234
Paroxysmal Sympathetic Hyperactivity (PSH) **127**
PATCH trial 64
Patient-Controlled Analgesia (PCA) **224**
Pbto2 monitoring 256
Peak inspiratory pressure (PIP) 295
Pentobarbital 88
penumbral region 256
Periodic paralysis 133
Perioperative hypertension 156
Peripheral parental nutrition (PPN) 205
Peripheral vasoconstriction 88
Permanent hormone supplementation 163
Pharmacokinetics **216**
Pharmacological properties of sedative agents 213
Phase 2 randomized clinical trial 256
Phenylephrine 55

Phenytoin 156, 202

Picco 239

Pituitary adenoma 151

Pituitary Apoplexy **164**

Pituitary surgery 162

Pituitary tumors 182

Planned invasive procedure 62

Poliomyelitis 133

Polycystic kidney disease 190

Pontine hemorrhage *34*

Positive airway pressure ventilation 285

Post Stroke Complication **28**

Post Thrombectomy Care **25**

Post tPA Management **24**

Post-TBI **126**

Post-TPA Complication **23**

Posterior cerebral artery Contralateral 13

Posterior fossa structural lesion 133

Posterior fossa surgery, 161

Postoperative Care and Complications 159

Postoperative endocrinopathy 162

Postoperative hemorrhage **152**, **156**

Postoperative Infection **158**

Postoperative spine 231

Postsynaptic neuromuscular transmission 136

Pregabalin 225

Presentation of toxidromes 144

Pressure support ventilation (PSV) 294, **295**

Pressure Targeted Ventilation **292**, **295**

Pressure Ventilation **295**

Primary brain tumors 151

Primary injury 119

Primary or secondary prophylaxis 66

Production 162

Progressive injury 123

Prolactinoma 182

Prophylactic Anticonvulsant Use **50**

Prophylactic transfusion 61

Prophylaxis Thresholds **62**

Propofol 127, **210**, 212

Propofol (Diprivan) **216**

Propofol infusion syndrome (PRIS) **216**

Propranolol 127

Proprietary algorithm 248

Prostaglandins 159

Prostate 182

Protein Needs **199**

Proximate Cause of Coma **170**

Psychogenic symptoms 133

psychomotor activity 4

Pulmonary artery catheter 239

Pulmonary artery catheter (PAC) 240

Pulmonary artery occlusion pressure 240

Pulmonary artery occlusion pressure (PAOP) 241

Pulmonary artery pressure (PAP) 241

Pulmonary disease 231

Pulmonary Thermodilution **240**

Pulmonary tumors 182

Pulmonary vascular permeability index (PVPI) 242

Pulse contour analysis 239, **245**

Pulse Contour Cardiac Output (picco) **242**

PULSION Medical System **242**

Q

Qflow 500 Perfusion Probe **260**

Quantitative EEG (qeeg) 251, *252*

R

Radial artery site 26

Radiographic classification of hemorrhage transformation of ischemic stroke 24

Ramsay score 5

Ramsay sedation scale 6

Rebleeding **48**

Red Blood Cell Transfusion 59

Red Cell Transfusion **59**

refeeding syndrome *198*, **198**

Refractory Status Epilepticus (RSE) **116**

Regional Brain Tissue Oxygen Saturation (NIRS) **253**

Reliable assessment tools for sedation 211

Remifentanil 225

Renal Cell Ca 182

Renal clearance 67

Repetitive nerve stimulation 137

Respiratory Failure **285**, 286

respiratory failure (type 1 and type 2) 287

Resting energy expenditure (REE) 198

Reversible inhibitors of monoamine oxidase 146

Reversing anticoagulant 38

Rhabdomyolysis 217

Richmond agitation sedation scale 6

Richmond agitation sedation scale (RASS) 5, 86, 211–212

Right atrial pressure (RAP) 241

Right frontal hemorrhage *34*

Riker sedation agitation scale (SAS) 5

Riker sedation scale 7

Rivaroxaban 39, **66**, 67

Ruthenium luminophore 255

S

Schwannoma 151

Second medical therapy 114

Secondary injury 119

Sedation

– agents for 215

– assessment of **211**

– complications of **211**

Sedation **210**

Sedative, choice of **212**

SEDCOM study 218

Seizure prophylaxis 153, **156**

Sellar tumor **162**

Sequential compression devices 157

Serotonin releasing agents 146
serotonin syndrome 145
Serotonin Syndrome (SS) **142**
Serum ganglioside antibodies 134
Serum osmolality 183
Severe Chronic Mild-Moderate Hyponatremia **185**
Severe fat malabsorption 205
Severe gastric or intestinal motility disturbance 205
Severe infectious enteritis 205
Severe pancreatitis 205
Short bowel syndrome 205
SIADH Treatment **186**
Sickle cell disease 190
Single fiber electromyography 137
Skeletal muscle activity 88
Skull fractures 126
Slow growing tumors 150
Small bowel obstruction 205
Sodium Dysregulation **178**
Spasticity 234, **234**
Spinal cord 286
Spinal cord injury 73
Spinal cord injury (SCI) 119
Spinal dural arteriovenous fistulas (davfs) 279
Spinal epidural abscess 104
Spine Imaging **266, 279**
Spondylosis **233**
Spontaneous breathing 294
Spontaneous breaths 292
Spontaneous Intracerebral Hemorrhage **33**
Standard (intact protein) EN formulation 204
Standard propofol 216
Standing acetaminophen 29
Statins **53**
Status epilepticus (SE) 111
Stereotactic biopsies 156
STICH II trial 38
Stress-dose corticosteroids 162
Stress-dose steroids 56
Stroke 82, 182
Stroke Subtypes **12**
Stroke symptoms by vascular territory 13

Stroke volume (SV) 241
Stroke Volume Variation (SVV) **246**
Strokeworkup and Management **26**
Stunned Myocardium 51
Subarachnoid hemorrhage 181–182, **186**, 194
Subarachnoid hemorrhage (SAH) 45, 249
Subarachnoid hemorrhage, management of **47**
Subcortical Contralateral 13
Subcutaneous heparin (SQH) 70
Subdural empyema 103
Subependymoma 151
Subfalcine (Cingulate) herniation 81
Suboccipital craniectomy 30
Super Refractory Status Epilepticus (SRSE) **116**
Supplemental steroid administration 162
Supratentorial Tumors **152**
Surface or intravascular cooling devices 52
Surgical Management of Acute SCI **121**
Surgical management of stroke 30
Swan-Ganz catheter 240
Sympathomimetics 146
Symptomatic cerebral edema 159
Symptomatic Hyponatremia **179**
Symptomatic intracranial hypotension 160
Symptomatic pulmonary complications 51
Syndrome of inappropriate antidiuretic hormone secretion (SIADH) 163, 178, 180, **181**
Synthetic stimulants 146

T

T1-weighted **275**
T2-weighted FLAIR and GRE **275**

Tachycardia 127
Tachypnea 127
Targeted Control Variable **292**
Targeted temperature management (TTM) 204
TCD 250
Technetium Scan 175
Tension pneumocephalus 161
Therapeutic paralysis 204
Thermal diffusion and laser doppler flowmetry 250
Thiazide diuretics 180
Thomas Jefferson Algorithm
– for the management of hypertensive emergency in patients with hemorrhagic stroke 36
– for the reversing anticoagulants or antiplatelet 41
– for the management of hypertensive emergency in patients with acute ischemic stroke 22
Thomas Jefferson Algorithm , for the management of post-thrombectomy patients 25
Thomas Jefferson early management of acute aneurysmal subarachnoid hemorrhage protocol 49
Thoracic cage and pleura 286
Thrombin Inhibitors **67**
Thrombocytopenia **61**
Thrombocytopenia, medications associated with 61
Thunderclap headache 45
Tidal Volume (VT) **294**
Timing of Breath Delivery **293**
Tiracetam 156
Tolvaptan 186
Tonicity 178
Total parentral nutrition (TPN) 205
Toxoplasmosis 99
Tramadol 225
Transcranial Doppler (TCD) 249, **252**
Transcranial doppler velocities 54
Transcranial Dopplers 175, 267
Transfusion Medicine **58**

Transfusion Requirements in Critical Care (TRICC) 60
Transfusion-associated graft-versus- host disease (TA-GVHD) 59
Transpulmonary thermodilution (TPTD) 241
Transsphenoidal resection 161
Transverse myelitis 133, **234**
Traumatic Brain Injury **122**, 182
Traumatic brain injury (TBI) 119, 210, 249
Treatment for spinal epidural abscess 105
Treatment of botulism 140
Treatment of myasthenia crises 138
Triphasic response of diabetes insipidus *164*
Trivalent equine serum botulinum antitoxin 140
Tumor Classification **151**
Tumors by location 151
Twist-drill burr hole. 261

U

Ultrasonography **281**
Ultrasound 267
Ultrasound-based trans-cranial Doppler (TCD) 281
Uncal herniation 81
Unfractionated heparin 39, **70**

Uniform Determination of Death Act 169
Unpleasant sensory 222
Unstable hemodynamics 242
Unsuccessful thombectomy 26
Upper airway 286
Upward herniation 81

V

Vancomycin+ceftriaxone 106
Varicella-zoster virus (VZV) 96
Vascular endothelial growth factor (VEGF) 159
Vascular malformations 33–34
Vasoconstriction 84
Vasogenic edema 81, 159
Vasopressors 238
Vasospasm **53**
Vasospasm Treatment **54**
Venography **277**
Venous congestion 159
Venous sinus thrombosis 33
Venous thromboembolism 70, 72
Venous thromboembolism (VTE) **157**
Ventilation **285**
Ventilation Strategies in Neuro-ICU **285**
Ventilator Parameters **289**
Ventilator Problems **295**, 296
Ventriculitis **97**

Ventriculoperitoneal shunt 102
Ventriculoperitoneal shunt (VPS) **98**
Ventriculostomy 261
Venturi mask 288
Versed **217**
Vertebral endplate Modic changes 279
Vertebral osteomyelitis 106
Viral Meningitis **96**
Vocalization 235
Volume Assessment and Management **51**
Volume targeted ventilation 292, **294**
Volume-based feeding protocols 202

W

Warfarin 39, **64**, 202
Washed RBC **59**
Water intoxication 82, 180
Weaning from Ventilator **295**
Wedge pressure 240
Withdrawal Symptoms **219**
World Federation of Neurological Surgeons Grade **47**
Worsening cerebral edema 159

Z

Zinc supplementation 216